To Ron P____
Best Wishes,
Zol____
1/3/96

Return to the
Joy of Health

ZOLTAN P. RONA MD MSc

Natural Medicine & Alternative Treatments for All Your Health Complaints

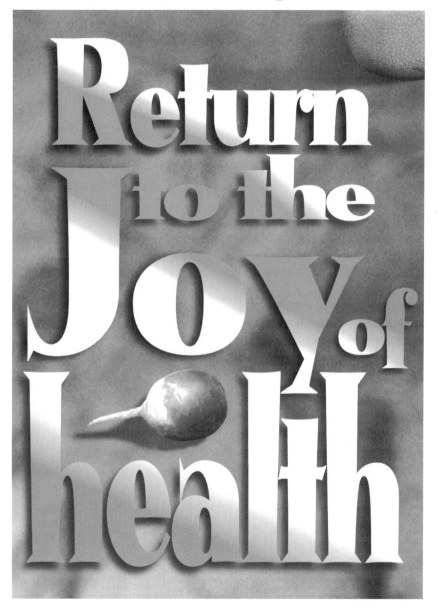

Return to the JOY of health

Healing Foods, Recipes & Nutrition Advice by JEANNE MARIE MARTIN

Published by
alive **books**
7436 Fraser Park Drive, Burnaby BC Canada V5J 5B9

Cover Design: Peter Virag
Typesetting: Peter Virag and Lisa Trommeshauser

First Printing – June 1995

Canadian Cataloguing in Publication Data

Rona, Zoltan P., 1952–
Return to the joy of health

Includes bibliographical references and index.
ISBN 0-920470-62-9

1. Alternative medicine. 2. Nutrition. 3. Diet therapy. I.
Martin, Jeanne Marie, 1951- II. Title.
RA784.R67 1995   613   C95-910586-7

Printed and bound in Canada

To Sharon, whose love sustains me and has been instrumental in my success and happiness. She has fought for the things that really matter in life. Sharon has shown me time and time again that optimal health depends on happy relationships. Wife and family come first and that is the real secret to returning to the joy of health.

To my two sons, Matthew and Darcy for their love, patience, wisdom, wit and support.

To my loving mother, Agnes and the memory of my father, George.

To my brother, Gabe and my grandmother, Icu for their love and support.

I would like to sincerely thank the following wonderful people who have, in many ways, made it possible for me to do what I do and publish this book:

Ms. Jess Borowets

Mr. Stewart Brown

Dr. Borys Chambul

Dr. William Crook

Mr. Harvey Diamond

Ms. Kris Drasutis

Mr. Sam Graci

Mr. Siegfried Gursche

Mr. Brian Hurst

Ms. Lori Imbert

Dr. Norbert Kerenyi

Ms. Jeanne Marie Martin

Ms. Rhody Lake

Ms. Marian Maclean

Mr. Bob McLean

Mrs. Willa McLean

Mr. David Paget

Mr. David Rowland

Dr. Robert Sager

Ms. Karin Shultz

Dr. Vivien Smith

Mr. David Wolf

Ms. Julia Woodford

Sincerely,

Zoltan P. Rona MD MSc

TABLE OF CONTENTS

CHAPTER 1 – THE MAJOR CONTROVERSIES

CHAPTER 2 – BOOSTING IMMUNITY AND ENERGY

Chapter 3 – The Heart and Circulatory System

Chapter 4 – Improving Digestion Naturally

Chapter 5 – The Brain, Nerves and Mind

CHAPTER 6 – WOMEN AND COMPLEMENTARY MEDICINE

CHAPTER 7 – SKIN, HAIR AND NAILS

CHAPTER 8 – MUSCLES, JOINTS AND LIGAMENTS

Chapter 9 – Healing Foods for Healing Diets
by Jeanne Marie Martin

Recipes:

Foreword

L ife is filled with circumstances that call for choices to be made. Some are insignificant and can be made with little or no effort, while others impact our lives in a big way and demand study and soul-searching before a decision is made. Obviously, choosing what color car you will drive pales in importance compared to choosing where to raise your children or what kind of work you will do.

At the top of the list of importance when it comes to making choices, are the ones you make that regard your health. Let's face it, when it comes right down to it, nothing is more important than your health. And making the right choices can determine how long you will live and how healthfully.

There is certainly no shortage of health philosophies—one can choose from the ideas of countless authorities from many varying disciplines. There are doctors (of many disciplines), nutritionists, dietitians, cooks, philosophers and lay people galore, all sharing their views. A never-ending parade of books are available at our bookstores and libraries. How on earth does one know what the right choices are?—especially in light of the fact that frequently we are propagandized into following a particular approach that may not even be in the best interest of our well being.

For example, hundreds upon hundreds of millions of dollars have been spent to condition people to think of meat and other animal products when they hear the word protein, or of dairy products when they hear the words calcium and osteoporosis. This flies in the face of the fact that the healthiest races of the world—the ones that live the longest and the healthiest—eat the fewest animal products. The most populated country in the world is China, with over a billion people. Yet, they have one of the lowest incidences of the so-called diseases of affluence—heart disease, cancer, diabetes, osteoporosis and obesity—while we in the west have one of the highest. The Chinese obtain seven percent of their protein from animal products: we obtain 70 percent from animal products. The Chinese have no liking for dairy products and do not eat them. There is not even a word for osteoporosis in their language!

There are many disciplines when it comes to health care: medical, chiropractic, natural hygiene, homeopathy, naturopathy, osteopathy, nutrition and dietetics, acupuncture and herbology. All have their rightful place and are appropriate in certain circumstances. None are appropriate all of the time or have all the answers for all situations. Yet, we have been systematically conditioned over the years to believe that the medical approach is best and everything else is somehow inferior, no matter what the circumstances.

The beleaguered consumer is deluged with propaganda praising medicine and denigrating everything else. You cannot watch TV without hearing the incessant refrain, "check with your doctor," as though doctors have all the answers to all aspects of health care. They don't! Wasn't it medical doctors who thought bloodletting was the cornerstone of scientific wisdom? Wasn't it medical doctors who appeared in commercials dressed in white smock and stethoscope proclaiming that more doctors smoke Camels than any other brand? Why, only a short decade ago, medical doctors attacked as irresponsible and dangerous the suggestion that diet was a major contributing factor in the cause and prevention of cancer. Today, there's hardly a person who walks upright that's not aware of that crucial link.

Medical care does have its place. When it comes to diagnosis, surgery, emergency and trauma, the medical profession is there, thank God. But when it comes to long-term, chronic illness, they're out of their league. Unfortunately, however, the medical profession, early in this century, gained a monopoly over health care and has been busy ever since trying to discourage you from utilizing the other disciplines, even though they may better serve you!

This brings us to Dr. Rona's work. Here is a man who has been raised in the medical framework. He is an M.D. and his father before him was a life-long M.D. But Dr. Rona, having a stronger allegiance to his patients than to his profession, made it his business to learn what the best possible treatment was for his patients, whether it was medical or non-medical. He has dedicated himself to disseminating that information and *Return to the Joy of Health* is his monument to that endeavor. Thanks to Dr. Rona's efforts, your choices in the all-important area of health care treatment will be a lot easier.

As we all make our way through this life, on occasion we are fortunate enough to cross paths with others whose integrity and desire to improve the human experience is exceeded only by their love and genuine caring. Such a man is Dr. Zoltan Rona, for whom I feel honored to write this foreword.

- Harvey Diamond, Author, *Fit for Life*

Introduction

The King of the Vitamins

"What an honor it is for me that 'the king of the vitamins' asks me for my vitamins."

Dr. George Rona
(1924–1993)

M y father, George Rona, said a lot of funny things to me during his lifetime. One of the most memorable was when he jokingly referred to me as "the king of the vitamins." This occurred on one of my trips to visit him a few years before his death. I had forgotten my vitamin supplements at home and asked if I could take some of his multiple vitamin and mineral pills.

George was a pathologist, a full professor at McGill University Medical School and a great believer in the "Church of Modern Medicine." So much a believer was he that when he was diagnosed as having bone cancer he willingly submitted himself to painful radiation and chemotherapy. Being more a proponent of natural remedies, I advised him against these poisonous and mutilating treatments since the success rates were so poor. I never won an argument with my father, and to this day I regret that I could do nothing to change his mind on the treatments. I shall probably always feel badly about the circumstances of his death and the indescribable suffering he must have endured. Whether following my advice would have made a difference will never be known. He died within two years of starting conventional cancer therapy.

The practice of conventional medicine has its greatest strength and value in the hospital emergency room. Acute crisis intervention demands the state-of-the-art in life-saving drugs and surgery. There is no alternative medical treatment for most of life's major traumas. Conventional medicine is the clear choice when it comes to the treatment of broken bones, lacerations, severed tendons, heart attacks and organ failures. On the other hand, conventional medicine leaves a lot to be desired when it comes to the treatment or prevention of chronic illnesses like arthritis, cancer, diabetes and heart disease.

Largely as a response to the failures of conventional medicine, the early 1990s has seen an explosion in scientific research and in interest in herbs, vitamins, minerals, amino acids and natural therapeutics. Unfortunately, it has also brought with it a great deal of myth, misinformation and angry political activity: official denouncements and ridicule by the medical profession, unprecedented intervention by various government agencies and the dissemination, by the mass media, of lies from pharmaceutical and food lobbies.

Why is there suddenly a great interest in reclassifying natural therapies as drugs? Why are health food stores, nutritional doctors' offices and food supplement manufacturers in the United States suddenly being raided by groups like the FDA? Why are some items like tryptophan banned?

The consensus of opinion is that all this negativity is a direct result of either economics or politics. As I tried to explain in my first book, *The Joy of Health*, rationality, common sense and scientific proof have been bypassed in order to protect the financial interests of the pharmaceutical and medical industries. Other authors—James P. Carter in *Racketeering In Medicine: The Suppression of Alternatives*, for example— have gone into great detail as to how this comes about. Medical associations and allied government agencies have been successful in preventing anyone from making a claim about any natural food supplement. For example, it is a crime to advertise the fact that beta-carotene supplementation can prevent cancer even though there are over 200 published studies showing that it can.

In 1993, published research indicated that more than one-third of the American public had either visited an alternative health care provider (e.g., chiropractor, herbalist, holistic doctor, homeopath, etc.) or had used at least one natural remedy to complement or replace conventional medical care. The reason for this relates to the failure of the medical profession to help the North American public prevent or cure cancer, heart disease, diabetes, arthritis and hundreds of other chronic illnesses.

One in every three North Americans will experience cancer during their lifetime. Despite the fact that billions of dollars have been spent on cancer research in the past two decades, cancer cases and deaths from cancer are increasing. The same is true for diabetes, heart disease, arthritis and a host of immune system diseases like AIDS and chronic fatigue syndrome.

Since the publication of *The Joy of Health*, I have continued writing regular columns for health magazines like *alive*, *Health Naturally* and *Natural Health Products Report* to help spread the good news about herbal and nutritional medicine. I even started contributing regular articles to mainstream publications like the *Toronto Star.* I have lectured in almost every major city in Canada and the United States. Consequently, over the past three years, I have accumulated a large amount of material which I would like to share with a larger audience. Everything you read in this book is a response to readers' questions about the natural approach to prevention and healing using nutrition and herbs. Some of the topics came from questions at public lectures. This information is not meant to replace conventional medical treatment but to complement it.

I am a great believer in freedom of choice in health care. To have this freedom you must have information. I also believe that responsibility for health does not belong to doctors, health care practitioners, insurance companies, lawyers or the government. It belongs to the individual. If that individual wants a doctor to decide a treatment, that individual should be free to do so. Alternatively, he or she should also be free to decide on a treatment that excludes the medical profession. Health care providers ought to be, for the most part, educators, not interveners, persecutors or dictators. Unfortunately, even in 1995, the opposite is largely true. This means that individuals must do a great deal more to educate themselves on basic prevention and wellness if they expect to have more control over their health; one cannot rely solely on the medical or dietetic profession.

If you need immediate help or education on a personal health matter, consult a naturopath or medical doctor familiar with nutrition and herbal medicine. There is a growing army of such practitioners. For names, addresses and phone numbers of organizations or associations that can give you a list of natural health professionals in your area, consult the resources section in the appendix.

Avoid trying to convert people to your way of thinking about health. That's almost as difficult to do as to convert a Jewish rabbi into a Muslim. The psychological and spiritual aspects of healing must always be taken into account, especially when asking anyone to make radical changes in diet and lifestyle. Natural therapies are not for everyone. Although it may be hard for you and other wellness-oriented folks to accept, some people are far better off with conventional medicine.

I have rarely seen any disease clear up when the patient had no belief in the treatment or the doctor. This is true of conventional medical treatment as well. If the patient is negative about the treatment, it usually will not work. Support the medical therapy of the person's choice, especially if the person has a lot of trust in it and in his or her doctor. Of course, you can always provide people with written information, videos and audiotapes of lectures, etc. It's up to them, however, to act on the information when and if they are ready to do so.

Prevention, wellness and health promotion have a great deal to do with things that are largely under your control, not your doctor's. Your lifestyle and eating habits may be crucial in determining your susceptibility to disease. As you will read in the pages that follow, there is a great deal more you can do to take health matters into your own hands. Hopefully, this book will be a good starting point in your return to the joy of health. Much of it updates and complements *The Joy of Health*. My sincere thanks to all of you who bought a copy of my first book. Thanks to the success of *The Joy of Health*, I am able to bring you this sequel. If you have any questions, comments or criticisms, please write to me in care of the publisher.

– ZR

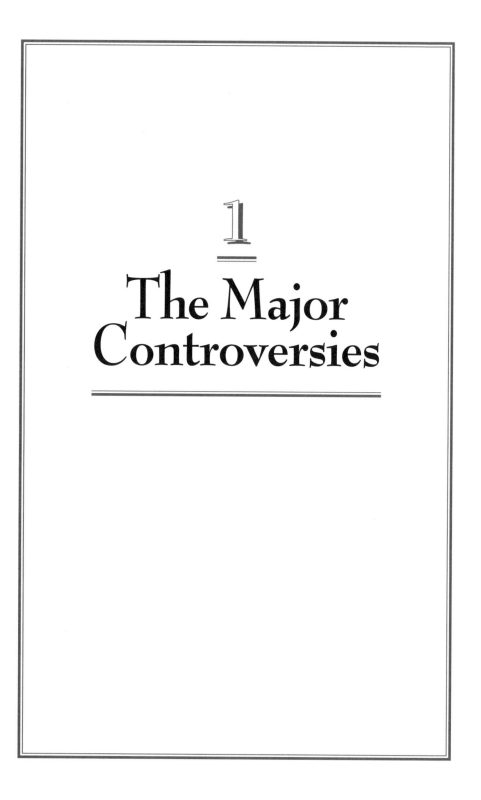

1
The Major Controversies

The Suppression of Medical Alternatives

The world of conventional medicine sees to it that there is a relentless battering of holistic doctors, naturopaths, homeopaths, chiropractors, acupuncturists, herbalists, osteopaths, colonic irrigationists, reflexologists, nutritionists and any practitioner not intimately affiliated with the medical monopoly. If you're the competition, keep your eyes peeled. As a past president of the Canadian Holistic Medical Association, I assure you that there is plenty of documentation to support this.

In publicly funded hospitals, dietitians, who are generally opposed to vitamin, mineral and herb supplements, are the food dictators while physiotherapists monopolize the manipulative arts. Ever wonder why chiropractors and naturopaths are not allowed to practice in hospitals? Why isn't acupuncture and biofeedback covered by Medicare when hundreds of scientific studies show them to be superior to physiotherapy for pain control? What about visualization or meditation therapy for cancer patients instead of the Catholic priest or Protestant minister? After all, why can't hospital patients who want a different approach to spiritual healing get it? Ever wonder why clinical ecology testing and treatments are not covered by Medicare even though many allergy sufferers find the results superior to those of conventional allergy treatments?

Alternative practitioners often have their offices raided, their equipment confiscated and their practices interrupted in other ways in the name of "protecting the public." If the usual bag of dirty tricks fails to intimidate the alternative practitioner, then pulling political strings and using the law to ban or eliminate the alternative treatment may succeed in putting him or her out of business. If you want proof that this is indeed going on in Canada, pick up a copy of Dr. James Carter's book, *Racketeering in Medicine: The Suppression of Alternatives*. It's a real eye-opener.

Carter discusses the plight of chelation therapy, one of the many treatments that is the focus of attack by medical associations and licensing bodies. In 1988, intravenous chelation therapy was banned in Ontario despite the fact that thousands of Ontario residents demanded it. There is a great deal of published information on the benefits of chelation and no objective evidence of any danger to the public. Residents of Ontario must now cross the border to receive chelation therapy legally. Over 20 million people worldwide have benefited from chelation without deaths or significant side effects. So, why did the Ontario government ban chelation?

According to Carter, the more than 30 years of harassment may have started as scientific arrogance but now seems to stem from chelation's threat to the very profitable business of coronary bypass surgery, angioplasty and related treatments. The average cost of coronary bypass surgery is $40,000 while the average cost of a series of chelation treatments is $3,000. Studies show that the more a medical procedure costs the insurance company, the more that company can charge in premiums. Hence, coronary bypass surgery is profitable; chelation therapy, on the other hand, threatens the profits of those who invested huge sums of money in surgical equipment and facilities. Currently, these investments are handsomely reimbursed by insurance companies including, in Canada, provincial Medicare.

Medical costs are spiralling out of control to such an extent that in Ontario, for example, the provincial Medicare plan can no longer afford to pay for the annual physical. Doctors now say that the annual physical is "unscientific." Sound familiar?

Natural treatments are less expensive, can be applied by non-medical practitioners, are well tolerated, with limited or no side effects, and have the potential of saving Medicare billions of dollars. It is time for us to take a more aggressive stand for natural therapeutics. It is time to put a stop to the disrespect for alternative training and knowledge and the suppression of the medicine of the future.

The "COPS" Come Out of the Closet

Less than a decade ago, the College of Physicians and Surgeons—the official provincial medical licensing bodies in our country—were an almost invisible group of bureaucrats. These professional organizations have the power to license doctors and a mandate to protect the public from medical incompetence and professional misconduct. The public seemed satisfied with their work or, at the very least, were not upset with any of their decisions regarding the health care system. Challenges to the dominant power of physicians in health care were easily defeated and went unnoticed by both the public and the mass media.

Toward the end of the 1980s, however, large numbers of Canadians, disenchanted with conventional medicine, began turning to non-drug, non-surgical alternatives. Practices such as nutrition therapy, chelation therapy, homeopathy, chiropractic and acupuncture grew in popularity. The *New England Journal of Medicine* reported that at least one in three Americans sought the services of alternative practitioners with or without the approval of their medical doctors. In Canada, the figure is closer to one in five.

Nothing happens by coincidence, especially in the escalating war between conventional medicine and its perceived competition. In reaction to the explosive popularity of complementary health services, the medical "COPS"—the College of Physicians and Surgeons—have come out of the closet; the pressure is on them to protect a turf that has long been assumed to be solely their own. In a detailed letter to all B.C. provincial legislators, Lorna J. Hancock, executive director of Health Action Network Society (HANS), presents evidence for "Project 2000," a political strategy designed to eliminate any competition to the established medical system. Project 2000's impact will be felt not only across Canada, but globally as well.

Although the drama is unfolding differently in each province, there are some common characteristics to the struggle. In each province where the College of Physicians and Surgeons has attempted to suppress alternatives, the public has risen up and engaged them in political, legal and media battles. In the 1990s, organized public dissent against these provincial groups is a powerful force.

In Nova Scotia, the cases of Drs. Baker and LaValley set a precedent for grass roots public confrontation with the College of Physicians and Surgeons. Covert attempts by the "COPS" to harass these popular homeopaths led to the birth of Citizens for Choice in Health Care—a grass roots advocacy group. Headlines in publications across the country, appearances on TV talk shows, embarrassing medical journal editorials and heavy lobbying of elected government officials by the public forced the College of Physicians and Surgeons of Nova Scotia to retreat and give in to the demands of the public. Not only did the embattled doctors speak up against the college, but so did a very angry public, frightened by the prospect of losing homeopathic services. As public servants, the College of Physicians and Surgeons had no other choice but to back off and serve the public.

In British Columbia, naturopaths and massage therapists are partially covered under Medicare. Recently, the B.C. Medical Association and the College of Physicians and Surgeons of B.C. have come out swinging against these supplementary services, claiming that Medicare could no longer afford such "non-essential," "unscientific" therapies. Of course, these same doctors say nothing about the millions of tax dollars spent by B.C. on "essential" benefits like disability and malpractice insurance for doctors.

Since the late 1980s the College of Physicians and Surgeons of B.C. has vigorously opposed intravenous chelation therapy and has made it next to impossible for doctors to provide this alternative to bypass surgery. Snide, arrogant and erroneous quips to the media about complementary medicine did not go unnoticed by those who felt insulted by a group perceived to be abusing their power. The public opposed the college through the efforts of groups like Health Action Network Society (HANS) and the EDTA Chelation Lobby Association of B.C. As in Nova Scotia, the war of words is intensifying.

In Ontario, the College of Physicians and Surgeons has managed to create a situation which could result in the extinction of doctors practicing nutrition, environmental medicine or any other complementary medical therapy. On December 13, 1993, the Ontario Legislature passed Bill 100, a law aimed at curtailing sexual abuse of patients by health care practitioners. No one is opposed to any bill designed to prevent patient abuse, but an eleventh hour amendment by the College of Physicians and Surgeons, aimed at "re-educating" physicians who deviated from conventional medical practice, raised the ire of dozens of professional and public groups. If this amendment is approved by the health minister, it would give the college, through a proposed "Quality Assurance Program," unprecedented power to eliminate any or all unconventional medical practices. At the very least, it would frighten new physicians away from even considering a career in complementary medicine.

The Ontario Medical Association and at least 24 other professional colleges have angrily opposed the amendment. Three new groups have formed to fight this issue: Freedom of Choice in Health Care, Coalition for Access to Preventive Medicine and Coalition of Physicians for Responsible Medical Democracy. Several thousand people have signed petitions demanding that the health minister repeal the amendment and allow the public the freedom to choose the type of health care they want. The amendment is currently under review.

Governmental agencies, pharmaceutical companies and professional organizations like the College of Physicians and Surgeons are attempting to discredit complementary medical practices and de-license any practitioner who strays from the status quo. Thus, although more people are demanding natural therapies, fewer physicians will be available to deliver the goods. I know of at least four complementary medical doctors who have left to practice in the United States as a direct result of intimidation such as that suffered by the Nova Scotia homeopaths. Provincial health plans do not cover many alternative practitioner services. The good news is that there are fewer Canadians satisfied with standing on the sidelines watching vested interest groups undermine the availability of complementary medicine.

It's Time to Clean Up Dirty Medicine

"The most effective way to put an end to alternative and complementary medicine is to criminalize its practitioners and supporters."

Martin J. Walker
Dirty Medicine

Since 1990, Freedom of Choice in Health Care groups have been popping up across Canada in growing numbers. They have been formed out of necessity to protect the public's right to have access to alternative and complementary medicine. Ironically, these groups, organized and run by members of the general public, are waging war against the very organizations empowered by governments to protect the public, namely each province's College of Physicians and Surgeons and the Federal Health Protection Branch (HPB).

The colleges, HPB, provincial medical associations and big-business pharmaceutical companies are all intensifying their efforts to suppress medical alternatives. This is evident in the harassment of doctors of complementary medicine, especially practitioners of environmental medicine.* It is also evident in the creation of repressive laws banning effective treatments like chelation therapy. The targeting for elimination of 64 herbs from Canadian health food store shelves is yet another example of how these groups have conspired to eliminate their perceived competition.

Why is all this happening and why now? Martin J. Walker, author of *Dirty Medicine*, presents evidence for the existence of an organized campaign to stop complementary and alternative medicine. He feels this conspiracy has accelerated in the past few years owing to the need for pharmaceutical firms to defend their products and profits from the competition. Natural medicine in its many forms is expanding and becoming popular beyond all expectations. Drug firms may very well be reacting to this perceived threat. The AIDS drug AZT, for example, alone produces yearly profits of over $400 million. It is amazing that a drug like AZT can make such incredible profits when research is proving that AZT has never cured a single case of AIDS.

Another reason for the conspiracy is that alternative health care practitioners like naturopaths, homeopaths, herbalists and chiropractors are, as Walker puts it, "eroding the mystique which presently defends the profes-

---

* Environmental (or ecological) medicine is a specialty devoted to the treatment of allergies caused by chemicals, drugs, food, eletromagnetic pollution and other elements of a polluted environment. It was originally called clinical ecology, but in recent years has been renamed "environmental medicine."

sional monopoly of allopathic medicine." Power over treatment options and modalities is gradually shifting from the orthodox medical doctor or surgeon to the patient or client. Alternative or holistic medicine nurtures an understanding of the inner workings of the body, mind and spirit as opposed to the allopathic approach of "fixing" the body with drugs and invasive techniques. Losing the monopoly is clearly making the pharmaceutical kingdom nervous. Drug companies may no longer be able to rely on their puppets—the medical profession—to generate fortunes for them through their prescription pads.

> *"Investigations against alternative practitioners follow a pattern of arrogance, dogmatism, deprivation of constitutional rights and a might-makes-right attitude."*
>
> James P. Carter
Racketeering in Medicine

What is this dirty medicine? It is the bogus patient, sent to the offices of alternative health care practitioners by various government agencies, claiming to have symptoms for an illness and demanding a diagnosis. It is the tapped phone lines, the sabotage of office equipment, the vilification by press release, the slander by poison-pen letters to academic and civic organizations, the harassment of office staff and the setting up of bogus research projects purposefully carried out with a complete disregard for scientific procedure. It is the investigation of an alternative health care practitioner by orthodox doctors for no specific reason other than the fact that the practitioner's treatment philosophy is different from the status quo.

Cleaning up dirty medicine may be a difficult task. Some inroads, however, have already been made in Canada. Most notable of these is the successful campaign waged by the citizens of Nova Scotia on behalf of Dr. William LaValley, an M.D. and homeopath who was under investigation by the College of Physicians and Surgeons simply and only because he was a homeopath. It was recently my honor to speak at the second annual conference of the South West Nova Citizens for Choice in Health Care based in Yarmouth, Nova Scotia. I was most impressed by the fact that the local provincial member of parliament, Allister Surret, came to speak before the group, offering his government's support in the fight to bring about legally recognized alternatives in health care. Similar sentiments are being expressed by the Ministry of Health in Ontario. New Freedom of Choice in Health Care groups are forming in New Brunswick and other provinces. Encourage people to join and support these groups. It's time to clean up dirty medicine.

Scientific Medicine, the Placebo Effect and Health Fraud

"Scientific matters cannot possibly ever be decided upon in court. They can only be clarified by prolonged, faithful bona fide observations in friendly exchanges of opinion, never by litigation."

Ivan Illich, 1976

History will attest to the fact that many doctors practicing natural medicine have had to spend a large amount of their time and money in court, defending the scientific validity of various diagnostic and treatment modalities, before doctors who knew little and could care less about natural therapeutics. Conventional, drug-oriented doctors, despite the advice of scholars like Ivan Illich, are not terribly interested in "friendly exchanges of opinion." They attack alternative physicians for, among other things, prescribing vitamin and mineral supplements, recommending herbal or homeopathic remedies and using intravenous vitamin therapy.

The dogmas of conventional medicine are guarded ferociously by powerful medical associations and licensing groups. Although this medical monopoly claims to operate strictly on the basis of science, in reality, "scientific" medicine depends on the whims of politics and on the dictates of big-business pharmaceuticals. Treatments that fail to conform to the belief systems of the drug cartels are derogatorily referred to as "placebo medicine" or "quackery." If they become too popular, they get attacked and eventually eliminated. One example is the removal of tryptophan from health food stores. This coincided with the appearance of Prozac, a megamoney maker. If you think this was a coincidence, think again.

In November 1989, there was a nationwide recall of L-tryptophan by the U.S. Food and Drug Administration (FDA). This was in response to reports of over 900 cases of tryptophan-related eosinophilia myalgia-syndrome (EMS). Symptoms included severe muscle and joint pain, fever, weakness and a marked elevation of white cells. By June of 1990, several thousand cases had been reported to the Center for Disease Control from across the United States and Puerto Rico. There were several hundred fatalities, and L-tryptophan was banned entirely from the shelves of health food stores in the United States. There have as yet been no fatalities reported in Canada.

I was quite surprised when I read these reports since I had never seen any significant side effects to L-tryptophan in my 17 years of practice. L-tryptophan is an amino acid (a building block of proteins) and can be used safely and effectively to treat depression, insomnia, premenstrual syndrome, migraine headaches and eating disorders. Until a few years ago, it was available without prescription in Canada. Currently, you need a doctor's prescription to get it from a pharmacy.

There are no studies that prove that L-tryptophan can cause EMS. In over 30 years of use and 30 million users, no indication of EMS had been noted. It is known, however, that people who suffer from adrenal insufficiency, vitamin B6 deficiency and liver dysfunction may develop eosinophilia when they supplement with high doses of L-tryptophan. Anyone known to be suffering from these conditions should be carefully monitored by a physician if they are also supplementing with L-tryptophan. Eosinophilia is usually considered to be a sign of allergy, infections caused by parasites or fungi and certain adverse drug reactions.

In an article in the January 1990 issue of the *Townsend Letter for Doctors*, Drs. Alan Gaby, Jonathan Wright and Jonathan Collin write: ". . . the FDA has misled the public by implying that an elevation of blood eosinophils resulting from an allergic reaction is related to any of the serious eosinophilic syndromes. It is also misleading to call eosinophilia a 'blood disorder' when it is usually a natural response to contact with an allergen." These authors speculated that it was more likely that "a manufacturing error resulted in a contaminated tryptophan product, with eosinophilia the consequence of the contaminant."

As of 1994, consensus in the medical literature is that the reported EMS cases were caused by a single batch of contaminated tryptophan. Even the FDA now admits that a contaminant in tryptophan capsules and tablets from Japanese suppliers was the source of the problem. L-tryptophan supplements currently available from suppliers in Canada are free of contamination. The amino acid remains unavailable in the United States.

In a similar way, contaminated Tylenol caused several poisoning deaths. The capsules were taken off the market and swiftly replaced by uncontaminated Tylenol. Uncontaminated L-tryptophan, although available in many countries, has not been allowed back on the shelves in U.S., not even by prescription. Many holistic practitioners who were major prescribers of L-tryptophan suspect that it was kept off the market to make way for the newly released antidepressants known as serotonin reuptake inhibitors (Prozac, Zoloft, Paxil and others). In case you haven't heard, these drugs are now the most widely prescribed antidepressants on the market. L-tryptophan works biochemically in a very similar way to these drugs, increasing brain levels of the neurotransmitter serotonin.

One of the many ploys used by medical monopolists when manipulating the mass media or when lobbying politicians, is to argue that naturopaths, chiropractors, homeopaths and other health care professionals use treatments that have never been proven scientifically. The phrase, "Where are your double-blind studies?" is a common quip employed by arrogant physicians intent on discrediting natural treatments. We would all like to believe that the practice of medicine is based on scientific principles, but at least 80 percent of currently used conventional medical/surgical procedures (like the coronary bypass) have never been subjected to either controlled clinical trials or double-blind, placebo-controlled studies. Yet, no licensing board has ever disciplined a doctor for using worthless allergy tests, prescribing drugs that have been proven to make a disease worse or failing to practice effective prevention.

How scientific is conventional medicine anyway? Allow me to illustrate. Physicians who have been in practice for over a decade have had numerous opportunities to evaluate the accuracy and reliability of the skin scratch test for food allergy diagnosis. Despite the fact that this test has been proven to be next to worthless in the diagnosis of food allergies, conventional allergists continue to use this test. And dissatisfied patients wander from allergist to allergist in an attempt to get an accurate diagnosis. One patient I saw recently had been to five allergists. Each did skin scratch tests and each diagnosed a different set of allergies and recommended different treatments. One found no allergies and referred the patient to a psychiatrist. This is science?

Non-steroidal anti-inflammatory drugs (NSAIDS) have been shown to worsen osteoarthritis. Yes, they provide temporary pain relief, but studies show they accelerate the disease process. In addition, these drugs have been documented to cause over 25,000 cases of gastrointestinal hemorrhage each year. When the arthritis patient bleeds to death from these drugs, does the doctor get hauled up before disciplinary committees? No way. After all, he practices "scientific" medicine.

Another conventional medical behavior that passes for scientific medicine is the treatment of heart disease. Despite overwhelming scientific evidence supporting the benefits of diet and antioxidant supplementation in the prevention and treatment of heart disease, conventional cardiologists continue to do little more than prescribe a shopping bag full of drugs with side effects too numerous to list. One particularly detailed book, written by Dr. Joe Goldstrich, a cardiologist who worked for the Pritikin Center, lists over 200 pages of medical references on the benefits of diet, exercise and food supplements. Cardiologists, by and large, continue to ignore this research while licensing boards continue to persecute doctors who apply this latest research to their patients. In the past month alone I saw six new cardiac patients who were basically told by their cardiologists to eat anything they wanted. I submit to you that this is the real health fraud that needs to be addressed, not a holistic doctor's vitamin prescriptions.

Medicine has always been more of an art than a science. Should physicians who deviate from the conventional scientific dogmas, whatever they may be, be punished even if no harm is done to the patient? It is not a question of whether any specific healing philosophy is scientific, but whether science itself should be such a dominant force in the art of medicine.

In Defense of Expensive Urine

Prescribing vitamin and mineral supplements is not scientific medicine. At least that is what groups like the National Council Against Health Fraud (NCAHF) state repeatedly in their newsletters. The NCAHF is perhaps the most vocal of the groups opposed to chiropractors, homeopaths, acupuncturists, chelators and holistic doctors, branding them time and again as dangerous quacks.

I am sure that many of you have heard medical "experts" claim that any practitioner who prescribes vitamins or other food supplements is not only creating expensive urine, but is defrauding the public. Is there any truth to this? Are natural health care practitioners really guilty of practicing unscientific medicine?

The term "scientific" has been used successfully this century to sell the legitimacy of the medical profession to the public. The practice of medicine, however, is no more scientific than the use of tarot cards. Medicine is an art. Calling it scientific is, at best, wishful thinking. After all, the United States Office of Technology Assessment estimates that 80 to 90 percent of all conventional medical procedures have no scientific validity. Scientific studies, for example, have proven that coronary bypass surgery is no better than conservative medical care for the treatment of hardening of the coronary arteries. Other studies by people like Dr. Dean Ornish go so far as to say that coronary artery disease can be reversed by diet and lifestyle changes alone. Despite this, a record number of bypass surgeries are done year after year by advocates of scientific medicine.

The cost of coronary bypass surgery runs into the millions of dollars annually, money that could be better spent on health promotion programs. The NCAHF has said nothing about such public ripoffs by so-called scientific medicine. A similar story is true for the prescription of hundreds of commonly used drugs, cancer chemotherapy and dozens of surgical procedures like routine episiotomies at baby deliveries. The science to back them up is simply not there. The public accepts most drugs and surgery as valid on the say-so of the doctor. It's time to start questioning expensive scientific medicine and not the people and procedures opposing this sham. The NCAHF is certainly not doing anything about the real fraud in health care delivery.

What about vitamin and mineral supplements? We are told by the purveyors of scientific medicine that people can get all the essential nutrients from food alone. A lot of scientists disagree. The quality of food grown today does not meet the standards of the medical/dietitian system. With over 70,000 new chemicals added to our environment since the 1940s, our food supply is not what it used to be. Hundreds of studies indicate that our daily vitamin and mineral needs are not met by food alone. Deficiency-related diseases are more frequently reported in medical journals. Hospitals, with their dietitian-supervised meals, have been shown to increase the incidence of vitamin and mineral deficiencies in patients. Studies show that the longer one stays in hospital, the greater the risk of developing a nutritional deficiency.

"On its way from the garden to the gullet," writes Dr. Emmanuel Cheraskin of the University of Alabama School of Medicine, "the food on your table has had 50 percent of its nutrients removed." Countless others echo this leading nutrition researcher's findings: up to 80 percent of food's value is lost through processing, transportation, freezing, storage, cooking, spraying and chemical additives. In order to get the same amount of vitamins and minerals from food alone that your grandparents did in the early part of the twentieth century, you would have to consume six large meals per day. Since this would overload you with calories, it is far better to either grow your own food organically or take vitamin and mineral supplements. Some have argued that one of the reasons for the epidemic of obesity, fatigue, immune system disorders and mental illness in the population is micronutrient deficiency.

Supplemental vitamins and minerals protect the body against the toxic effects of a polluted environment. Over the past decade, extensive research has been done on the subject of free radical pathology. Knowledge of free radical pathology is so widespread that even formerly conservative groups like national cancer societies preach the merits of beta-carotene, vitamin C, vitamin E and selenium in combating disease. Many reputable scientists and medical doctors believe that free radical pathology is at the root of cancer, allergies, heart disease, immune system disorders and a long list of degenerative diseases.

Free radicals are highly reactive molecules (containing an unpaired electron) that can cause damage to the body. They can be offset by antioxidants (vitamins, minerals, enzymes). Free radicals come from drugs, radiation, pesticides, herbicides, food additives, cigarette smoke, hydrocarbons from car exhausts, industrial waste products and many other sources. The gradual deterioration of the ozone layer and stress in general play a part. All of this necessitates even greater protection with antioxidant nutrients like beta-carotene, vitamin A, B vitamins (especially B3 and B6), vitamins C and E, bioflavonoids, selenium, zinc, silicon, amino acids, enzymes like superoxide dismutase (SOD), coenzymes and essential fatty acids.

If you are a practitioner involved in health promotion and disease prevention, rest assured that the prescription of vitamin and mineral supplements is supported by sound science. Vitamin- and mineral-rich urine, expensive or not, is a legitimate marker for health promotion and real preventive medicine.

The Scandal of Hospital Malnutrition

The important role of nutrition in the prevention and treatment of disease is gaining credibility not only with the general public but with a growing segment of the medical community. Unfortunately, the conclusions of hundreds of scientific studies have not yet been implemented in the majority of Canadian hospitals.

In the late 1980s, several scientists and clinicians reported that the poor quality of food served to hospitalized patients was contributing to their illnesses. One 1987 report in the *Medical Post* claimed that "up to 40 percent of patients in Canadian hospitals are suffering from clinically significant malnutrition that is more life-threatening than the disease or operation they were originally hospitalized for." Others echoed these sentiments, warning that the longer one stays in hospital, the more likely it is that he or she will suffer the effects of one or more nutritional deficiencies.

The American Dietetic Association recently concluded that at least half of all hospitalized elderly suffer from malnutrition. Long-stay patients are especially victimized and are described in published studies as having "gross undernourishment." Food and beverages provided to patients evaluated in these studies did not satisfy basal metabolic demands according to the recommended dietary allowances.

Why is this happening? Malnutrition in hospitals is caused, by and large, by the neglect of basic nutritional principles. It can be seen when protein (albumin) levels and lymphocyte counts drop below acceptable levels. Aside from protein and calories, hospitalized patients may not be receiving adequate amounts of calcium, potassium, zinc, folic acid and vitamins A, D, E and B6.

Often, hospital menus create the malnutrition of excess. For example, contrary to some hospital food philosophies, a pepperoni pizza, cola and donut are not a good idea as a first meal after coronary bypass surgery. Similarly, colitis patients should not eat "anything they like," and hypoglycemics do not benefit from jello and cookies. And why is it that tonsillectomy patients are fed dish after dish of ice cream when it is a documented fact that high sugar consumption suppresses immunity?

Recently, I received copies of weekly menus from two Ontario hospitals. One was a large community hospital in Toronto and the other was a teaching hospital in Ottawa. The Toronto menu was given to me by a patient, while the Ottawa menu was provided by the hospital. A computerized nutrient analysis was done on both seven-day menus using Food Processor II, a diet evaluation software program used by thousands of dietitians, nutritionists and doctors across North America. The Toronto menu was found to be deficient in 11 out of 30 nutrients, while the Ottawa menu was below the recommended dietary allowances in 16 out of 30 nutrients. Both menus were lacking in dietary fiber, essential fatty acids, zinc, copper, selenium and several B vitamins. The Toronto diet had 31 percent of the calories coming from fat, while the Ottawa fat count was 28 percent of the diet.

Understandably, hospital departments of nutrition and food services are defensive about the quality of food provided to hospitalized patients. Eight out of nine hospitals contacted refused to provide a copy of their menus. Hospital spokespersons claimed to follow the *Canada Food Guide to Healthy Eating* to ensure that patients receive adequate nutrients during hospitalization. There is no evidence that this is actually taking place. Hospital spokespersons also had a great deal of difficulty explaining why fast food chains like Tim Horton's and Macdonald's are starting up businesses in Canadian hospitals.

One hospital employee, who wished not to be identified, explained: "We try to follow the Canada Food Guide, but if chicken fingers or ice cream is all they want, something is better than nothing. Whatever we can get into them, we do. When they get better, we worry about the Canada Food Guide."

Under-staffing, a shortage of nutritional experts, hospital staff ignorance of proper nutrition, interdisciplinary rivalries and the medical profession's negative attitude and denial about the role of nutrition in health and disease are some of the reasons cited for the poor quality of hospital nutrition. Years of nutritional ignorance have led to the entrenchment of microwaved, degraded, devitalized hospital diets packaged in styrofoam.

Money and cutbacks are often blamed for substandard food in hospitals. This is a smokescreen—food in Canadian hospitals was substandard many years before any cutbacks. Secondly, common sense tells us that longer hospital stays cost the system more money. Since malnourished patients do not recover from their illness or surgery as quickly as do patients fed a diet that at least conforms to RDA levels, the money excuse makes no sense.

Suggested Solutions

Although doctors tend to oppose diet supplementation, and dietitians prefer to recommend dietary changes before advocating nutritional supplements, to date, neither attitude has been proven effective in eliminating hospital malnutrition. Therefore, if the patient can swallow a pill, and provided it is not medically contraindicated, I recommend that all hospitalized patients take at least a multiple vitamin and mineral supplement. Nutritional evaluations should be mandatory for all hospitalized patients, and diets tailored to specific individual nutrient needs.

If you are hospitalized, or have a loved one in hospital, ask the doctor if supplements are allowed, or, at the very least, have nutritious food ordered into the room. On the other hand, if your hospital menu includes donuts, cheeseburgers, milk shakes and French fries, you don't really need permission from anyone to improve your nutrient intake. Order in plenty of fresh fruits, vegetables, whole grains and legumes, along with a multiple vitamin and mineral supplement. Most importantly, write a letter of complaint to your provincial member of parliament and to the minister of health demanding an investigation into the scandal of malnutrition in Canadian hospitals.

Fighting the Penicillin Mentality

Nothing in conventional medical practice is as revered as the antibiotic prescription. Penicillin, tetracycline, erythromycin, sulfa drugs and dozens of other antibiotics are so commonly prescribed by doctors that most of us hardly give it a second thought. Antibiotics have no impact whatsoever on viral infections. They are misused and abused when they are prescribed without diagnostic cultures or other lab tests and when they are taken for the flu, the common cold and other self-limiting viral infections. They are also abused when prescribed for "prevention" of real or imagined infectious diseases and chronic conditions like acne. Not all antibiotics are prescribed by doctors. Many over-the-counter lotions, creams and drops contain generous amounts of broad-spectrum antibiotics and are available, no questions asked, from any pharmacy.

As one of the major sacraments of the Church of Modern Medicine, the use of antibiotics is seldom questioned or criticized. Even when studies show that antibiotics for middle ear infections in children have no advantage over a placebo (sugar pill), family doctors and pediatricians continue to dole them out. Antibiotics are firm dogma, the "magic bullets" of orthodoxy. Farmers and food processors eagerly feed antibiotics to commercial animals as if these chemicals were essential vitamins. Subsequently, they appear in milk, dairy products, beef, chicken, pork and other animal products. It is time to rethink our penicillin mentality.

Antibiotic Use May Cause:
- Antibiotic-resistant bacteria
- Immune suppression and chronic fatigue syndrome
- Food allergies or intolerance
- Yeast colonization and superinfection
- Chronic gastrointestinal diseases
- Return of tuberculosis
- Nutritional deficiencies
- Liver damage

The late 1980s and early 1990s witnessed some alarming effects from long-term antibiotic exposure. Antibiotic-resistant bacteria strains are just one of these emerging problems. Many strains of streptococcus, E. coli and haemophilus influenza are not only resistant to penicillin, but to broad- spectrum cephalosporin and sulfa antibiotics as well. The more antibiotics used by a given individual, the more likely the development of resistant infections. The reemergence of diseases like tuberculosis, once nearly eradicated in North America, is just one of the many newly recognized dangers of antibiotic overuse.

Antibiotics weaken the immune response. Studies show that the more antibiotics are used, the higher the rate of infection. Dr. Carol Jessop, clinical professor at the University of California at San Francisco, claims that 80 percent of her patients with chronic fatigue syndrome have a history of multiple antibiotic treatments as a child, adolescent or adult. The more one uses antibiotics, the less the body will be able to fight infections.

Dr. Leo Galland, a well-known author and specialist in internal medicine, links antibiotic use to the development of food allergies and food intolerance: "Several times a week I see a new patient whose allergies appeared or became much worse after a course of antibiotics." The use of tetracycline for months or even years on end for acne, chronic prostatitis or chronic bronchitis leads not only to the development of food allergies, but to chronic gastrointestinal disease (e.g., colitis, chronic diarrhea or irritable bowel syndrome).

One of the mechanisms by which antibiotics suppress immunity is through the destruction of friendly bacteria in the small and large intestines. Lactobacillus acidophilus and bifidobacteria protect us against infections not only in our bowel but in areas like the skin. Overuse of antibiotics, as well as use of the birth control pill, wipes out these friendly organisms and renders the body more susceptible to bacterial, viral, yeast (candida), fungal and parasitic infections. According to several authors, susceptibility to HIV infection and AIDS is increased by the frequent use of antibiotics in high risk groups.

Beneficial bacteria are also involved in either the synthesis or the bioavailability of many vitamins and minerals. Antibiotics can therefore lead indirectly to a long list of vitamin and mineral deficiencies. The most important of these are the B-complex vitamins, vitamin A, zinc and magnesium. The end result may be anemia, chronic fatigue and other nervous system symptoms (memory loss, depression, anxiety, worsening premenstrual syndrome, fibromyalgia and insomnia).

When laboratory culture reports indicate the presence of a bacterial infection, and if signs and symptoms warrant it, prescription antibiotics are valid treatment options. In such cases, a supplement of a friendly bacterial culture (e.g., L. acidophilus and bifidus) would certainly be a logical measure. One or more of a long list of natural antimicrobials (see list below) could be used while waiting for the results of throat, urine, vaginal or other cultures. If cultures prove negative, there is no legitimate reason to take a prescription antibiotic. If cultures show a bacterial infection, and antibiotics are prescribed, it is still valid complementary therapy to use garlic, vitamin C, zinc and herbal remedies along with the acidophilus supplement. Herbs, vitamins, minerals and probiotics help the immune system work better, compensate for some of the side effects of prescription antibiotics and, in the long run, speed recovery from infectious disease.

While one remedy may work better for some than others, singly or in combination, the common denominator of all these natural vitamins, minerals, herbs and probiotics is that they have no negative, long-term effect on the immune system. For a personalized program, see a naturopath or holistic doctor for assessment and counselling.

Natural Antibiotics and Immune System Boosters:
(Note: This is a partial list; missing is a list of homeopathic remedies, which are also valid options. See a homeopath for an individualized program.)

Aloe vera	Licorice
Astragalus	Lomatium
Beta-carotene	Lactobacillus acidophilus
Calendula	and bifidobacteria
Capsicum	Mullein
Coenzyme Q10	Propolis
Colloidal silver	Reishi, maitake and shiitake mushrooms
Echinacea	Suma
Essiac (a combination of sheep sorrel, burdock, slippery elm and Turkish rhubarb)	Saccharomyces boulardii
	Selenium
Goldenseal	Tea tree oil
Garlic	Vitamin A
Grapefruit seed extract	Vitamin C
Germanium	Vitamin E
St. John's wort	Zinc

The Organic "Immaculate" Deception

Organic foods and supplements have gained a lot of popularity over the past decade for many political, economic and health reasons. Natural health care practitioners and health enthusiasts are leaning toward organic because of growing concerns over the safety of commonly available commercial foods. According to the United States Environmental Protection Agency (EPA), the average child receives four times more exposure than an adult to at least eight widely used cancer-causing pesticides in foods. Also, 60 percent of all herbicides, 90 percent of all fungicides and 30 percent of all insecticides are carcinogenic. They can also cause nerve damage and genetic mutation and are implicated in birth defects as well.

Unfortunately, another potential area of hype and deception centers around the concept of organic certification. What is organic food, and what are organic products? According to the Organic Crop Improvement Association (OCIA), one of the oldest certifying agencies, organic farm products must meet the following criteria:

1. No synthetic herbicides, pesticides or chemical fertilizers can be used for three years prior to initial certification and thereafter.

2. Livestock must be fed 100 percent certified organic feeds and must receive no hormones, growth promoters, medicated feeds or indiscriminate medications.

3. All manure fertilizers must be composted a minimum of six months prior to use.

4. All animals must be raised in a humane fashion: no battery cages, small pens or physical mutilations are allowed.

5. Food processors must not use chemical rinses or other synthetic materials to produce their foods.

Other recognized, independent certifying agencies include Farm Verified Organic (FVO), Quality Assurance International (QAI) and California Certified Organic Farmers (CCOF). Any product claiming to be "certified organic" must have the certifying agency's logo on the produce or packaged products. If it does not have this logo, its organic authenticity can be traced by an audit trail—a list of farmers, processors, transporters and wholesalers who have handled the product. Consumers and health care practitioners have a right to this type of information. If such information is unavailable, or if the product is certified independently, there is no assurance whatsoever that the product is organic. A manufacturer that claims to certify its own products should be suspected of a lot of hype, at the very least. In the very important area of fresh-pressed, organic vegetable oils, several leading brands are actually deficient with respect to legitimate organic certification.

The Best Water

I'm often asked about the best type of drinking water. There still seems to be a great deal of controversy surrounding the subject. In *The Joy of Health*, I recommended spring water and distilled or reverse osmosis filtered tap water. Distilled water and reverse osmosis filtered water (i.e., soft water) are the cleanest of all the different types of drinking water, but both are deficient in trace minerals. After doing blood and hair mineral analysis on over 1,000 individuals, I've discovered that people who drink distilled or reverse osmosis filtered waters exclusively have a generally low level of minerals. Those who drink spring water, charcoal-filtered tap water or various bottled mineral waters (including club soda) have far fewer problems with trace mineral deficiencies. Important minerals like calcium, iron, copper, zinc, manganese, magnesium, silicon, and boron are seemingly leached out of the body by chronic use of soft drinking water. On the other hand, for short term detoxification from excess body burdens of toxic heavy metals like lead, cadmium, arsenic, aluminum, mercury and others, distilled or reverse osmosis filtration water is ideal. However, exclusive consumption of soft water increases the risk of heart disease, arthritis, osteoporosis and other conditions where optimal mineral levels provide protection.

If it's available to you where you live, use a good spring water for daily drinking purposes. If you live in a big city and have limited or no access to spring water, the best alternatives are bottled mineral waters or filtered tap waters (activated charcoal filters). A combination of charcoal-filtered and ozonated tap water is the best of both worlds. Ozonation destroys or inactivates all bacteria, fungi and parasites as well as most chemicals (e.g., chlorine), while the activated charcoal eliminates the majority of the larger impurities and carcinogenic substances. As the price of home ozonation/filtration units come down, affordability and availability will no longer be the issues they are now.

Herb Toxicity: The Real Story

Many people are concerned about the toxicity of certain herbs, in particular ma huang, also known as Mormon tea, ephedra or desert tea. Since all the seemingly credible horror stories about ma huang come from respected sources like family doctors, dietitians, pharmacists and government bureaucrats, there is a need to respond to these fears.

If you isolate one of its dozens of chemical constituents, concentrate it and purify it as a drug, there could indeed be toxicity with ma huang. It must be remembered, however, that herbs are not meant to be used in this fashion. Only pharmaceutical manufacturers use herbs in this way, and, as a result, get toxic effects with resulting deaths. Over 1,000 deaths occur each year as a direct result of over-the-counter cough and cold pharmaceuticals alone.

ASA and other anti-inflammatory, FDA-approved drugs, kill over 2,000 people in the United States each year as a result of stomach or intestinal hemorrhage. At least 25,000 hospital admissions each year are a direct result of this family of FDA-approved drugs. In 1991, the total number of poisonings from pharmaceuticals (prescription and over-the-counter) was 9,805. These fatalities were attributed to various analgesics (2,669), antidepressants (517), antihistamines (412), antimicrobials (953), cough and cold drugs (1,526), asthma therapies (257), cardiovascular drugs (370), gastrointestinal preparations (619), hormones and hormone antagonists (488), anti-anxiety/anti-psychotics (888) and topicals (1,106). Please note that each and every death was the result of "safe and effective" FDA-approved drugs. The total number of deaths in 1991 as a result of ma huang (or all herbs for that matter) was zero. For the years 1983 to 1990, statistics show a gradual rise in the number of deaths caused by FDA-approved drugs and zero deaths caused by vitamins, minerals or herbs. These statistics were reported by Donald Loomis from information supplied by the National Capitol Poison Center of the United States.

Let's take a closer look at ma huang. When one uses the whole herb, balanced by nature, or uses it synergistically with other herbs, toxicity is extremely rare. Ma huang *(Ephedra sinica)* is a whole herb. Ephedrine is simply one of ma huang's many components and is sold as a drug. It is the chemical responsible for the side effects frequently whined about by critics of herbal medicine. Take enough ephedrine on its own and death is possible. Please note, however, that ephedrine on its own does not have the same properties as ma huang. Any claim to the contrary is false, or misleading at best.

I have used ma huang in my practice for over 12 years. It is effective in the treatment of colds, flus, chronic fatigue, poor stamina, asthma, allergies, slow metabolism, depression, digestive problems and obesity. Yes, there are some people who cannot tolerate its stimulating effects, but such individuals are rare and frequently deficient in antioxidant vitamins and minerals. The majority of the population (99 percent or more) tolerates ma huang well.

It is said that people with high blood pressure, heart problems and prostate problems should not take ma huang. Nonsense. Coffee and tea are more likely to cause such people problems than ma huang. For those with heart or blood pressure problems, ma huang should be taken in low doses to begin with and gradually increased as tolerated. For those with prostate problems, ma huang can be combined with saw palmetto and bee pollen. This will prevent problems with the urinary flow, and help shrink a swollen or enlarged prostate. In large doses, ma huang can prevent weight gain and, for this reason, it is not recommended during pregnancy. However, once the baby is born, the mother can go back to using ma huang to help lose the weight accumulated during pregnancy.

Statistics aside, any substance, including water and oxygen, can become toxic if the dosage is high enough. Although extremely rare, cases of water poisoning have been reported in psychotic patients who drank gallon after gallon of water until they drowned. Similarly, excessive oxygen can cause tissue damage so severe as to lead to organ destruction (e.g., blindness due to oxidative damage to the retina). It's simply a question of amount. Since most mentally balanced people do not guzzle 80 gallons of water in one sitting, it is reasonable to assume that water is a safe nutrient supplement. The same can be said for most vitamins, minerals and herbs. When taken in the traditionally recommended dosages, ma huang is safe. When used in conjunction with white willow bark, ginseng, saw palmetto, ginger and other synergistic herbs, it has potent health-enhancing effects that have been well-documented for centuries.

It's time we demanded real proof of toxicity from high profile doctors, dietitians, pharmacists, the FDA and government bureaucrats before allowing them to force natural remedies like ma huang off the market or under the medical prescription umbrella.

Herb, Vitamin and Mineral Addiction

Believe it or not, some critics of vitamin, mineral and herb supplementation have suggested that it is possible to become addicted to natural remedies. The most common reason cited for this purported addiction is the fact that taking supplements causes people to have increased energy, which disappears when the supplements are discontinued. If high energy is addictive, why isn't this a positive thing?

It is virtually impossible to become physically addicted to any natural remedies. There are small amounts of caffeine in herbs like kola nut, but the potential for addiction to kola nut is less than the potential for addiction to coffee. It is possible, however, to become psychologically addicted to any substance. We are all familiar with addictions to sugar, coffee, tea, chips, junk food, television, aspirin—the list goes on. There are also workaholics, chocoholics and saltaholics. These people may or may not need psychotherapy, depending on your belief system. Unfortunately, many of the people who get psychotherapy for these "addictions" become addicted to the therapy or therapist. Perhaps, as more and more people take supplemental vitamins, minerals and herbs, there will, at some point, be healthaholics.

Vitamin A Problems

Some people seem to have a low threshold for vitamin A. They must carefully monitor their daily intake so as to avoid symptoms of toxicity: headache, dry and itching skin, abdominal pain and bruising, among others. This is a condition known as hypervitaminosis A. Studies indicate that daily intakes of 25,000 to 50,000 IU of vitamin A may produce adverse side effects in some individuals. On the other hand, there are people who can easily tolerate 300,000 IU per day without side effects of any kind.

In cases where vitamin A toxicity occurs with intakes lower than 10,000 IU per day, there is almost always a history of liver disease associated with drugs, alcohol, viral hepatitis or protein/calorie malnutrition. Pregnant women and children also have a greater sensitivity to vitamin A at doses of 10,000 IU per day. Anyone who has a history of almost any kind of liver disease, or who has been on long-term drug therapy, should be cautious in their use of vitamin A.

Hypervitaminosis A is reversible by stopping any vitamin A supplementation and improving liver health with a vegetarian diet. Great benefits may be derived from following a raw vegetable and fruit diet for several weeks. Short-term juice fasting is also beneficial. Since the 1950s there have been several reports on the benefits of supplementation or infusion of vitamin B12, folic acid and vitamin C. The basic effect of these nutrients is to reduce the mean duration of hepatitis. Supplementation with the bioflavonoid cianidanol (catechin) is also effective in reducing the damage seen in hepatitis.

Milk thistle extract (silymarin) helps most liver disorders. So does coenzyme Q10, black radish, red clover, dandelion, B-complex vitamins and the amino acids L-methionine and L-cysteine. Injections of raw liver extract and vitamin B12 may be dramatically effective in some cases. Many patients can learn to give themselves regular injections until the liver has had a chance to repair and rebuild itself. Dosages for all these remedies depend on individual patient tolerance and disease severity. Supervision by a health care practitioner (medical doctor or naturopath) is strongly recommended.

Vitamin A may not cause any deaths, but doesn't vitamin A supplementation lead to birth defects? There has never been a study demonstrating a clear cause-and-effect relationship between women using massive doses of vitamin A during pregnancy and the appearance of birth defects. Certainly, the amount of vitamin A in multivitamins or cod/halibut liver oil (10,000 IU or less) has no effect on the fetus. One recent study by Johnson et al. proved that such doses do not even raise blood levels of vitamin A, let alone cause birth defects or abnormalities in liver function tests. The same cannot be claimed for synthetic (adulterated) forms of vitamin A used in the treatment of acne (i.e., isotretinoin). Synthetic, prescription forms of isotretinoin do indeed cause birth defects, even at low doses. Let us not confuse these drugs with naturally occurring vitamin A in multivitamins or fish oil capsules.

Vitamin toxicity is rare and only theoretically possible. The most common vitamin toxicity reported in scientific journals is hypervitaminosis A.

The dose required to produce toxicity is highly variable. One study claims that 1 million IU taken daily for five years did not lead to toxicity in a series of patients. Others claim toxicity with daily intakes of 25,000 to 50,000 IU for several months. These discrepancies can be reconciled by understanding that low doses are more likely to produce toxicity in those whose liver function has already been compromised. In those with normal liver function, even massive doses fail to have a toxic effect.

It is essential that health care practitioners put things in proper perspective so as not to scare patients who are practicing sound preventive medicine. If a pregnant woman has normal liver function, there is absolutely no evidence to suggest that taking a multivitamin containing vitamin A will do any harm. On the contrary, she is helping to prevent birth defects, blindness, infections and a large number of other afflictions seen all too often in newborns whose mothers are unaware of sound nutritional practices.

If vitamin A was a dangerous nutrient one would expect cases of vitamin A toxicity to be increasing, given that a significant number of people are now supplementing with this vitamin. This is not the case, however. Worldwide, vitamin A toxicity is rare—estimated at only 200 cases annually. And the condition is reversible if the supplement is discontinued. Incidences of toxicity occur far more frequently with the over-the-counter drugs often recommended by doctors for pregnant women (e.g., acetaminophen, ASA, anti-nausea drugs, antibiotics, etc.).

What are some of the signs of vitamin A toxicity? According to published reports, signs of chronic vitamin A toxicity include fatigue, malaise, lethargy, headaches, abdominal pain, constipation, insomnia, restlessness, night sweats, hair loss, brittle nails, irregular menses, emotional lability, mouth fissures, dry, scaly, rough, yellowish skin, superficial retinal hemorrhages, exophthalmos, gout attacks, peripheral edema, abnormal bone growth in children, and increased intracranial pressure with headaches, nausea and vomiting. In the majority of cases, however, most of these symptoms are relieved within a few days to a week of discontinuing vitamin A. Full recovery usually follows within weeks or months. However, cirrhosis and bone growth abnormalities caused by vitamin A toxicity are irreversible. Since nausea is likely to occur long before any significant liver damage sets in, most people will see this as an obvious reason to stop or decrease their intake of vitamin A supplements. This built-in safety mechanism is not one hundred percent foolproof, so periodic lab tests to assess liver function are a good idea, especially in those who take more than 25,000 IU daily for any extended period of time.

Public Deceived
by Vitamin E and Beta-Carotene Study

In the past decade, over 200 published medical studies have reported the cancer-preventive effects of antioxidant vitamins, minerals and amino acids. It was, therefore, a shock to read that a new Finnish study, published in the prestigious *New England Journal of Medicine* (April 1994), claimed that beta-carotene and vitamin E have no impact on cancer prevention.

The study also concluded that these vitamins may actually cause cancer. The *New York Times*, *Toronto Star* and the major media around the world jumped on the news and, with sensationalized headlines, warned the public about the potential dangers of taking vitamins. Can we really believe the conclusions of this study? There are some glaring problems with the credibility of the information reported and used to fuel a smear campaign against vitamins:

1. All the subjects of the study had smoked an average of 20.4 cigarettes per day for 35.9 years. The average age of the male participants was 57.2 years. No study has ever made the ridiculous claim that taking vitamins at any dose could compensate for the harmful effects of smoking a pack of cigarettes daily for over 35 years. It is highly probable that such individuals would develop lung and other cancers; attempting prevention through vitamin therapy is meaningless without cigarette cessation.

That it may take twenty or more years for cancer of the lungs to develop in smokers was not accounted for by the study. It is possible, therefore, that a large number of these heavy smokers already had cancer before the supplements were taken. The measly dose of two antioxidants would have little, if any, impact on an established cancer.

2. The study was carried out at many different medical centers around the world for periods varying from five to eight years. This is hardly a long enough period of time to make such strong conclusions about long-term vitamin safety and efficacy, especially in potentially diseased smokers. Since cancer takes more than five to eight years to become clinically noticeable, the study time is meaningless. This point is supported by an editorial in the same issue of the *New England Journal of Medicine*. In it, Hennekens, Buring and Peto point out that a "lack of significant benefit in the ATBC trial, which had a median duration of only six years, does not necessarily preclude the finding of a significant benefit in substantially longer trials." On the other hand, despite overwhelming published evidence to the contrary, these same authors conclude that the benefits of antioxidant vitamins have not yet been proved.

Additionally, to quote directly from the fine print, "all formulations were colored with quinoline yellow." Quinoline yellow is an artificial food dye with known cancer-causing properties. This gross error in methodology may very well have been another reason for the higher than expected cancer rates.

3. The study did not account for important nutritional variables like selenium. Finland has extremely low levels of selenium in the soil, and it is known that vitamin E requires selenium in order to have antioxidant effect. Nutrition intervention trials done in China using a broader spectrum of antioxidants, including selenium, showed cancer reduction rates as high as 21 percent.

What about alcohol intake? It is well known that alcohol interferes with the activity of both beta-carotene and vitamin E. It is also a fact that the Finns have one of the highest rates of alcohol consumption in the world.

4. The study agents were synthetic dl-alpha-tocopherol and synthetic beta-carotene. The biological activity of synthetic vitamin E has been proven to be significantly lower than the corresponding natural form.

Vitamin E is also known as alpha-tocopherol. Whether natural source or synthetic source, all forms supply the body with at least some vitamin E activity. The natural forms of vitamin E are d-alpha-tocopherol, d-alpha-tocopheryl acetate, d-alpha-tocopheryl succinate and mixed tocopherols. The synthetic forms are dl-alpha-tocopherol, dl-alpha-tocopheryl acetate or dl-alpha-tocopheryl succinate. Studies indicate that the most biologically active are the esterified natural forms—d-alpha-tocopheryl acetate and d-alpha-tocopheryl succinate. Both have been found to provide full antioxidant activity in the body and are the ones recommended by top authorities on vitamin E.

In addition to the fact that the least active form of vitamin E was used in the Finnish study, the vitamin E dosage used (50 mg per day) is anywhere from one-eight to one-fortieth the dosage of vitamin E used in at least 20 other studies that show a lower rate of lung cancer in smokers supplementing with vitamin E. The beta-carotene dosage of 20 mg daily is one-tenth the dosage usually recommended for lung cancer prevention in smokers.

When one reads the Finnish study in detail, and compares it to the results of hundreds of other scientific reports, the credibility gap is obvious. Unfortunately, most of the general public does not make a habit of reading the *New England Journal of Medicine*. Many will believe the negative headlines in the mass media and will discontinue their supplements.

The press has already reported that some doctors are advising their patients to stop taking beta-carotene and vitamin E supplements on the basis of this negative study.

Why would any responsible scientist put his or her name after such blatantly misleading data? The answer lies in the field of politics and economics, not science, altruism or social conscience. The tobacco industry leaders, for example, claim that nicotine is not addictive. They made this claim before a U.S. congressional committee the same week the Finnish study appeared. If the tobacco moguls could convince the public and the government that cigarettes are non-addictive, it would obviously be to their financial advantage. Similarly, it is advantageous for the pharmaceutical lobby group to persuade the public that vitamin supplements are dangerous. Remember that the Finnish study was published in a medical journal heavily dependent on the drug industry for its advertising support and long known for its bias against vitamin therapy. Believe its conclusions at your own risk.

Calcium Confusions

The need for calcium supplementation for women at any age is questionable. Vegetarian women who do not consume dairy products or take calcium supplements of any kind have a significantly lower incidence of osteoporosis than non-vegetarian women. If animal protein intake is low, calcium supplementation need will also be low. The more you eat animal products (including dairy and eggs), the more phosphorus you are putting into your system. Phosphorus stimulates calcium loss through the kidneys. In other words, cut down on animal products. Your need for calcium supplementation will be zero or close to zero.

Dairy products are a calcium source, but by no means the only source. Contrary to popular belief and the dogmas of the Dairy Bureau, women do not need milk or dairy products to be well nourished with respect to calcium. Other excellent sources include dulse, almonds, figs, filberts, asparagus, broccoli, cabbage, collards, mustard greens, parsley, and other green leafy vegetables. If you consume a large variety of these calcium sources, there is no need to use dairy products.

Calcium also has a very important relationship with silicon. According to Passwater and Cranton, silicon is concentrated in the body in sites of active calcification in the bones. In their book, *Trace Elements, Hair Analysis and Nutrition*, they state: "Calcium and silicon are probably concurrently necessary for bone formation." Silica is, in fact, necessary for calcium absorption.

Calcium citrate is the best absorbed of the different calcium products. This is the finding of a study reported by Dr. Jean Harvey. The most recent research indicates that taking calcium supplements with meals increases absorption slightly. Liquid or capsule forms are superior to tablets or caplets.

Chronic calcium deficiency can occur as a result of hormonal imbalances, thyroid disease, parathyroid disease, kidney disease, gastrointestinal malabsorption, food allergies (milk being a very common one), inactivity, excessive fat intake, vitamin D deficiency, drugs such as diuretics, cigarette smoking, excessive alcohol intake, excessive sugar intake and stress.

A diet high in oxalic acid (e.g., soybeans, kale, spinach, rhubarb, beet greens, chard and cocoa) may interfere with calcium absorption. Excess zinc, magnesium, fiber and iron can also interfere with calcium absorption. High phosphorus sources, such as red meats, soft drinks and refined grains (e.g., white bread), are common calcium inhibitors.

Patients over 60 usually have a hard time with protein digestion and trace mineral absorption because of low secretion of hydrochloric acid in the stomach. Comprehensive stool and digestive analysis, as well as hair mineral analysis, can be done by a naturopath. The tests will assess how well various nutrients are being absorbed from the diet and should confirm the acid deficiency problem. Appropriate digestive aids (e.g., stomach bitters, apple cider vinegar, citric acid, betaine, pepsin HCL) can then be prescribed based on the degree of hypoacidity. Not all women require digestive supplements: before taking any further supplements, check with a natural health care practitioner.

How to Give Nutritional Advice Legally
(Non-medical practitioners and salespeople take note.)

Problem #1
It happens all the time. A reporter posing as a customer asks the sales clerk at a local health food store about natural remedies for AIDS. The sales clerk, with great enthusiasm, provides the "customer" with a long list of vitamins, minerals and herbs, with detailed explanations as to effective dosages. The hidden tape player records it all. The sale is made and all seems well. A few days later, a feature story appears in the local newspaper detailing how health food stores are places where claims are made for quack cures for AIDS.

Problem #2

It happens on occasion. Dr. Nat Preventive recommends that her patient visit the local health food store to buy antioxidant vitamins, minerals and herbs to help prevent cancer. The patient, now customer, visits the health food store and provides the sales clerk with the list. "What's all this for?," asks the clerk. "It's to help my immune system fight cancer," says the customer. The clerk winces, frowns and says, "Well, it looks all right but I think you really need to take this bowel detoxification program for the next six months before you can start all those other supplements. I've got it on special this week." Six months later the patient returns to Dr. Preventive and tells her what happened. After advising the patient that the program was unnecessary, both the doctor and patient are upset with health food stores.

Problem #3

It happens rarely. But when it does, it makes major headlines and headaches for all of us. Mrs. Matilda Whiner visits a health food store on her way to the pharmacy. Her family doctor, Dr. Morty Conventional, has just prescribed antibiotics for her three-year-old daughter's pneumonia. Upon hearing this, the health food store owner advises Mrs. Whiner against antibiotics, as they may lead to candida. Instead, he says, "Start giving your daughter lots of freshly-squeezed carrot juice. Mix in some vitamin C and zinc. Give her this homeopathic remedy; it won't cause candida." Two days later the child is dead of pneumonia, and two months later a well-publicized coroner's inquest places the blame on "quack remedies."

What Doctors Expect from Health Food Stores and Distributors

Most doctors, naturopaths, chiropractors and homeopaths like to establish a good working relationship with their local health food stores or independent distributors. However, health care practitioners have some basic expectations of proprietors:

1. Leave the diagnosis and treatment of all diseases to doctors. Never recommend dosages. Although the advice you give may be correct, you may be giving it to an undercover government inspector, a reporter or an under-employed lawyer with an axe to grind. They may interpret your actions as providing a medical service, something for which a medical license is required.

2. Do not offer any diagnostic services (iridology, muscle testing, hair analysis, etc.) that suggests the use of a particular food supplement. You are there to retail, not investigate. For more information, read *How to Give Nutritional Advice Legally*, by David Rowland.

3. Do not make claims for any nutritional supplements. If customers ask for product information, steer them toward health books, articles and flyers on various supplements. Unless you are a pharmacist and are familiar with counselling guidelines within the scope of your profession, say as little as possible and provide written references often. If customers are overly demanding, refer them to a local natural health care practitioner. If you are not too sure of what to do, it's always a good policy to call a practitioner for advice before you act.

4. Never recommend that anyone leave his or her doctor or stop taking prescription drugs. This is a sure-fire way of creating negative working relationships with local doctors and other authorities.

5. Keep up to date on new supplements and on political changes in the health care industry. Read as many of the books you sell as possible. The more you know about natural medicine, the better you can communicate with health care practitioners.

"It's All in Your Head"

Over the past 17 years I have seen an increasing number of people in my private practice who present themselves with several dozen different symptoms. The most common of these symptoms are listed below:

- Fatigue, lethargy, poor memory, numbness and tingling of the extremities (hands and feet), burning anywhere (especially mouth, stomach and skin)
- History of frequent infections and prescriptions for antibiotics
- Persistent prostatis, vaginitis, cystitis or other genito-urinary infections
- History of use of birth control pills and/or cortisone-like drugs
- Reactions to perfumes, tobacco and chemicals
- Athlete's foot, ring worm, jock itch, chronic fungal nail or skin infections
- Chronic rashes or itching, psoriasis, hives
- Cravings for sugar, breads or alcoholic beverages
- Insomnia, muscle aches, weakness, paralysis, joint pain or swelling, dry mouth or throat, rash or blisters in mouth, bad breath
- Nasal congestion or post-nasal drip, nasal itching, sore throat, recurrent cough, bronchitis, laryngitis, wheezing, otitis or otalgia
- Abdominal pain, bloating, gas, diarrhea/constipation
- Rectal itching, heartburn, food hypersensitivity, mucus in stool
- Impotence, loss of libido, endometriosis, infertility, premenstrual syndrome
- Anxiety, depression, irritability, cold extremeties, drowsiness, incoor-

dination, mood swings, headaches, dizziness, foot, hair or body odor not relieved by washing

Usually, these multi-symptomed victims make the rounds of general practitioners and specialists and after much conventional medical testing are told, "It's all in your head." People who suffer from multiple symptoms often escape a clear diagnostic label. Candidiasis is appealing as an explanation. So is stress. There are, however, many other possibilities.

In the late twentieth century, a health care practitioner must be willing to unravel the myriad clues presented to him or her each day by a poly-symptomed clientele. To assume that these people suffer from a strictly "psychosomatic" or "functional" illness, or from "burnout," is dangerous. New diseases are becoming more common due to the changing ecological environment: natural disasters bring plagues and other physical ailments; pollution, depletion of the ozone layer and the population explosion are also factors.

The all-in-your-head patient ultimately appears at the offices of alternative health care providers. The naturopath or holistic medical doctor is usually last on the list of practitioners who have attempted to resolve complex, chronic health problems. Careful physical investigation often reveals that these people have hidden biochemical and immunological imbalances. Although testing may be tedious and sometimes expensive, it usually leads to the physical source of the symptoms. Quickie drug prescriptions based on signs and symptoms, or the explanation that it's all in your head, are not only intellectually unsatisfying but frequently false.

If treatable medical conditions have been ruled out by doctors, the following is a list of things to consider as potential sources of chronic, intractable problems:

- Stress-related illness, psycho-neurosis, spiritual/relationship problems, etc.
- Viral neuromyasthenia, chronic fatigue syndrome, fibromyalgia or other chronic viral illnesses
- Hypothyroidism, Wilson's syndrome
- Heavy metal toxicity or hypersensitivity (e.g., mercury in dental amalgams)
- Subclinical vitamin deficiencies, especially of B-complex vitamins (Some patients are so deficient that injections are required before some B vitamins like folic acid can be absorbed from the gastrointestinal tract.)
- Mineral deficiencies or imbalances (zinc, copper, selenium, calcium, magnesium, chromium, manganese, silicon, boron, iodine, and others)

- Essential fatty acid and essential amino acid deficiencies or imbalances
- Masked food allergies and delayed hypersensitivity
- Hyper/hypoglycemia
- Chronic parasitic infections (usually missed through inappropriate or poor medical testing)
- Chemical or environmental allergies
- Other endocrinological disorders: adrenal, gonadal dysfunction
- Gastric hypochlorhydria (low or absent stomach acid), pancreatic insufficiency (low pancreatic digestive enzyme secretion)
- Candidiasis syndrome; other chronic undiagnosed gastrointestinal infections

The human being is a composite organism of body, mind and spirit. Wellness enhancement must take all three components into consideration. From the physical point of view, a variety of special testing can be considered to uncover underlying biological imbalances. These include dietary intake analysis, comprehensive stool and digestive analysis, vitamin and mineral analysis, endocrine organ testing, amino acid analysis, testing for food and environmental allergies and hair mineral analysis. If you are not convinced that your chronic health problems are just in your head, find a complementary medical practitioner in your area willing to spend the time to unravel the mystery that is uniquely you.

The Yeast (Candida) Syndrome

We all have various bacteria and fungi living in our large bowel as part of what's called our "normal flora." Ideally, there should be a balance between the yeast, the fungi, the beneficial bacteria and the more harmful ones. These micro-organisms are helpful in digestion, in the synthesis of vitamins and enzymes and in the prevention of both infections and cancer. Ordinarily, candida is benign and lives in balance with the other microbes in the bowel. There is no debate about these facts.

When we disrupt this flora balance with such things as antibiotics (penicillin, tetracycline, erythromycin, sulfa drugs and many others), steroid drugs such as estrogens, the birth control pill, progesterone and cortisone, we create an imbalance in the bowel that favors the growth of yeast. Consuming large amounts of refined carbohydrates (candies, chocolates, cakes, cookies, chips, soft drinks, white breads, donuts, etc.), alcohol and caffeine also leads to excessive growth of yeast in the bowel. Diabetics frequently suffer from the effects of an overgrowth of yeast, particularly when blood sugar levels are not under control. Yeast infections are also associated with diseases that compromise the immune system. Candida seems to thrive whenever the immune system has been weakened by drugs, disease or a poor diet. In addition, stress, chemical additives and nutritional deficiencies create an overpopulation of yeast in the colon; the yeast then spreads up the digestive tract into the small intestine, stomach, esophagus and oral cavity.

Benign yeast can convert into the more invasive fungal form of candida when host defenses are weakened. Candida can invade the bloodstream and spread to practically all organs and tissues in the body. Over-colonization of candida in the digestive tract causes changes in the permeability (degree of penetrability of substances from the gut to the bloodstream) of the bowel, allowing undigested or partially digested proteins to enter the circulation. Normally this would not happen. When it does, many foods start to behave as if they were food allergies.

Candida secretes an identifiable toxin into the bloodstream that produces an array of central nervous system symptoms – fatigue, confusion, irritability, mental fogginess, memory loss, depression, dizziness, mood swings, headaches, nausea, burning sensations, numbness and tingling, etc. This candida toxin has been isolated and described by the Japanese scientist, Dr. K. Iwata.

Candida overgrowth and invasion and the subsequent accumulation of toxins results in a condition known as the yeast syndrome. There is no uniformity of opinion even on what to call the syndrome itself. People usually identify themselves as "having candida." This is because no two people with candidiasis share exactly the same symptoms. Usually there are multiple symptoms—some people have 30 or more—and they are generally the same symptoms that lead many doctors to tell a patient that its all in their head (see the section "It's All in your Head"). Doctors who treat the condition prefer the term "candida related complex." It must be stressed that candida problems are secondary to other primary imbalances related to the general health of the immune and endocrine system. Treating candida may help relieve a number of symptoms but may not necessarily relieve the primary problem (e.g., diabetes, adrenal insufficiency, vitamin and mineral deficiencies, immune dysfunction, heavy metal poisoning, hypothyroidism, etc.).

The yeast syndrome manifests itself in five areas of the body:

1. The digestive system: Symptoms include bloating, gas, cramps, alternating diarrhea with constipation, multiple food allergies (the individual may feel allergic to all foods, i.e., pan-allergic).

2. The nervous system: Symptoms include anxiety, mood swings, drowsiness, memory loss, depression, insomnia, mental fogginess, etc. In extreme cases, hallucinations and violent behavior can occur.

3. The skin: Symptoms include hives, psoriasis, eczema, acne, excessive sweating and nail infections.

4. The genito-urinary tract: In women, common problems include pre-menstrual syndrome (depression, mood swings, bloating, fluid retention, cramps, craving for sweets, headaches prior to menstruation), recurrent bladder or vaginal infections and a loss of interest in sex. In men, common problems include chronic rectal or anal itching, recurrent prostatitis, impotence, genital rashes and jock itch.

5. The endocrine system: An intimate relationship exists in the body between the immune system, the nervous system and the endocrine system. The thyroid and adrenal glands in particular may be involved.

Since candida toxin can travel to virtually all organs and tissues in the body, the syndrome has been associated with practically every medical condition, including multiple sclerosis, AIDS, asthma, arthritis, chronic sinusitis, recurrent flus, middle ear infections, alcoholism, addictions, diabetes, eating disorders, hypoglycemia and many other less common conditions. In most of these diseases, candida is a secondary "opportunistic" infection.

The most troublesome aspect of this syndrome is the diagnosis. Doctors, skeptical of its existence, frequently point out that there have been no objective tests done to verify its existence. Some conservative members of the medical profession accuse practitioners who believe in the yeast theory of being quacks. Medical journals are filled with anti-yeast pronouncements, yet the general public is growing more and more aware of the condition and is seeking out treatment for their symptoms from an ever-growing contingent of sympathetic doctors.

There is a blood test for candidiasis called the Elisa/Act test. This test can detect candida antibodies in the IgG, A and M families as well as immune complexes. In another aspect of this blood test, lymphocytes are challenged with candida to evaluate inhibition of lymphocyte blastogenesis and natural killer cell activity. In cases where candida is not a factor in symptom production, the results will be negative. The test has an accuracy rate of close to 100 percent.

When the test is positive, treatment can be started using a low carbohydrate diet, garlic, lactobacillus acidophilus, pau d'arco, caprylic acid, psyllium seed powder, digestive enzymes, essential fatty acids, gentian, berberine, grapefruit seed extract and wormwood. In more severe, chronic or disseminated cases, prescription drugs like nystatin, ketoconazole, fluconazole and itraconazole may need to be used. See the resource section in the appendix for contact information on the Elisa/Act test.

Yeast Wars

In the 1970s and early 1980s, people who complained of fatigue, mood swings, memory loss, concentration problems and had a craving for sweets were labeled as having "hypoglycemia." Whether a glucose tolerance test was done or not, most of these people improved by giving up sugar and simple carbohydrates, eating frequent small meals instead of three large ones and by following a high protein diet or a high fiber, high complex-carbohydrate diet.

Most hypoglycemics took supplemental vitamins and minerals as well as food supplements like brewer's yeast, nutritional yeast and other yeast-containing health food store products. For the most part, these people improved to the point where no medical treatments were necessary. Carlton Fredericks, Adelle Davis and Paavo Airola were the health movement gurus of the day. All advocated yeast supplements for their rich content of B vitamins, chromium, selenium, other trace minerals, amino acids, enzymes, essential fatty acids, nucleic acids and anti-stress, hormone-like polypeptides.

Many published studies verified the ability of these yeast products to control blood sugar, improve energy levels, and enhance the immune system. Brewer's yeast and other yeast-derived products are effective remedies for menopausal hot flashes, weakened immunity, neurasthenia, anxiety and diabetes. They help replace nutrients destroyed by prescription antibiotics and other drugs.

As the label "hypoglycemia" went out of fashion in the mid-1980s—to be replaced by "candidiasis" and the "yeast syndrome" for the same set of signs and symptoms—there was a strong movement to eliminate yeast, and anything containing yeast, in foods and supplemental vitamins and minerals. Suddenly, there was a population of "yeast-allergic" patients who had to give up yeast anywhere and everywhere in order to recover from candida. I often wonder how, from one day to the next, there suddenly emerged this army of people allergic to yeast. I also wonder how a terrific product like brewer's yeast could disappear from the market virtually over night.

The 1990s epidemic of "chronic fatigue syndrome," said by physician and author William Crook to be related to candida, caused many more to fear anything containing yeast. Even worse, since most homeopathic remedies and herbal tinctures contained, by necessity, alcohol, and since alcohol was associated with yeast, it was proclaimed by the anti-yeast movement that candida victims could not use these products. Sales of anything containing yeast or alcohol in health food stores declined. Misinformation in popular health books on diet and candida further fueled the fires of the yeast paranoia. The era of yeast-free breads, cookies, pastas and supplements had arrived.

But is this all really necessary, and is there really such a thing as "yeast free"? The answer is no, not likely. Harmless yeasts, including candida albicans, are everywhere—in our oral cavity, gastrointestinal tract, skin and hair. This is a normal fact of life. Yeast can be found growing on practically all ripened fruits, vegetables, breads, baked goods, seeds, nuts, herbs and anywhere mold grows, including yeast-free bread. It cannot be eliminated entirely, and even those who take prescriptions of nystatin, keto-conazole, fluconazole and other antifungals can never claim to completely eradicate all yeast, ubiquitous in our environment as well as our bodies.

There is also little, if any, evidence to suggest that anyone suffering from candida syndrome must eliminate yeast from the diet in order to clear up symptoms. The minute quantities of yeast and/or alcohol found in hundreds of herbal, nutritional and homeopathic supplements have never been proven to harm candida sufferers or anyone else. In fact, many health care practitioners have advocated the use of supplements like brewer's yeast and nutritional yeast to successfully treat candida overgrowth naturally. I fear we have been misled on this yeast-free issue; it is time we reconsidered the use of these low-cost, high nutrient supplements.

Admittedly, there are rare individuals with a strong sensitivity to yeast-containing foods, molds and fungi, but the number of these unfortunate individuals is too small to justify the mass yeast paranoia we see reflected both in our "well-read" patients and on health food store shelves.

Dr. William Crook, author of *Chronic Fatigue and the Yeast Connection*, agrees that most sufferers of candidiasis can keep yeast-containing foods and supplements in their diet. This message, however, does not seem to be getting through. Whether one suffers from candida-related problems or not, keeping yeast out of the diet is next to impossible and has not been demonstrated to be of any health benefit. In fact, based on all the credible research on yeast supplementation, a case could be made for the harmfulness of yeast-free anything.

How to Choose Your Complementary Medical Practitioner

Finding the right alternative practitioner depends on many factors. The primary factor for most people is their own belief system of health care. Other determining factors include the nature of the health problem, the degree of responsibility one wishes to take for health care and the compatibility of the personalities involved. For example, many people still have a great deal of confidence in some aspects of conventional medicine, but are also interested in preventive nutritional programs, detailed biochemical testing, determination of food allergies and of vitamin and mineral deficiencies and nutritional therapeutics, including intravenous chelation therapy. Such a person would be looking for a doctor who practices nutritional medicine or "complementary medicine." Another term that describes this type of practitioner is "orthomolecular" doctor. Orthomolecular therapy is based on the theory that health status can be controlled by restoring optimum amounts of substances normally present in the body. Linus Pauling and Dr. Abram Hoffer are the fathers of orthomolecular medicine.

"Holistic" doctors are very difficult to describe since there is little uniformity in the services offered. The common denominator seems to be that holistic physicians treat individuals as partners in health care. They acknowledge the body/mind/spirit relationship to health. Some holistic doctors offer nutritional medicine, but many do not. There are even some holistic doctors who discourage the use of vitamin and mineral supplements. Some offer psychotherapy, while others focus on providing different forms of visualization therapy, yoga, meditation, acupuncture, homeopathy and a long list of at least 30 other modalities. Before you choose the practitioner, look carefully into his or her philosophy of health care.

If you are more interested in a completely non-medical approach to health care, a naturopath is the right practitioner to consult. Naturopathy can be defined as a system of treating disease that avoids drugs and surgery and emphasizes the use of natural agents. Naturopaths believe that disease happens when natural defense mechanisms are overpowered by stress, poor lifestyle and poor nutrition. They believe that the body has to be allowed to heal itself without drugs or surgery. Although most naturopaths are willing to work in cooperation with medical doctors (allopaths), the reverse is usually not the case. Holistic medical doctors can usually be counted on to work with naturopaths, if necessary. Most naturopaths in Canada have a chiropractic degree plus an N.D. (naturopathic doctor) degree and practice different forms of hands-on therapy (e.g., massage, spinal manipulation, applied kinesiology). All are licensed as "drugless practitioners." Some naturopaths are experts in nutritional therapeutics, herbology, homeopathy, colonic irrigation, acupuncture, hydrotherapy, and iridology. All have had training in these modalities, but most specialize in just one or a few of them.

Before you make a commitment, check the credentials of anyone with the label holistic practitioner, wellness counselor, iridologist, reflexologist, homeopath, acupuncturist and any other without the initials M.D., N.D., D.C. or R.N. Many who claim to do natural therapeutics are not accredited as an M.D., nurse, chiropractor or naturopath. Such lay practitioners may have only taken a weekend seminar in nutrition, iridology or homeopathy. Their intentions may be good, but their training is not at a professional level. While it is true that some of these practitioners are wise beyond their training, this is not the general rule. If you are looking for an alternative practitioner, consult a professional and not just a weekend seminar graduate or one with an impressive mail order degree from a diploma mill.

Beware of an ever-growing army of lay practitioners dispensing advice on natural therapeutics. Please remember that what took a naturopath or medical doctor five years or more to learn cannot be obtained from a weekend seminar or a paperback health book. If you listen to a lay practitioner's advice, at least verify it with your doctor, chiropractor or naturopath. It is well within your rights to question any practitioner about his training and licensing background.

There are several very helpful resource groups across Canada and the United States that can give you more information on the availability of various therapies or practitioners. Some of these groups can even help you find a practitioner in your area. See the appendix in the back of this book.

The Hostile Doctor and Vitamin B12 Shots

One of the most rewarding procedures in the field of nutritional medicine is the B12 injection. When conventional treatments have failed, many chronic health problems respond to B12 given intramuscularly. These include fatigue, chronic fatigue syndrome, depression, burn-out, non-specific stress and memory loss. Aside from these neuropsychiatric disorders, inexplicable hair loss, tendinitis, numbness, tingling, multiple sclerosis, heel spurs and even asthma have been reported to benefit from B12 injections. The pill or the intranasal form of vitamin B12 may work for some people, but not for the majority of those who suffer from chronic illness. These people need the injectable form because of hereditary factors (a low output of stomach acid, an absence of intrinsic factor) or because of parasites, candida, food allergies, chemicals in food or interference by drugs.

Standard lab tests for vitamin B12 deficiency are unreliable and miss a large number of people with this problem. For this reason, most natural health care practitioners will use a trial therapy with a few vitamin B12 injections. If the response is favorable, it is usually recommended that patients either give themselves the B12 shots (as simple as self-injection with insulin) or receive a series of them from their family doctor. Dosage, frequency of injections and length of treatment all depend on the bio-chemical uniqueness of the individual.

Unfortunately, few conventional doctors have been willing to give patients the injections despite obvious evidence of benefit. One example that comes to mind from my own practice is the case of a 55-year-old resident of a nursing home whose depression and short-term memory loss lifted after a single 3,000 mcg vitamin B12 injection. The attending doctor at the nursing home refused to give any further injections on the grounds that it was "unconventional." Within a few weeks the patient had a severe relapse and never did get out of the nursing home.

Why the medical hostility toward B12 shots? When patients ask their family doctors for vitamin B12 injections, some of the more common responses include:

"You can get all the vitamin B12 you need from food. You don't need injections."

"Your tests for vitamin B12 do not show a deficiency. The Schick test is negative. You don't need injections."

"There is no proof that vitamin B12 works for depression, fatigue or any other condition except pernicious anemia. If it does help, it's just a placebo effect."

"High doses of vitamin B12 can be toxic. You're probably only going to be making expensive urine. If B12 makes you feel better, it's all in your mind."

"Vitamin B12 injection for anything other than pernicious anemia is quackery. There are no double-blind studies that support vitamin B12 injections for any other reason."

All these, by the way, are real quotes from family doctors of patients who had the audacity to request B12 shots. How valid are such statements? If one uses scientific studies as the sole criteria for legitimizing any treatment, it is safe to say that conventional medicine would have to abandon 85 percent of all currently used drugs and surgical procedures. According to the Office of Technology Assessment of the U.S. government, that's the approximate percentage of therapies that have never been subjected to double-blind, placebo-controlled studies. Yet, despite this, conventional doctors continue to use unproven remedies like antacids, chemotherapy, coronary bypass surgery and bed rest. There are hundreds of others.

Are there any scientific studies supporting vitamin B12 for low energy and depression? Yes, there are quite a few. For example, a 1990 study by Carney, published in the *British Journal of Psychiatry*, reported that vitamin B12 deficiency can cause neuropsychiatric disorders such as depression despite the absence of pernicious anemia. Other studies by Carmel (1990 and 1992) recommend a therapeutic trial of vitamin B12 as the ultimate proof of deficiency since conventional lab tests miss a high percentage of deficiency cases.

Therapeutic trials with B12 are, at the very least, safe. There has never been a single reported case of toxicity arising from B12 shots. One physician jokes that about the only way you could get vitamin B12 toxicity is to fill your bath tub to the top with B12 and submerge your head for as long as it takes to stop breathing. Vitamin B12 is a fraction of the cost of the commonly prescribed anti-depressant Prozac. It is Prozac, and antidepressants like it, that are associated with expensive urine, not vitamin B12.

There are many myths about vitamin B12, generated for the most part by out-of-date physicians and dietitians. Physicians who cast a jaundiced eye at B12 shots and other non-drug therapies are often surprised to learn that there is a great deal of scientific documentation to support their use. Finding this documentation means keeping up with the most recent scientific literature and not blindly following the dogmas of aging professors and textbooks.

The New Four Food Groups

The new and controversial *Canada Food Guide* has been criticized by many doctors, dietitians and advocates of prevention. Dr. Neal Barnard, president of the Physicians Committee for Responsible Medicine (PCRM), summarized the problem with the new food guide in a letter to the editor of the *Toronto Globe and Mail* (December 7, 1992):

"The new Canadian food guide, like it's U.S. counterpart, includes the unfortunate suggestion that citizens eat both dairy products and meats. Fat and cholesterol are major components of meats and dairy products and are linked to the biggest killers of North Americans: heart disease, stroke, diabetes and some forms of cancer. In comparison, a plant-based diet is naturally low in fat, high in fiber and entirely cholesterol-free. A diet such as promoted by both of our governments may well be good for the economic health of dairy and cattle farmers but it will only hinder their—or anyone else's—physical well-being."

The PCRM, whose members include the world-renowned Dr. Benjamin Spock and Dr. Denis Burkitt, contends that animal products of any kind are "simply not necessary in the human diet." This position is supported by a very large and growing segment of scientific literature and has been popularized in recent years by authors such as John Robbins (*Diet For A New America*) and Dr. John McDougall (*McDougall's Medicine*).

Despite the propaganda of the dairy, beef and pork lobby, there is not a single scientific study that proves a) that animal products are necessary for any health reason; b) that animal products are necessary for a "balanced diet" or c) that elimination of animal products leads to nutrient deficiencies. On the contrary, recent research by Dr. Dean Ornish and others proves that coronary artery disease is reversible by following a completely plant-based diet.

The PCRM has published a booklet promoting improved health and disease prevention by following an eating plan using only the "New Four Food Groups": whole grains, legumes, vegetables and fruit. This excludes fish, seafood, beef, pork, chicken and other poultry, eggs, dairy products and other animal products.

If one follows the new food group guidelines, and provided adequate calories are consumed relative to the degree of physical activity, a child or adult, male or female, can meet all their daily nutrient requirements for protein, carbohydrates, fat and fiber, as well as all vitamin and mineral requirements, including calcium, iron, zinc and vitamins A, B12 and D. All information to the contrary is just hype, rumor, speculation or scare tactics designed to encourage meat, egg and dairy product consumption.

Four Food Group Guidelines:

Whole Grain Group: Includes whole grain breads, pastas, cereals and burgers; brown rice, corn, spelt and quinoa; psyllium and flax seed; rice milk and rice products. Five or more servings daily is recommended.

Legume Group: Includes navy, kidney and lima beans; lentils and chick peas; nuts and nut products (almond milk and almond butter); soy products (soy milk, soy burgers, tofu, miso, tempeh). Note: Soy products can be made to taste like beef, pork, ham, chicken, cheese and other mainstream North American artery-cloggers. Two or more servings daily are recommended.

Vegetable Group: Includes all starchy (potato, etc.) and non-starchy (tomatoes, peppers, carrots, onions, lettuce, etc.) vegetables. Three or more servings daily are recommended.

Fruit Group: Includes apples, peaches, pears, plums, berries, etc. Three or more servings daily are recommended.

These guidelines lead to a relatively low protein intake. Some individuals with digestive disturbances may have a problem. For most people, however, the guidelines have several advantages, including reduced calcium loss from the body and a lower risk of osteoporosis despite an absence of dairy products. Calcium is abundant in a large variety of plant and plant products. Some studies indicate that dairy product consumption may actually hasten the development of osteoporosis. It is also a fact that the more animal protein one consumes—and this includes dairy products—the more calcium is eliminated by the kidneys. Osteoporosis is almost unknown in parts of the world where there is little or no intake of meat and dairy products. Population studies have repeatedly verified these facts.

A lower intake of animal protein also means a lower intake of sodium, antibiotics, hormones, parasites and other chemicals that generate free radical tissue damage. It is therefore no surprise to learn that populations following the New Four Food Groups' guidelines have a significantly lower incidence of stroke, cancer, arthritis, diabetes, high blood pressure and coronary artery disease.

Vitamin B12 and Vegetarians

Some doctors and dairy industry-financed dietitians will attempt to scare people into eating animal products by warning them of the danger of vitamin B12 deficiency for those who follow the New Four Food Groups' guidelines. This is nonsense. B12 deficiency is usually not caused by inadequate intake. It is more likely to be caused by a lack of intrinsic factor and/or low or absent hydrochloric acid secretion. In fact, in my practice, I see far more B12 deficiencies in meat eaters than in strict vegans.

Many people still believe that animal-derived foods are the only nutritional sources of B12. Recent studies, however, have shown that some sea vegetables contain substantial amounts of vitamin B12, more than enough to meet one's nutritional needs. These sea vegetables include arame, wakame, kombu, hijiki, alaria and nori.

Tempeh, tamari, pickles and sauerkraut also contain significant amounts of B12, as does miso, provided it is unpasteurized and prepared with traditional miso cultures. For those who find these foods unpalatable or unavailable, I suggest the following natural food supplements, which are rich in vitamin B 12: blue-green algae, chlorella, barley green and spirulina. These and many others are widely available at most health food stores. The Recommended Daily Allowance for vitamin B12 is: 2 mcg for infants, 3 mcg for children, 6 mcg for adults and 8 mcg for pregnant and lactating women. Check labels to make sure you are getting this minimum level from any supplement. By the way, vitamin B12 is non-toxic and has been used therapeutically in doses several hundred thousand times the RDA without side effects.

Food intake guidelines of any kind should be based on scientific data and the most recent research, not on the lobbying efforts of various agribusiness groups and their quasi-scientific henchmen. I encourage everyone to write to their members of parliament demanding a complete revision of the cholesterol- and fat-laden *Canada Food Guide.*

Vitamin B12 and Low Back Pain

In some cases, low back pain can be relieved by a series of vitamin B12 injections. If you do not have access to a doctor who will provide this service, purchase some sublingual vitamin B12 and take 3,000 mcg (3 mg) daily. It's harmless and worth taking for at least six weeks to see if there is any impact on the back problem.

People with back pain should consider the possibility of nutritional imbalances of calcium, magnesium, copper, zinc, manganese, vitamin C, vitamin E and other B vitamins, especially B6. Ask your natural health care practitioner to do a nutritional evaluation that includes hair mineral analysis. Consider hidden digestive problems (e.g., parasites) and delayed food allergies as well. Tests such as the comprehensive stool and digestive analysis (CSDA), and various blood tests for food allergies will address these concerns.

In women, low back pain may be a reflection of a hormonal imbalance. A natural progesterone cream (from an extract of Mexican wild yam) applied to the skin will allow the body to absorb enough hormone to rebalance the system. Premenstrual pain or chronic pelvic irritation is thus relieved. Progesterone cream is available from any health food store and is very safe to use. If the body does not require progesterone, excesses will be eliminated.

Some low back pain is psychogenic and helped by yoga, relaxation techniques, biofeedback, magneto-therapy, meditation and other mind-control modalities. Physiotherapy, posture therapy and muscle strengthening exercises help many cases.

Yet another option is to use safe and effective natural analgesics like feverfew, devil's claw, white willow, wood betony, St John's wort, evening primrose oil, L-tryptophan and DL-phenylalanine. High doses of echinacea (well above therapeutic antibiotic levels) is another good pain killer. Discuss all these with your doctor or naturopath.

Butter: The Better Choice

Which is better, butter or margarine? As a health care practitioner and nutritional consultant I get this question asked of me on an almost daily basis. I have said elsewhere that margarine is nothing more than "plastic butter." This description of margarine is not without merit, since under the microscope a hydrogenated fat molecule from margarine or vegetable shortening looks the same as a plastic molecule. Why well-intentioned doctors and dietitians continue to recommend edible plastic as a butter substitute may depend more on financial and political considerations than on science.

Health writer John Finnegan pulls no punches in his book *The Facts about Fats: A Consumer's Guide to Good Oils* when he quotes extensive research documenting the fact that margarine is a "lifeless, devitalized poison, packed with carcinogens (cancer-causing chemicals), fit only for lubricating the front wheel bearings of your car." The brand of margarine is irrelevant; all brands are potentially toxic.

How dangerous can margarine be? A study by Malhotra, published in 1967 in the *American Journal of Clinical Nutrition*, compared two populations in India where the only difference in the diet was the type of fat consumed. The population that used margarine instead of butter had a heart disease rate that was fifteen times greater than that of the population that used butter. A follow-up study twenty years later reported the same findings.

There is no question that people who suffer from heart disease and high cholesterol levels need to revise their diet and lifestyle. This does not mean, however, that they ought to replace butter with margarine in their diets. The only healthy butter substitutes that I can confidently recommend are olive oil, flax seed oil, hazelnut oil or canola oil. Butter and ghee (clarified butter) have been used by man for thousands of years without any indication that it leads to or causes any particular ailment. In large amounts, butter, and any high fat animal product, will lead to obesity and a long list of medical problems. It's simply a question of amounts and of a person's hereditary tendency to develop high blood-fat problems and coronary artery disease.

What is margarine? In simple terms, it is nothing more than hydrogenated vegetable oil. Hydrogenation is a process whereby vegetable oils are hardened. Partial or complete hydrogenation ruins the nutritional value of the oil. Margarine companies claim that their products are safe because they contain no trans-fatty acids. This information gets twisted somehow to imply that margarine does not contain "hydrogenated fats." Unfortunately, it does. Studies also indicate that the supposedly safe cis-fatty acids in margarine go through a transformation process. According to one source, the transformation of cis- to trans-fatty acids in margarine may be as high as 40 percent.

In *Fats that Heal Fats that Kill*, fat and oil specialist Udo Erasmus says that trans-fatty acids "compete for enzymes, produce biologically nonfunctional derivatives and interfere with the work of the essential fatty acids in the body." Trans-fatty acid consumption causes high cholesterol levels in the long run. Do not be fooled into thinking that you are buying something that is health enhancing simply because the margarine label reads "high in polyunsaturates" or "low in saturates." You may very well be buying something that is actually a contributor to the overall level of toxins in the body.

Dr. G. J. Bisson, professor of nutrition at Laval University in Quebec, has been an outspoken critic of the hydrogenation process in the production of margarine. He was recently quoted by John Finnegan as saying that it "would be practically impossible to predict with accuracy either the nature or the content of these new molecules [produced by hydrogenation]. Between the parent vegetable oil sometimes labeled 'pure' and the partially hydrogenated product, there is a world of chemistry that alters profoundly the composition and physiochemical properties of natural oils."

Your choice of oils in your diet may be more important than you think. All your body cells have membranes that are made up of the essential fatty acids. The body must get these from the diet since it cannot synthesize them from other nutrients. If you use margarine regularly, you may be unwittingly replacing your essential fats with defective or chemically altered fatty acids ("plastic butter"), leading to abnormal cell function, dry skin and hormonal imbalances. As many responsible nutritionists have pointed out, we have only just begun to scratch the surface of all the essential fatty acid imbalance conditions (PMS, eczema, obesity, psoriasis, allergies, arthritis, heart disease, autoimmune disease, immune system impairment, mental illness, etc.). Could margarine be involved? The consensus of the world medical literature says yes. If you have to choose between butter and margarine, go with butter. It really is the better choice.

The Myth of Harmless Sugar

The only people saying that sugar is harmless are those involved in the sugar industry. According to British researcher Dr. John Yudkin, studies refuting the negative health effects of sugar are flawed. In 1983, the United Kingdom National Advisory Committee on Nutrition Education recommended a 50 percent reduction in sucrose consumption. According to Dr. Stephen Davies, author of *Nutritional Medicine*, this report was opposed by "certain quarters" intent on preserving the "good name" of sugar. The sugar controversy has nothing to do with science; it is strictly a political debate, similar to the one involving the association between cigarette smoking and lung cancer that raged in the 1950s and 1960s. It may take another decade before the powerful sugar lobby takes the same battering that is presently being taken by the tobacco industry. Until then, dietitians and scientists on the payrolls of various segments of the sugar industry will be trying to sweet-talk the public into buying sugar.

Study after study demonstrate that sugar consumption is directly or indirectly associated with poor health. The volume of supporting literature is staggering. A partial list of health conditions associated with high sugar consumption follows:

Obesity	Allergies
Eating disorders	Immune suppression
Stuttering	Premenstrual syndrome
Eczema	Recurrent infections
Alcoholism	Reactive hypoglycemia
Drug abuse	Candida syndrome
Cardiovascular disease	Depression
Atherosclerosis	Anxiety
High blood pressure	Chronic pain syndromes
Increased platelet stickiness	Hyperactivity in children
Adult-onset diabetes mellitus	Learning disabilities
Dental caries	Criminal behavior
Gallstones	Gastrointestinal disease
Kidney stones	(diverticulosis, irritable bowel
Kidney failure	syndrome, etc.)

Sugar hinders the body's immune system and predisposes people to infections and allergies. The shape, activity and number of white cells are adversely affected by heavy sugar consumption. Sugar is the single most underrated cause of immune system impairment.

Sugar goes by many names, including sucrose, fructose, brown sugar, invert sugar, dextrose, maltose, lactose, candies, carob, chocolate, xylitol, sorbitol, honey and molasses. Products made with white flour are not sugar in themselves, but are quickly converted to simple sugars in the body (e.g., one slice of white bread is equivalent to one teaspoon of sugar).

Sugar is hidden in many commercially available foods. For example, one tablespoon of ketchup contains one teaspoon of sugar. Some soft drinks contain up to 12 teaspoons of sugar per eight fluid ounces. Jelly beans and marshmallows have 100 percent of their calories derived from sugar. Regular and diet soft drinks, besides being loaded with caffeine, glucose and fructose, are derived mainly from corn sources and are extremely high in phosphorus, thereby promoting calcium loss from the skeleton. This may lead to kidney stones, osteoporosis and osteoarthritis. Even some unsweetened fruit juices contain the equivalent of ten teaspoons of sugar and should be avoided by diabetics, hypoglycemics and those with high triglyceride blood levels. Mayonnaise, cereals, breads, mustard, relish, peanut butter, gravies, sauces, TV dinners and even drugs are hidden sources of large amounts of sugar.

Sugar and sugar equivalents such as white bread rapidly raise blood glucose and insulin levels shortly after ingestion. The more sugar consumed, the more insulin that must be made by the pancreas. Eventually the pancreas gets overworked. If sugar intake remains excessive and frequent, blood glucose levels crash below acceptable levels, producing transient, low blood sugar attacks (hypoglycemia). These may be experienced as anxiety, panic, headaches, sudden fatigue, sleepiness after eating, mood swings and a craving for more sweets. The adrenal glands—the body's anti-stress glands—in turn get over-stressed, leading to chronic fatigue and a situation which has been loosely termed "burn-out." Other terms used to describe the symptoms of nutritional stress caused by sugar are idiopathic post-prandial syndrome, nutritionally induced chronic endocrinopathy (NICE) and adrenal insufficiency. One endocrine gland after the other may become involved (i.e., thyroid, pituitary, ovaries, etc.). Full-blown diseases such as diabetes, hypothyroidism and Addison's disease result after years of unabated nutritional stress caused by a high sugar intake.

It is a well-known fact that sugar is an appetite stimulant. Frequent consumption of high sugar junk food causes insulin levels to be chronically elevated, leading to overeating and weight gain. Triglycerides, the storage form of sugar, may become chronically elevated in the blood of obese individuals.

Honey and molasses are no different from table sugar in composition and have no nutritive value that cannot be derived from other sources. The highest quality, unrefined honey is 48 percent glucose and 52 percent fructose. Table sugar is 50 percent glucose and 50 percent fructose. The levels of vitamins, enzymes and trace minerals in honey or molasses are negligible. The only advantage of honey or molasses over regular sugar is that people tend to use less because they taste sweeter, teaspoon for teaspoon, than regular sugar.

There is no universal agreement as to the safety of sugar substitutes like saccharine, cyclamates or aspartame. Toxicity studies have involved extremely large intakes in animals. At the level of one to two teaspoons per day, there is little evidence of harm to healthy people. In some cases, aspartame has been associated with headaches, hyperactive behavior and mood control problems. This is because of reactions to phenylalanine, one of aspartame's ingredients. Although a natural amino acid, in large amounts and when isolated from other amino acids, phenylalanine is converted into other compounds that have a stimulating or toxic effect. Children suffering from hyperactivity or other behavior problems may be adversely affected by aspartame in large amounts. An allergy may also be responsible for bad reactions to this sweetener. Reactions to aspartame are not universal, but those suffering from any neuro-psychological problems (e.g., eating disorders) should avoid it.

There is documented evidence that aspartame can cause seizures and tremors. Aspartame is also suspected as either a cause or a contributing factor in multiple sclerosis and brain cancer. The sharp rise in the incidence of brain tumors coincides with the increasing appearance of aspartame—now found in over 4,000 products available at the supermarket or drug store.*

The ideal solution would be to get out of the sugar rut altogether. People who do not use sweeteners find they grow accustomed to the natural taste of foods. Few realize their taste buds become anesthetized by sugar over the years. By using a sugar substitute, the cravings for sweetness will be perpetuated and the enjoyment of natural foods will still be blunted. Although artificial sweeteners are lower in calories, they promote a craving for sugar, which encourages the consumption of high calorie foods.

---

*Dr. H. J. Roberts has published an article on this, and you can request a copy by writing to: H. J. Roberts, M.D., Palm Beach Institute for Medical Research, 300 27th St., West Palm Beach, Fl 33407.

Like it not, sugar can become an addiction. Breaking the sugar habit is difficult for most long-time addicts to do. Supplementing the diet with B vitamins (especially vitamin B5 and B6), vitamin C, chromium, manganese, magnesium and zinc will help cut down the cravings. The use of natural, high-fiber foods (vegetables, whole grain breads, cereals, pastas and starchy beans in particular) to replace the junk will produce a "full" sensation that cuts appetite. Increasing whole fruit (not juice) intake will also cut down on sugar cravings. The moderate use of licorice or ginseng herbal tea will keep energy levels high and sugar cravings low.

Some cases fail to respond to these simple approaches and may require special tests to determine whether or not there are problems with food allergies, heavy metal toxicities or chronic gastrointestinal infection. Biochemical individuality dictates appropriate dietary or supplement remedies for different people. A holistic doctor, naturopath or qualified nutritionist can help you sort out the problem if you are unsuccessful in kicking the sugar habit on your own.

Why Take Vitamins?

The most common question I hear as a health care practitioner is, "Do you recommend that everybody take vitamin and mineral supplements?" The answer to this question is an unequivocal "yes."

Supplemental vitamins and minerals protect our bodies against the toxic effects of a polluted environment. Over the past decade, extensive research has been done on the subject of free radical pathology. Many reputable scientists and medical doctors believe that free radical pathology is at the root of cancer, heart disease, immune system disorders, and a long list of degenerative diseases. Free radicals are highly reactive molecules (containing an unpaired electron) that can cause damage to the body. Their damage, however, can be offset by antioxidants (vitamins, minerals and enzymes). Free radicals come from radiation, pesticides, herbicides, cigarette smoke, drugs, food additives, hydrocarbons from car exhaust, industrial waste products and many other sources. The gradual deterioration of the ozone layer also plays a part. All of this necessitates even greater protection with antioxidant nutrients like beta-carotene, vitamin A, B vitamins (especially B3 and B6), vitamins C and E, bioflavonoids, selenium, zinc, silicon, amino acids, enzymes like superoxide dismutase, coenzymes and essential fatty acids.

It would be ideal to have a preventive health care system that tested individuals for vitamin, mineral and enzyme deficiencies. Specific nutrient supplements could then be prescribed to promote wellness on the basis of biochemical individuality testing. Unfortunately, we have a "disease care" system that ignores the value and importance of prevention, natural treatments and nutrient supplementation. This is gradually changing, but until a true health care system emerges, what can the average person who has no access to wellness doctors and nutritional testing do?

First of all, even in the face of less-than-ideal food quality, eating a healthier diet is possible. Most importantly, lower the intake of saturated fat and cholesterol by eliminating red meats from the diet. Keep high-fat dairy products, especially cheeses, to a minimum. Cultured dairy products such as yogurt or buttermilk in small amounts are fine, as long as they are low in fat. Avoid coffee, regular tea, alcohol, sugar and white flour products. The more vegetarian your food selection, the better.

Next, take some broad-spectrum antioxidant supplements. The two worry-free supplements I recommend are bee pollen extract and blue-green algae. This combination provides a perfect mixture of the richest, maximum-spectrum antioxidants available in tablet or capsule form. Some scientists have called both bee pollen extract and blue-green algae nature's most perfect foods. Together they contain a very well balanced supply of all the essential amino acids, vitamins, trace minerals, essential fatty acids, RNA, DNA, plant enzymes, coenzymes and prostaglandin precursors. Blue-green algae is one of the few palatable vegetarian sources of vitamin B12.

Aside from fulfilling daily essential vitamin and mineral needs and providing antioxidant protection for life extension, both these products can be used to enhance work and sports performance. The use of bee pollen by professional and Olympic athletes for physical endurance and power is well documented. Naturopaths and medical doctors have also had excellent results prescribing bee pollen in high doses to treat coronary artery disease, high blood fats and nocturia (the need to urinate at night caused by an enlarged prostate). The medical literature attests to the benefits of bee pollen extract for a number of chronic conditions: anemia, depression, chronic fatigue, premature aging, poor memory and concentration, obesity, insomnia, arthritis, senility, menopause and prostatitis. Blue-green algae, on the other hand, has been demonstrated to help in both the prevention and treatment of all viral conditions including chronic fatigue syndrome and AIDS. Testimonials as to its energy-enhancing properties are legion.

There have been no reports of side effects or toxicity with blue-green algae or bee pollen, even in children, and even after thirty years of broad-scale use. For those who want a safe and effective way of optimizing health, preventing illness and living longer, these whole food supplements may very well be the answer.

High Energy Survival Antioxidants, Minerals and Herbs

The following is a list of supplemental nutrients that can be taken without side effects by most healthy people who just want to feel better, look better and have more energy. The primary reason for their effectiveness is due to the fact that most North Americans are deficient in minerals or one or more of the many nutrients contained in these supplements. Whenever possible, use whole food concentrates rather than single nutrient tablets or capsules; isolating a single component from a given food results in the loss of many of the benefits of the whole food.

Bee Supplements

Royal jelly is a supplement that must be combined with honey to preserve its potency. It has been touted as something that benefits a wide range of health conditions. This is because royal jelly contains all the B-complex vitamins, high concentrations of vitamin B5 (pantothenic acid) and vitamin B6, acetylcholine, minerals, enzymes, hormones, amino acids, immune boosting substances and vitamins A, C, D, and E. Most healthy people tolerate it well without any side effects.

Bee pollen contains complex carbohydrates, calcium, carotene, copper, enzymes, iron, magnesium, manganese, polyunsaturated fatty acids, sodium, potassium, vitamin C and plant sterols. Proponents of bee pollen supplements claim that they helps combat fatigue, infections, cancer, bowel disorders, prostate problems and depression. There is no known toxicity, but the rare individual may be allergic to pollen and experience symptoms similar to hay fever.

If you are a well-controlled diabetic or have hypoglycemia (low blood sugar), taking either supplement should not affect your blood sugars noticeably. If, on the other hand, your sugar level is poorly controlled, these supplements might upset the apple cart for you.

Beet Powder

Beet powder is particularly high in carotenes, iron, calcium, potassium, niacin, copper, vitamin C, folic acid, zinc, manganese, magnesium and phosphorus. Beet powder enriches the blood and is also a good general tonic.

Kelp

Kelp is a seaweed high in sodium alginate, calcium, phosphorus, magnesium, iron, sodium, selenium, potassium, iodine, sulfur and vitamins C and B12. Kelp is an alkaline-forming food that replenishes glands and nerves, particularly the thyroid. It is a good source of trace minerals and has traditionally been used in the complementary medical treatment of goiter, hypothyroidism, anemia, emaciation, impotence, nervousness, a weakened immune system and hair loss.

Boron

Boron is a trace mineral that is essential in the prevention of osteoporosis and arthritis. An adequate intake of boron ensures a healthy balance between male and female hormones in both men and women. Many people are deficient in this mineral simply because of poor soil quality.

Chromium Picolinate

Chromium picolinate is the most bio-available (best absorbed) form of chromium. It is essential for the prevention and the complementary medical treatment of diabetes, heart disease, atherosclerosis, high blood cholesterol, obesity and other eating disorders. It is a general tonic that improves energy, cuts cravings for sweets and normalizes blood sugar levels.

Fo-Ti

Fo-Ti is a Chinese herb useful in the treatment of arthritis, rheumatism, atherosclerosis, insomnia, impotency, senility, constipation and early menopause. It also helps improve circulation and energy levels. Fo-Ti is also a mild anti-diabetic agent and has been shown to possess anti-tumor activity in animals. It has both antispasmodic and antibacterial properties.

Ginger

This herb is best known for its soothing affect on the gastrointestinal tract. It is particularly effective for nausea associated with pregnancy (morning sickness), anorexia, gas and flatulence, gastric and intestinal spasms, acute colds, painful menstruation, joint stiffness and cold extremities. It is also helpful for serious conditions like colitis and diverticulitis. Ginger is a cardiac tonic, eases uterine pain, decreases cholesterol and helps poor circulation. Ginger inhibits platelet aggregation much like ASA and thus prevents blood from clotting excessively. Along with ginkgo biloba, it is an effective remedy for tinnitus.

Ginkgo Biloba

Ginkgo biloba is a strong antioxidant that can produce relaxation of blood vessels, inhibit platelet aggregation, increase peripheral and cerebral blood flow and act, in general, as a cardiovascular and brain tonic. It has traditionally been used in the complementary medical treatment of arterial insufficiency, ischemic heart disease, peripheral vascular disease (it affects both arteries and veins), memory loss, other failing mental faculties, almost any neurological condition, asthma, tinnitus and high blood pressure. Ginkgo biloba improves blood supply to the brain. It increases the rate at which information is transmitted at the nerve cell. Ginkgo biloba is an effective free radical scavenger and may improve oxygenation of tissues and enhance tissue repair.

Hawthorn Berries

This herb is best known for its use in cardiac weakness, valvular murmurs, shortness of breath, mitral valve regurgitation, chest/angina pain, anemia associated with heart irregularity and nervous exhaustion. Hawthorn has traditionally been used in the complementary medical treatment of coronary artery disease, angina pectoris, arrhythmias, arteriosclerosis and other circulatory weaknesses. Hawthorn reduces cholesterol, dilates coronary blood vessels and thereby increases blood flow to the heart muscle. It prevents and reverses plaque formation. It has a potent synergistic effect with the digitalis cardiac glycosides and should be used with caution by people taking prescription cardiac drugs.

Kola Nut

Kola nut is a natural antidepressant, gastrointestinal stimulant, astringent, diuretic and pain reliever. It has traditionally been used in the complementary medical treatment of depression, nervous irritability of the stomach, chronic diarrhea, migraines, tremors, insomnia and constipation.

Licorice Root

Licorice root has been used since very ancient times as a flavoring agent and in the treatment of coughs and colds. It is anti-inflammatory and increases the effectiveness of the body's production of cortisone. It helps liquefy mucus in the lungs and bronchial tubes. Licorice root treats peptic ulcers by reducing stomach acid production and protecting the lining of the stomach from damage by acid and bacteria. Licorice has been traditionally prescribed for conditions as diverse as colitis, eczema, stress, hypoglycemia, muscle spasms, weakened immunity, irritated and inflamed mucous membranes, menopausal hot flashes and a long list of autoimmune diseases like lupus, rheumatoid arthritis and thyroiditis.

Ma Huang

Also known as ephedra, Mormon tea or desert tea. It stimulates the sympathetic nervous system, decreases bronchial spasm, works as a natural decongestant, increases energy and helps curb appetite. It has traditionally been used in the complementary medical treatment of asthma, allergies, fatigue, colds, flu, eating disorders and obesity. Studies also indicate that it can boost thermogenesis, the body's natural ability to burn fat.

Parsley

This common herb has natural anti-viral, anti-bacterial, expectorant and diuretic effects. It has traditionally been used in the complementary medical treatment of viral infections, sore throats, bronchitis, coughs, fluid retention and infected cuts and wounds. Parsley aids digestion, gets rid of intestinal gas, treats prostate problems and is a good source of iron, carotene and vitamins B1, B2 and C. In high doses, parsley is effective as a uterine stimulant and helps normalize menstrual flow. It will disguise the odor of garlic and works synergistically with other herbal antibiotics like echinacea, goldenseal and chaparral. Parsley also contains a substance in which tumor cells cannot multiply.

Passion Flower

Passion flower is a very popular European remedy for emotional upsets. In large doses, it has sedative, antispasmodic and tranquilizing properties. Many nerve conditions and neurological problems can be helped by passion flower. Some of these are seizures, hysteria, neuralgias, headaches, insomnia, muscle spasms, asthma and Parkinson's disease.

Saw Palmetto

This herb works as a diuretic, nerve sedative, expectorant, general nutritive tonic, urinary antiseptic, gastrointestinal stimulant, muscle builder and circulatory stimulant. Saw palmetto has traditionally been used in the complementary medical treatment of prostate conditions (benign prostatic hypertrophy, prostatitis), enuresis (bed wetting), stress incontinence, infections of genitourinary tract and muscle-wasting diseases of any kind.

Siberian Ginseng

This general tonic is a circulatory stimulant that fights stress, debility, exhaustion, depression, poor memory and a low sex drive. Studies show that long-term use may increase both physical stamina and IQ. Along with ma huang, it is a booster of thermogenesis, the body's ability to burn fat naturally. Siberian ginseng is a very useful supplement for children, adults and the elderly.

White Willow

The bark of the white willow tree is a powerful remedy because of its content of salicin and tannins. It has anti-inflammatory, antipyretic, analgesic, antiseptic and astringent properties. Studies also indicate that it can boost thermogenesis. White willow has traditionally been used in the complementary medical treatment of pain, arthritis and rheumatism, connective tissue inflammation, headaches, muscle aches, fevers and infections of all types. It works synergistically with ma huang and Siberian ginseng.

Yerba Maté

This herb is used as a stimulating beverage throughout much of Latin America. Yerba maté is a central nervous system stimulant, but has some calming properties as well. It is antispasmodic, helps control excessive appetite and, if taken only during daytime hours, helps induce a restful sleep at night. Yerba maté contains caffeine (0.2 to 2 percent) but significantly less than coffee or tea. It also contains iron and may help with iron deficiency anemia. Yerba maté enhances the healing power of other herbs and has been reported to be effective in the treatment of arthritis, headache, hemorrhoids, fluid retention, obesity, fatigue, stress, constipation, allergies and hay fever. It has diuretic properties, but is non-toxic if used in moderation. In sensitive individuals, excessive consumption may cause anxiety, insomnia and diarrhea. In small amounts, however, yerba maté is well worth using for its health-promoting qualities.

Aloe Vera

Many of you know that aloe vera is an ingredient in cosmetics, pharmaceuticals, gels, lotions, shampoos, creams, toothpastes, juices, and nutritional supplements. Some use aloe topically for its antibiotic properties, some internally for its antioxidant and anti-aging effects as well as its bowel-cleansing action.

Aloe vera is gaining credibility even with the conservative medical profession: more and more doctors are turning to this plant for its cleansing, soothing, healing and immune-boosting properties. The medical and scientific literature supports its primary or complementary use, topically or as a juice, for practically all conditions, especially the following:

Acne

Bleeding and hemorrhage

Bites (bee stings, other insect bites)

Boils

Bruises

Burns

Cancer (aloe contains several anti-carcinogenic compounds)

Canker sores

Constipation
(Note: Avoid as a laxative during pregnancy unless anthraquinone content is known to be low)

Eczema

Heartburn and indigestion

Inflammation and infections

Stomach problems

Sunburn

Ulcers

How can aloe vera be effective for so many different conditions? The answer lies in the nearly one hundred ingredients contained in the leaf of the healthy aloe plant. These include numerous antioxidant vitamins and minerals. Antioxidants are natural substances, either manufactured by our bodies or obtained from the diet, that protect us from free radical damage. Free radicals are everywhere: they include chemicals from pollution, tobacco smoke and drugs; radiation from x-rays and the sun and self-produced poisons (auto-toxins) stemming from poor digestion and poor elimination from the bowel.

Free radicals cause damage in our bodies similar to the rust we see on our cars as they age. The cell damaging effects of free radicals lead to degenerative diseases like cancer, heart disease, arthritis, diabetes as well as premature aging. Aloe vera contains many free radical scavengers and immune system enhancers. These include beta-carotene, vitamin B complex, vitamin C, selenium, silicon, zinc, boron, calcium, chromium, magnesium, manganese, potassium, polyphenols, essential fatty acids, saponins and large molecular weight polymeric sugars (e.g., acemannan).

One of the many reasons why aloe vera is so effective for digestive problems is its content of natural digestive enzymes and co-factors. Aloe contains amylase, lipase, oxidase, catalase, bradykinase, glucomannan and fiber – all of which help reduce inflammation, soothe ulcers and stimulate better digestion of protein, carbohydrate and fat.

Beta-Carotene

The best source of beta-carotene is whole carrots. Eating carrots is therefore better than just drinking carrot juice, which in turn is better than just taking a beta-carotene supplement. Carrot juice contains beta-carotene as well as small amounts of protein, carbohydrate, fat, fiber, potassium, vitamin C and a long list of other essential nutrients.

Carrots and carrot juice are alkaline-forming foods. They lower the risk of cancer, especially smoking-related cancers like cancer of the lung, and help lower blood cholesterol. Carrots and carrot juice are excellent complementary treatments for all skin disorders, as well as for respiratory problems like asthma and bronchitis. They may also be of help for gastrointestinal problems like colitis, enteritis and ulcers. I am not saying that beta-carotene capsules are a bad idea, just that it is better to eat the whole food and/or its juice—you will get far more nutritional value.

Vitamin E

Vitamin E is otherwise known as alpha-tocopherol. Studies indicate that supplementation with as little as 200 IU daily can reduce the risk of a heart attack by 46 percent for men and 26 percent for women. The natural forms of vitamin E are d-alpha-tocopherol, d-alpha-tocopheryl acetate, d-alpha-tocopheryl succinate and mixed tocopherols. The synthetic forms are dl-alpha-tocopherol, dl-alpha-tocopheryl acetate or dl-alpha-tocopheryl succinate. All forms supply the body with at least some vitamin E activity.

Studies indicate that the most biologically active are the esterified natural forms: d-alpha-tocopheryl acetate and d-alpha-tocopheryl succinate. Both have been found to provide full antioxidant activity in the body, and are the ones recommended by the top vitamin E authorities at the Shute Institute and Medical Clinic in London, Ontario.

Vitamin C

Vitamin C is an antioxidant that helps prevent atherosclerosis and all degenerative diseases. Vitamin C directly promotes the breakdown of cholesterol and triglycerides. It has an essential role in collagen formation, making it indispensible for joints, muscles, ligaments, tendons and bones. Vitamin C is essential for preventing and treating infections of all kinds.

Selenium

Low selenium levels are associated with an increased risk of atherosclerosis. Selenium is an antioxidant that works in conjunction with vitamin E to protect vascular tissue from damage by toxins. Selenium helps in both the prevention and complementary medical treatment of cancer, arthritis and a long list of degenerative diseases.

Fear of Microwave Cooking

In my frequent discussions with naturopaths, homeopaths, acupuncturists and practitioners of other holistic disciplines, the consensus is that microwave cooking should be avoided because it devitalizes food. But I have yet to see any credible documentation to support this point of view. The available scientific literature presents an entirely different viewpoint.

No matter how carefully we may cook food, any kind of cooking destroys some nutrients. The longer one cooks food at high temperatures, the more nutrients are lost, irrespective of the type of cooking process used. According to recent scientific journals, stir frying, steaming and microwaving are the healthiest methods for cooking. For positive health benefits, however, the best thing is to eat as much of your diet as possible in its natural raw form. Until proven otherwise, microwave cooking does not appear to damage food any differently than other types of cooking.

Body Fat Percentage and Weight

The bathroom scale may be deceptive: only 20 percent of the population conforms to the averages on standard height and weight charts. Unless you know your exact frame size, muscular development and other important variables, these charts will mislead you about your optimal weight. In other words, is your weight problem the result of big bones, well-developed muscles, excess water retention or too much fat? Body weight is the sum of lean tissue, fat tissue and water. Optimal health requires a proper balance of lean, fat and water. Having the "right" weight according to height and weight charts does not guarantee this balance.

For example, a 5'10" male may weigh 200 pounds. The height and weight chart says he should weigh about 165 pounds if he has a large frame. However, if this individual is a world-class body builder with 10 percent body fat (the average is 18 percent for a male), would you say he's overweight? Most trim body builders would be considered overweight based on standard height and weight charts alone. This is because, pound for pound, muscle is heavier than fat. To get an accurate reflection of ideal body weight the balance of lean, fat and water must be taken into account.

Optimal body fat percentages have been established according to age and sex. For example, if you are a female between the ages of 30 and 39, your ideal body fat percentage is between 20 and 24 percent. For a male in the same age bracket, the ideal body fat percentage is between 16 and 20 percent. Optimal lean body percentage, lean body mass and total body water levels have also been established for men and women according to age groups.

In any weight loss program it is desirable to lose fat as opposed to lean body mass or water. Diets that claim weight losses of 10 or more pounds the first week usually fail to say that most of this weight loss is water and lean body mass, not fat. Low carbohydrate diets (e.g., Atkins diet) cause rapid loss of water and lean body mass, not fat. Knowing what type of weight you are losing on any weight control program is a definite health advantage.

The most popular methods of testing for body fat percentage in the past have been with a skin fold test and underwater weighing. Although these techniques are reasonably accurate, they are cumbersome and difficult to conduct. There are portable (slightly larger than a hand-held calculator) body composition analyzers available from many different distributors. These are computerized gadgets that measure total body electrical impedance and, according to Henry Lukaski et al., are "by far the most accurate of all laboratory and clinical methods" used to determine body fat percentage, lean body mass and total body water. Computerized body composition analyzers can also determine basal metabolic rate (BMR). This refers to the calories used by the body during a normal resting state.

Many doctors, dietitians and fitness clubs use body composition analyzers in their offices. Anyone on a long-term weight reduction program should get their body fat percentage, lean body mass, total body water and BMR checked weekly, along with their weight. The safety and effectiveness of the weight control program must be judged on all these factors and not just on weight loss alone.

Correcting Weight Disorders

Approximately 80 million people in North America are plagued by weight problems. Studies indicate that this is a life-long problem for 95 percent of these people. The weight loss industry has sales of over 33 billion dollars per year and continues to increase its profits despite a 95 percent failure rate.

A five percent cure rate may sound discouraging, but suggests that the problem does have a solution for at least some people. Studies show that the majority of the five percent who are able to lose weight permanently do so with common sense self-care or self-directed programs. Did these people do it by dieting? Did they do aerobic exercises? Did they take special supplements advertised in the latest tabloids?

Dieting

Diets don't work. Diets are nothing more than an exercise in self denial where one is usually being asked to give up foods that seem to satisfy deep psychological or emotional needs. To many with longstanding weight problems, dieting not only feels restrictive but also punitive.

Whether it's an 800 calorie diet, a doctor-supervised diet with special injections, the no-carbohydrate diet, a hospital-directed program, a weight loss clinic with a "system," a liquid meal replacement program or any number of calorie counting meal plans, the result is always the same. Weight is lost in the first few weeks but is eventually gained back—and then some.

For a variety of reasons, people on diets cheat, or at least bend the rules. Moreover, the more one diets, the lower one's metabolism goes and the more weight is gained. This is because dieting always lowers metabolic rate and establishes a set point for burning off calories lower than before the diet was started. It is very common for victims of dieting to have average daily body temperatures lower than 98.6° F.

Reducing calories is not the answer. And contrary to popular belief, fasting is also not the answer. Skipping meals slows metabolism. When one drastically lowers metabolism and caloric intake, the body goes into a "starvation" or "conservation" mode, meaning that the body starts storing fat and burning off glycogen (stored carbohydrate) in muscles. With each cycle of dieting, the net result is a an increase of body fat relative to muscle mass. In other words, dieting causes fat gain.

To lose weight, one must increase metabolic rate by stimulating the body to burn fat, not lean tissue. In addition, there has to be a way to enhance waste elimination, enzyme activity and hormone function (especially of the thyroid, adrenal and pituitary). One needs to permanently leave the conservation mode. This involves eating regular meals, making healthy food and beverage choices, correcting nutrient deficiencies or metabolic imbalances and having a positive mental attitude.

Exercise

By itself, exercise is an ineffective way to lose weight. Further, studies show that the wrong type of exercise leads to weight gain, not weight loss. For example, overweight individuals who go on a six-month program of jogging or rigorous aerobics will expend a great deal of energy but will usually end up gaining weight because of a concomitant increase in food intake. The right type of exercise is one which stimulates metabolism, improves the breakdown of fats in the body, stimulates circulation and enhances lymph flow. The right type of exercise—power walking, bicycling, using a treadmill or rebounder—also improves muscle tone and helps burn fat even when one is not exercising. This occurs best at a fixed rate of 30 to 35 percent of capacity and includes exercises like walking slightly above normal pace and using a rebounder (a home mini-trampoline). For optimal effects, exercise should be done before eating a meal of complex carbohydrates, or several hours after the last meal has been completely digested.

Metabolic and Nutritional Balancing

Brown fat—representing about two percent of all the fat in the body—is responsible for a considerable amount of thermogenesis, the burning of calories from fat stores in the body. Brown fat metabolism can only be stimulated by that which activates the sympathetic nervous system. This could include caffeine, essential fatty acids, herbs (e.g., Siberian ginseng, kola nut, yerba maté, ma huang, white willow, yohimbe and kelp) and regular physical activity. It may sound hard to believe, but overweight people tend to have low essential fatty acid levels; thus, supplementation is important to achieve permanent weight loss.

Certain vitamins, minerals and amino acids are important co-factors for the manufacture of neurotransmitters, active thyroid hormone, growth hormone and adrenal hormones. These include vitamin B complex, vitamin C, zinc, copper, iodine, selenium, chromium, manganese, carnitine, glycine, methionine, tyrosine, phenylalanine, tryptophan, arginine and ornithine.

Weight problems have more to do with what people eat than with how much. Studies indicate that you can eat all you want and still lose weight as long as you eat less fat and eliminate sugar and simple carbohydrates. Other studies indicate that hidden food allergies may play a role in suppressing metabolism. Such allergies are usually to common foods like milk, wheat, corn, eggs, chocolate and yeast. Eliminating unsuspected food allergies may be crucial to some individuals.

The herb *Garcinia cambogia* contains the organic compound hydroxycitrate, which has a beneficial effect in regulating body fat metabolism. It can block fatty acid synthesis from glucose by inhibiting a liver enzyme. It also controls appetite, especially a craving for sweets.

A high fiber intake of raw fruits and vegetables (at least 60 percent of daily intake) is crucial for permanent weight loss because complex carbohydrates stimulate thermogenesis. Also, fat burning works better when waste material in the large bowel is eliminated. If you do not have at least one large bowel movement for every meal you eat, you cannot expect to lose weight in an efficient manner.

A large intake of spring water (at least eight glasses daily for a healthy adult) plus fruit or vegetable juices (e.g., elderberry, carrot, grapefruit, etc.) are absolutely essential. There are a large number of high fiber foods and herbal supplements that may be used to help the body eliminate waste more efficiently. Some of these include psyllium seed powder, oat bran, fruit pectin, aloe vera, cascara sagrada, senna, buckthorn, uva ursi, parsley and other herbs with a mild laxative/diuretic effect.

In some cases, treatment of subclinical hypothyroidism with a trial of liothyronine (T3) or desiccated thyroid is a treatment option. In cases of subclinical hypothyroidism, the usual lab tests for thyroid are in the normal range, but average body temperatures may be below 98.6° F. Short-term supplementation with liothyronine or desiccated thyroid (the dosage adjusted to bring average body temperatures to normal) will help improve metabolic rate. This treatment is not an alternative; to be effective, it must be done in conjunction with the other measures mentioned earlier, and under the supervision of a medical doctor.

Lastly, we must not ignore the fact that weight problems are often directly related to deeper mental, emotional and social stresses. Although supplemental vitamins, minerals, amino acids and herbs are of great help to a large number of overweight people, they will not, by themselves, offset poor eating habits, sedentary lifestyle or deep-seated emotional problems. It is also important to note that some people do not tolerate even tiny doses of nutritional supplements due to allergies or individual hypersensitivities. The help of a psychotherapist or natural health care practitioner may be required.

Healthy Weight Gain

Much has been written about how to lose weight by eating healthily, but it's difficult to find information on how to gain weight while maintaining a nutritious diet. Let's take as an example a woman who is 5'5" tall, has a small frame and weighs about 98 pounds. She has always been too thin—the most she has weighed is 105 pounds, when, as a teenager, she practically lived on junk food. She is now 32 and does not want to return to a regimen of French fries, chocolate bars and potato chips in order to put some weight on. She is also leery of following a fat-free, fiber-full diet for fear of becoming even thinner. What is the answer for such a woman?

First of all, one does not have to eat a junk food diet to gain weight. It can be done by following a healthy diet that gets approximately 65 percent of the calories from complex carbohydrates, 20 percent from protein and 15 percent from fat. This could be called a high complex carbohydrate, high fiber diet.

According to the calculations listed below, one would need to consume at least 1,768 calories daily to maintain a weight of 98 pounds. If activity is moderate or heavy, calories would have to be proportionately higher. If the diet is increased by about 500 calories daily of the right kinds of foods, you should gain about one pound per week, provided one has a normal metabolism and digestive function.

If one does not gain weight according to these guidelines, a number of sub-optimal health conditions should be considered. These include thyroid, gonadal and adrenal glandular imbalances; malabsorption syndromes caused by deficiencies in hydrochloric acid and/or pancreatic digestive enzymes; hidden parasitic infections; hidden candida/yeast infections;

unsuspected food allergies; an imbalanced bacterial flora in the digestive tract; amino acid deficiencies and vitamin and mineral deficiencies. These can all be assessed by a naturopath or holistic medical doctor familiar with appropriate testing and natural treatment programs.

A nutritional assessment can help determine whether or not there is a greater need for certain vitamins, minerals, essential fatty acids, digestive enzymes and amino acids. For example, amino acids like carnitine, arginine and ornithine are essential to help build greater lean muscle mass (i.e., weight) and might need to be supplemented in selected individuals. The same can be said for a long list of other nutrients and metabolic boosters. If simply increasing the intake of healthy foods does not work, look into these other possibilities with the help of a health care practitioner.

Profile: **A. B. RDA**
Age: **32**   Weight: **98 lbs.**   Activity Level: **Light**
Sex: **Female**   Height: **5 ft 5 in**

Calories	1768 *	Vitamine B6	1.6 Mg
Protein	33.4 G	Vitamine B12	2 Mcg
Carbohydrates	256 G **	Folacin	180 Mcg
Dietary Fiber	17.7 G #	Pantothenic	7 Mg *
Fat-Total	58.9 G **	Vitamin C	60 Mg
Saturated	19.6 G **	Vitamin E	8 Mg
Mono	19.6 G **	Calcium	800 Mg
Poly	19.6 G **	Copper	2.5 Mg *
Cholesterol	300 Mg **	Iron	15 Mg
A-Carotene	RE	Magnesium	280 Mg
A-Preformed	RE	Phosphorus	800 Mg
A-Total	800 RE	Potassium	2000 Mg *
Thiamin-B1	1 Mg	Selenium	55 Mcg *
Riboflavin B2	1.2 Mg	Sodium	2400 Mg *
Niacin B3	13 Mg	Zinc	12 Mg

* Suggested values within recommended ranges
** Dietary Goals   # Dietary Fiber = 1 gram/100 calories

Source: The Food Processor II, Nutrition and Diet Analysis System. Available for Macintosh and IBM-compatible personal computers from ESHA Research.

2

Boosting Immunity
and Energy

Fatigue is the most common complaint of people seeing doctors in the late twentieth century. In mild cases, fatigue prevents enjoyment of life and interferes with optimal performance at work. In severe cases of chronic fatigue syndrome, fatigue can be incapacitating for several years at a time. It is estimated by well-known author Dr. William Crook that about 15 percent of the population suffers from fatigue severe enough to require medical attention. The majority of these victims of low energy are diagnosed by conventional medical doctors as having psychosomatic illness or depression. A fewer number of cases are diagnosed with more severe illnesses such as cancer or AIDS. If no organic explanation can be found for fatigue, victims are often referred for psychiatric care or prescribed antidepressants and told to live with their symptoms. I have often been told by my patients that conventional doctors told them that "it's all in your head."

Fatigue is not just in your head. There is growing awareness among scientists and natural health care practitioners that fatigue is simply a reflection of weakened immunity. The immune system consists of many organ systems—an army of white cells, antibodies, lymphatic channels, glands, hormones and chemicals. Vaccinations, prescription antibiotic drugs, ionizing radiation, electromagnetic fields and at least 70,000 inorganic chemicals in our polluted environment contribute to the slow but sure breakdown of the immune system. Devitalized, processed, irradiated and otherwise adulterated foods further contribute to altered immunity and to fatigue. What can be done?

Anyone can enhance the body's resistance to viruses, bacteria, fungi, parasites, allergies, chemicals and other stressors by optimizing the levels of antioxidant vitamins and minerals in the body. Immunity, and hence energy, can also be increased by the use of safe and effective herbal remedies, green food factors, enzymes and amino acids. Detecting hidden food and chemical allergies, eliminating parasites, clearing candida overgrowth in the gastrointestinal tract and normalizing the bowel flora are also important. This chapter focuses on natural solutions to boosting immunity and energy.

Food Allergies and Allergy Testing

Food allergies can produce a long list of symptoms and are a puzzling and sometimes frustrating cause of illness. The symptoms evoked by foods can be the essence of individuality. A bacterium or virus may trigger very similar symptoms in each person it infects. A food allergy, on the other hand, may produce different symptoms from one individual to another. In one person, food allergy leads to migraine headaches. In another, arthritic symptoms flare up. Some of the world's leading physicians have linked mental confusion, depression, migraine headaches, schizophrenia, arthritis, hallucinations, eczema, obesity, irritable bowel syndrome and many other physical conditions to hidden food allergies.

Most people think of a food allergy within the framework of the classic but rare case of an immediate response to an allergen: an individual eats lobster, strawberries or peanuts and immediately breaks out in hives or suffers an asthmatic attack. People with this sort of problem are lucky because they know exactly what foods they are sensitive to and, hence, what foods to avoid. The more common and serious problems, however, are seen with hidden (masked, delayed) allergies to wheat, corn, milk and other common foods. Symptoms associated with these foods are usually so chronic that they go unrecognized. The offending foods are so thoroughly enmeshed in the diet that the chances of avoiding them are virtually nil.

Masked food allergies can produce symptoms so diffuse and nebulous that they are easily dismissed by mainstream allergists as neurotic in origin. Hidden food allergy is the great masquerader of many symptoms striking adults and children alike. One clue to its existence is the presence of food cravings. Although it may sound unbelievable, most food cravings are in fact food allergies—it's just the way the immune system works sometimes. A food allergy is the body's response, through the immune system, to a food that it reacts to as foreign or toxic.

There are many good tests that help detect food sensitivities. Although considerable confusion exists about which is the best laboratory test, most agree with the accuracy and reliability of the elimination/provocation technique described by authors such as Drs. William Crook and Doris Rapp. This technique involves eliminating whole classes of foods for several days, then adding them back, noting reactions. Workable variations of this are the Coca pulse test, which does not require a practitioner, and sublingual food challenges, which are usually administered by clinical ecologists. Some of these procedures would not be appropriate for people suffering from severe pain syndromes, or those who do not have the time or stamina to experiment with their diets. On the other hand, there is something to be said for experiencing the effects of allergenic foods in reproducing symptoms. The elimination/provocation technique ultimately empowers sufferers to control symptoms with simple diet changes.

In the past decade of my practice, I have been using the elimination/provocation test, when appropriate, combined with the

Elisa/Act* test developed by Dr. Russell Jaffe. This test can determine hidden or unsuspected allergies to as many as 300 foods, chemicals and toxic heavy metals as well as to candida. In my opinion and experience, this is the state-of-the-art in food sensitivity detection. Please understand, however, that this in no way invalidates other forms of testing, which may work equally well for selected people.

The Elisa/Act test measures antibody reactions to foods from the IgG, IgA, IgM antibody families, as well as immune complex levels (combinations of antibodies and foods in the blood) and the effect of specific foods on the lymphocytes (white cells involved with the cell-mediated immune reaction). In terms of accuracy for delayed food hypersensitivity reactions, this test is superior (97 percent accuracy). Scratch skin testing for food allergies is only about 20 percent accurate. It is also a painful and sometimes dangerous procedure in that severe allergic reactions can occur. Skin tests are excellent, however, for picking up environmental (inhalant) allergies.

There are no conclusive studies comparing the accuracy and reliability of different types of food allergy/sensitivity tests. Electroacupuncture tests like VEGA and Interro, combined with professional counselling and the patient's personal experience with different foods, have been documented to improve the lives of countless thousands. Acupuncture and homeopathy work for a great majority, but there are people who do not benefit from any aspect of these methods of diagnosis. Continued research and practitioner experience will, in time, answer questions surrounding test validity and reliability.

Self-Help and Other Options for Chronic Fatigue Syndrome

Chronic fatigue syndrome (CFS) goes by many names. It has been called yuppie flu, chronic Epstein-Barr virus syndrome, myalgic encephalomyelitis and post viral neuromyasthenia. About 15 percent of the population now suffers from CFS. It is a poorly defined symptom complex characterized by chronic or recurrent debilitating fatigue. Various combinations of other symptoms may be present, including sore throat, lymph node pain and tenderness, headache, fibromyalgia (muscle pain), sleep disturbances, depression and arthralgia (joint pain). Many patients experience varying degrees of stomach and intestinal problems as well as

---

* Serammune Physicians Laboratories can provide more information on the Elisa/Act test, as well as a list of doctors in your area who can order it for you. See the resources section in the appendix for their address.

multiple food and chemical allergies. Chronic fatigue syndrome victims tend to be far more sensitive to prescription medications than the average person, with a high probability of having side effects to antidepressants, antibiotics and even herbal, vitamin and mineral remedies. Common to most sufferers is a frustration with the conventional medical system, which refuses to accept the validity of the diagnosis.

The Major Signs and Symptoms:

- Recurrent sore throat and flu-like episodes with general malaise
- Enlarged, tender lymph nodes, especially around the head and neck
- Recurrent headaches or sinus congestion
- Chronic low-grade fever
- Muscle and/or joint pain
- Inability to concentrate, short-term memory loss, "brain fog"
- Gastrointestinal upsets, alternating diarrhea and constipation (irritable bowel syndrome)
- Emotional upset and/or depression
- Allergies
- Insomnia, interrupted sleep
- Weight loss or gain, eating disorders

Chronic fatigue syndrome was once thought to be caused by the Epstein-Barr virus, but recent studies have proven that this virus is not responsible for the syndrome. Some believe that CFS may be caused by chemical poisonings, food and chemical allergies, hypothyroidism (e.g., low thyroid hormone function as seen with Wilson's syndrome), other viruses like cytomegalovirus, weak adrenal function, parasitic infections, amino acid deficiencies and even candida.

Despite research that proves otherwise, many patients I have seen in the past year are still being told by doctors that CFS is a form of depression or that "it's all in your head." Antidepressant drugs are usually ineffective. Stress reduction techniques such as biofeedback may be helpful in some cases. While there is no test that will diagnose or rule out CFS, there are some indicators: research done by doctors around the world shows that patients with CFS have measurable immune system abnormalities, particularly with respect to the numbers and ratios of different populations of white cells known as lymphocytes. And a psychological test called the Minnesota Multiphasic Personality Inventory (MMPI) shows a specific pattern in cases of CFS not found in any other disorder. This test, however, is not universally considered diagnostic for CFS.

If you have been told you have CFS, the good news is that there is a lot you can do to help yourself to a speedier recovery. It's important and even therapeutic to keep an open mind about CFS. Do not listen to negative people, medical or otherwise, who claim that nothing can be done, or that you need to see a psychiatrist. All cases of CFS improve or completely resolve with time (from a few months to a few years). Recovery rates are highly variable and very difficult to predict, but can be enhanced by complementary medical approaches. While there is no specific, recognized medical treatment for CFS, one can dramatically improve the function of the immune system through good nutrition, antioxidant supplementation and supportive herbal or homeopathic remedies. The immune system requires healthy levels of zinc, calcium, magnesium, potassium, selenium, germanium, silicon, iron, beta-carotene, vitamin A, vitamin C, vitamin E, B-complex vitamins (especially vitamins B5, B6 and vitamin B12) and all the essential amino acids, to name just a few. Testing for vitamin, mineral and amino acid levels may open the door to a speedier recovery.

Studies have also shown that refined carbohydrates (glucose, fructose and sucrose), have a depressant effect on the immune system as early as an hour after eating them. Removing sugar and white flour products from the diet is often helpful with most of the signs and symptoms of CFS. A hypoallergenic rotation diet with 70 percent of calories coming from complex carbohydrates (whole grains, fruits, vegetables and legumes) is best. It is also important to avoid caffeine, alcohol and processed foods. If possible, have an Elisa/Act blood test done.

Chronic fatigue syndrome sufferers who have irritable bowel symptoms (constipation, bloating, gas, diarrhea, mucous discharge, etc.), should ask their doctor to order a battery of tests called the comprehensive digestive and stool analysis (CDSA) combined with comprehensive parasitology. People suffering from chronic fatigue syndrome often have problems with digestive enzyme function, bowel flora balance and infestations of parasites, candida or other pathogenic microbes. For more information on the CDSA or comprehensive parasitology testing ask your practitioner to contact Great Smokies Diagnostic Laboratory. See the resource section in the appendix for their address.

A higher dietary intake of the omega-3-EPA oils (found in halibut, cod, mackerel, salmon, trout, shark and many others) and gamma linolenic acid (GLA) are of proven benefit to CFS. Despite what some may be saying about the relative merits or drawbacks of the various GLA supplements (flax seed, evening primrose oil, borage oil, black currant oil, etc.) I have noticed no significant difference in the results obtained from one source as opposed to others. I recommend experimentation with the different GLA sources before deciding on any specific brand.

Several herbs and whole food supplements help to boost immunity and control the symptoms of CFS. Some work better for given individuals than others, so it's best to avoid generalizations about any natural treatment. Many doctors and CFS sufferers have reported good results with the following natural supplements:

Adrenal extract
Astragalus
Baptisia
Blue-green algae, barley green, spirulina, green kamut and other whole green foods
Burdock, slippery elm, sheep sorrel, Turkish rhubarb combination
Carnitine
Chaparral
Coenzyme Q10
DHEA
DMG (dimethylglycine)
Echinacea
Garlic
Ginkgo biloba
Goldenseal
Kelp, dulse and other seaweeds
Kola nut
Lactobacillus acidophilus and bifidus

Licorice
Liothyronine
Lomatium
Ma huang
Methionine
Natural progesterone
Pau d'arco (Taheebo)
Pokeweed
Phenylalanine
Propolis, bee pollen, royal jelly
Pycnogenol
Red clover
Shiitake mushroom
Siberian ginseng
St. John's wort
Thymus gland extract
Tyrosine
Whole leaf aloe vera juice
Yarrow
Yerba maté

Natural Immune System Boosters and CFS Fighters:

Homeopathic remedies like ignatia, nux vomica, natrum muriaticum and cell salts often help CFS victims who are unable to tolerate vitamins, minerals and herbs. Consultation with a homeopathic physician is highly recommended.

Natural Treatments for Fibromyalgia

Fibromyalgia is a poorly understood chronic musculoskeletal pain syndrome associated with localized areas of deep muscle tenderness sometimes spread throughout the entire body. It is estimated that over six million people suffer from fibromyalgia in North America. The cause is unknown. Many doctors who treat patients suffering from chronic fatigue syndrome (CFS) believe that fibromyalgia may very well be a form of CFS. Patients complain of severe aching pain, usually with stiffness in the shoulders, hips, hands and feet. The characteristic feature upon physical examination is the presence of multiple, localized areas of tenderness over skeletal muscle groups.

Most patients complain of overwhelming fatigue, which may often be the chief complaint. Nearly all patients complain of poor, nonrefreshing sleep. Electroencephalographic (EEG) studies have documented a disturbance of the normal delta wave pattern in sufferers. Other symptoms seen frequently in patients with fibromyalgia include headache, irritable bowel syndrome, cold hands and feet, numbness and tingling in the hands and feet, depression and sensations of swelling (fluid retention). The severity of these symptoms varies with the individual victim.

Typical medical therapy is with low-dose antidepressant drugs. One recent medical journal article claimed a prompt and marked reduction of pain and stiffness when low dose antidepressants were used with lithium therapy. Another report claimed significant benefits with hypnosis. Cardiovascular fitness training, aerobic exercise programs and biofeedback training have all been found to reduce the severity of symptoms, but the disease often continues for many years. Complete remissions are rare and relapses can occur.

Although very little seems to be published on natural treatments for fibromyalgia, many nutrition-oriented physicians have reported success using approaches similar to those that are effective for several forms of arthritis and chronic fatigue syndrome.

Weight reduction may be very important, as losing weight alleviates some of the stress on the joints. Intake of refined carbohydrates (sugar and white flour products) and animal fats (especially those found in red meats) should be reduced as much as possible.

There are certain types of fats that may, in higher-than-average intake amounts, act in the same way as standard anti-inflammatory drugs. Examples of these include cold-pressed flax seed oil, gamma linolenic acid (GLA found in evening primrose oil and borage oil) and EPA (found in trout, cod, halibut, mackerel, salmon, shark, herring and other seafoods). Increasing these in the diet, or taking them in encapsulated supplement form, while decreasing the intake of saturated animal fats can have a remarkably good anti-inflammatory effect. There are several brands of essential fatty acid supplements available at most health food stores.

DL-phenylalanine is an amino acid that has been shown to help the body release its own natural opiates (endorphins), thus providing substantial pain relief naturally. It does what acupuncture does without the needles. DL-phenylalanine is only available in health food stores in the United States, but it may be imported without much difficulty.

Optimizing the body's trace mineral balance may be crucial. It is therefore necessary to avoid foods, such as bran, coffee and tea, known to interfere with mineral absorption. Minerals that may be important include iron, zinc, copper, manganese, calcium, magnesium, silicon, boron and selenium. Vitamins A, C and E, beta-carotene, bioflavonoids and B-complex vitamins can be supplemented in higher than RDA doses because of their antioxidant properties, which help prevent certain aspects of inflammation. The recommended doses for these nutrients must be determined for the individual by a qualified health care practitioner based on appropriate biochemical tests.

People with fibromyalgia have reported benefits from the use of certain herbs. Alfalfa, for example, has been extensively studied. It contains many important substances, including saponins, sterols, flavonoids, coumarins, alkaloids, vitamins, amino acids, minerals and trace elements. Aside from its ability to lower blood cholesterol levels, numerous clinical and anecdotal reports support its use for pain control.

Calendula is a natural antibiotic herb most often used as a topical cream for cuts, burns, rashes, infections and other injuries. (New mothers familiar with natural medicine are frequently astounded at how rapidly calendula cream will heal a baby's diaper rash.) Taken orally in fairly high doses, it has a profoundly positive effect in reversing the many signs and symptoms of fibromyalgia. Since there are no side effects, it is certainly one natural remedy well worth a therapeutic trial.

Other herbs that have been reported to have beneficial effects include devil's claw, burdock, licorice, red clover, comfrey, yucca and sassafras. Like vitamin and mineral supplements, herbs are not without their side effects and are best administered and supervised by an experienced health care practitioner.

Food allergies (hypersensitivities) are often associated with fibromyalgia. The Elisa/Act blood test can detect sensitivities to 300 unsuspected food, toxic heavy metal and chemical substances. (See section on Food Allergies and Allergy Testing.) People who are pan-allergic (i.e., react adversely to almost all foods), should also investigate the possibility of an intestinal tract parasitic or fungal (candida) infection. Such conditions must be treated before starting on a food allergy elimination program. Although one cannot say that parasites or candida cause fibromyalgia, many nutrition-oriented physicians and clinical ecologists have reported success in the treatment of fibromyalgia when the candida or parasitic infection was cleared first.

Assorted reports have claimed beneficial effects with supplemental niacinamide (vitamin B3), coenzyme Q10, DMSO and the New Zealand green-lipped mussel (because of its mucopolysaccharide content). Niacinamide seems to be the most effective: the usual therapeutic dose is about 3,000 mgs daily and it takes from three to six weeks to work.

Several practitioners have reported the benefits of a series of intramuscular injections of vitamin B12 and magnesium sulphate in the treatment of fibromyalgia. The injections seem to be especially effective against pain, insomnia and low energy symptoms. Recent research also validates the use of natural progesterone, liothyronine and DHEA—all hormones that improve energy, reduce inflammation and boost immunity. For more information, see *Wilson's Syndrome: The Miracle of Feeling Well*, by Dr. Denis Wilson, and *Natural Progesterone*, by Dr. John Lee.

Electroacupuncture treatments and oral supplementation with the amino acid tryptophan have also been reported to help fibromyalgia. It is interesting to note that one recent study reported that fibromyalgia sufferers have, in general, lower blood levels of tryptophan. Like many of the new SSRI (Selective Serotonin Reuptake Inhibitors) antidepressants (e.g., Prozac), tryptophan elevates the levels of the neurotransmitter, serotonin. Serotonin, in turn, has antidepressant and relaxant effects.

Many homeopathic remedies are also useful in fibromyalgia management. Since the right remedy for alleviating symptoms will vary from case to case, it is best to consult a homeopath; he or she will take a proper case history and prescribe the remedy on an individual basis.

One of the most important things to keep in mind with any alternative program is that treatment is long-term. There are no quick and lasting remedies that work in all cases. Patients should be prepared to actively involve themselves in all aspects of therapy and not just wait passively for something to happen. Any holistic approach requires a far greater degree of self responsibility than just taking aspirins. Occasionally, one hears of spontaneous remissions or overnight successes with the right remedy. However, the vast majority take from three to six months, or more, to stabilize. A holistic health care practitioner's guidance will help to ensure optimal results.

Aggressive Holistic Treatments for HIV and AIDS

Conventional treatments for people living with HIV and AIDS have significant limitations due to side effects like bone marrow suppression. Recent studies have also questioned the wisdom of using immunosuppressive drugs like AZT, DDI and others, when they have little, if any, impact on the course of the disease. Specialists who treat people with HIV and AIDS, continue, for the most part, to ignore the impact of diet, lifestyle and natural remedies. This is unfortunate. I would never question their attitude if the cures were there. They are not.

In recent years it has become increasingly evident that a holistic approach has a great deal to offer those infected with HIV. Published studies by scientists and natural health care consultants like Dr. Lark Lands support the use of a combination of several natural antivirals, immune system modulators and preventive agents. This is not to say that conventional treatments should be abandoned, but that they should be complemented by aggressive holistic supportive therapies.

In a recent paper, Dr. Lands states: "It now appears critical to address the autoimmune aspects of HIV disease. Currently, the best approach to this may be the use of the antioxidants and other nutrients that protect cell membranes and dampen the inflammatory response of the body to the infection (e.g., glutathione, coenzyme Q10, vitamins C, E and A, selenium, zinc, etc.)." Other natural remedies often promoted by Dr. Lands include St. John's wort extract, beta-carotene, N-acetyl-cysteine, DHEA, Siberian ginseng, acidophilus, wormwood, mathake tea, thymus gland derivatives and B-complex vitamins, especially vitamin B6 and vitamin B12.

Lands' recommendation of several dozen nutritional supplements, drugs, injections and other therapies is in sharp contrast to the use of intravenous ozone therapy and peroxide therapy. Studies in Germany and other European, Caribbean and South American countries report hundreds of HIV positive cases that have been converted to HIV negative through treatments with intravenous ozone alone.

DHEA (dehydroepiandrosterone) is the most abundant androgen (male hormone) produced by the adrenal cortex. DHEA has weak androgenic activity and can be found in almost any organ, including the testes, the ovaries, the lungs and the brain. In animal studies, DHEA has been shown to reduce body weight without food reduction. It can lower cholesterol, stimulate the immune system and inhibit tumor growth. Animal studies also suggest that it prevents aging. Laboratory studies (in vitro) demonstrate that DHEA can block infection with HIV-1 although the mechanism by which this takes place is unclear at present time. Interestingly, researchers have reported that DHEA levels are markedly lower in AIDS patients. Clinical trials are now underway to test DHEA's use in the treatment of HIV infection.

Ozone and Hydrogen Peroxide Therapies

A great deal of interest has been generated of late by different types of oxygen therapies, including ozone, hydrogen peroxide, dioxychlor and coenzyme Q10. To say that these are controversial therapies would be an understatement. Many Canadian and American physicians and clinics that offered these treatments have been forced out of practice by various government agencies. There is a great deal of confusion and misunderstanding surrounding the subject. For the most part, both ozone and hydrogen peroxide therapies are available only in Mexico, some Caribbean countries (the Bahamas, Cuba and the Dominican Republic) and Europe, (particularly Germany and eastern Europe). The reasons for this are not medical or scientific, but political.

One of the best sources of information on ozone ($O3$) and hydrogen peroxide ($H2O3$) therapy is *Oxygen Therapies: A New Way of Approaching Disease* by Ed McCabe. Another excellent general source is Jane Heimlich's book, *What Your Doctor Won't Tell You*. Yet another general source of information on these therapies is the International Bio-Oxidative Medicine Foundation (see the appendix for their address).

Both hydrogen peroxide and ozone therapies deliver more oxygen to cells, tissues and organs. Both therapies have been used outside Canada and the United States by conventional and alternative medical doctors alike in oral and intravenous forms. In general, both therapies can be used for the same purposes. There is an optimal dose for a given person and illness, below which there is no noticeable effect and above which there are toxicity problems. There seems to be no advantage of one therapy over the other, and no long-term hazardous effects have been documented for either therapy. Many practitioners use and advocate a combination of both oxidative therapies with or without conventional and alternative medical approaches.

If inhaled in large quantities, ozone can be toxic. The same is true of hydrogen peroxide, oxygen, water and any other nutrient. To categorically say that ozone is toxic or that hydrogen peroxide is toxic is almost as ridiculous as saying that water is toxic. Toxicity is a matter of degree. It is a biochemical fact that the body manufactures its own hydrogen peroxide under certain conditions. For ozone, hydrogen peroxide, oxygen and water to become toxic, huge amounts (far more than the levels used in therapy) would have to be consumed. By and large, the medical use of oxidative therapies is safe and effective for a broad range of conditions.

In many European countries, ozone, instead of chlorine, is used to purify water because it does not produce carcinogenic by-products. Chlorine does. Chlorine is linked to countless chronic diseases, including cancer. The city of Los Angeles has replaced chlorination of drinking water with the largest ozone water purification system in the world. Other major North American cities will soon follow suit.

Both ozone and hydrogen peroxide break down in the body and produce extra oxygen. They destroy viruses, bacteria, fungi, pyrogens and, according to some, cancer cells. There is no bacteria, virus, fungus or spore that can survive in the presence of ozone or peroxide. This explains their benefit in chronic viral conditions and candidiasis.

Cancer cells are killed by ozone or peroxide, yet healthy cells are unaffected. The theory is that cancer is a plant cell that can be killed by its waste product, oxygen. An increasing volume of scientific research supports the fact that extra oxygen supplied by ozone or peroxide therapy can help in the treatment of both infectious and degenerative diseases. These include AIDS, chronic fatigue syndrome, herpes, venereal diseases, hepatitis, mononucleosis, circulatory diseases, cardiovascular disease, diabetes, skin ulcers, infected wounds, gangrene, burns, colitis, psoriasis and almost all skin disorders. The availability of oxidative therapies in Canada and the U.S. will hinge more on increasing public demand and grass roots political action, than on further acceptance by the scientific community.

Chronic Bronchitis Alternatives

It has long been known that the liver can regenerate from a severely diseased state without drugs or heroic medical intervention. We now have evidence that all types of heart disease, including coronary artery disease, can be reversed by diet and lifestyle changes alone. Since the lungs are just another organ like the heart and liver, I see no reason why chronic obstructive lung disease (chronic bronchitis and emphysema) should be any different in terms of a positive response to natural therapies.

Most patients with chronic obstructive lung disease benefit from supplemental antioxidants. These vitamins, minerals, enzymes and amino acids protect lung and bronchial tissue from damage and help in tissue repair and healing. They include the following: vitamin A, beta-carotene, vitamin B complex, vitamin C, bioflavonoids (rutin, hesperidin, quercetin, pycnogenol and catechin), vitamin E, selenium, zinc, coenzyme Q10, L-arginine, L-ornithine, L-cysteine and N-acetyl-cysteine. Daily dosages should be several multiples of the RDA and be determined for you by a naturopath or holistic medical doctor.

Other helpful natural food supplements that speed recovery from chronic obstructive lung disease include rose hips, red clover, wheat grass, blue-green algae, spirulina, cod liver oil, lactobacillus acidophilus, Siberian ginseng, capsicum, echinacea, goldenseal, astragalus, ginger, germanium, pau d'arco, yarrow, chaparral, liquid chlorophyll, garlic, licorice root, ganoderm, lycium, peony, polygala, ligustrum, schizandra, atractylodes, St. John's wort, lomatium, chickweed, barley juice and the combination of burdock, slippery elm, sheep sorrel and Turkish rhubarb. For the most part, these herbs are immune system boosters and blood purifiers.

Chronic obstructive lung disease is caused by frequent irritation of the lungs, usually as a consequence of cigarette smoking or air pollution. Allergies may be at the root of some cases, and most sufferers complain of incessant coughing, mucous build-up, chest pain and difficulty breathing. Even if you do not smoke, watch out for second hand smoke. Passive smoking may be very dangerous for people susceptible to chronic obstructive lung disease. Look into purchasing an air purifier for your home. There are a number of excellent commercial products on the market that would be of help to anyone suffering from the effects of air pollution.

If you have not already done so, get yourself tested for food, chemical and environmental allergies by a qualified health professional. Skin testing by an allergy specialist may be helpful with respect to grasses, trees, pollens and other inhalants. However, food and chemical allergies are best diagnosed by blood tests (i.e., Elisa/Act). Many medical doctors, naturopaths and osteopaths use these tests regularly.

Allergies, infection and excess mucus in the respiratory tract can be helped by a combination of echinacea, goldenseal, myrrh, chaparral, propolis and capsicum. Coltsfoot, mullein, horehound, licorice, lobelia, borage, ephedra and cayenne open up the airways to improve breathing.

A comprehensive nutritional program that includes allergy control, supplemental vitamins, minerals, amino acids and herbs often reverses symptoms of obstructive lung disease in a matter of a few weeks or months. At the very least, it reduces reliance on repeated prescriptions for antibiotics, bronchodilators, steroids and the negative attitudes of some doctors.

Clearing Mucus

Excessive mucus can be caused by any number of things, including heredity, cigarette smoking, drugs, food and environmental allergies, nutrient deficiencies and toxic heavy metal accumulations in the body. Dairy products, red meats, grains and refined carbohydrates (sugar and white flour products) can cause some susceptible people to produce more mucus. A thorough nutritional assessment by a health care professional can often help pinpoint the source of the problem.

The most effective remedy for eliminating, or at least reducing, phlegm from the respiratory tract is an amino acid derivative called N-acetyl-cysteine. This mucolytic agent, which is also a powerful antioxidant, can be taken in oral capsule form. It actually dissolves the mucus by cutting up mucoprotein molecules into smaller, less viscous fragments. It is also an excellent oral chelation agent. In other words, it can hook up with toxic heavy metals such as lead, mercury, copper, aluminum, arsenic and cadmium in the body and remove them through the kidneys. I have personally witnessed this remarkable product rid obstructing mucus from the respiratory tract of a chronic bronchitis sufferer within a week. It's certainly worth a trial since it has a very low toxic potential.

There are several nutrient and herbal supplements that can be taken to help both boost immunity and prevent mucous buildup. Cod liver oil is one such nutrient. Most adults can tolerate a tablespoon, two or three times daily. To get a proper balance of all the essential fatty acids, add one tablespoon daily of flax seed oil. With an increase in fatty acid intake, it is also important to take extra vitamin E. Buy some 200 IU natural vitamin E capsules, break open the capsules and add the contents to each dose of either the cod liver oil or the flax seed oil. Next, add 1/4 teaspoon of vitamin C crystals (with bioflavonoids) to your favorite juice daily. Gradually increase the dose by 1/4 teaspoon a day until bowel movements become loose (not diarrhea). This is referred to as "taking vitamin C to bowel tolerance."

Zinc gluconate lozenges (25 mgs of zinc per tablet) should also be a part of the program. Most adults can take up to ten of these daily. Some brands may taste better than others, so try different ones to see which ones are best tolerated. One recent study in adults showed that taking about ten zinc lozenges per day reduced the length of recovery from the common cold from an average of 10.8 days to 3.9 days. One of the reasons for this may be because zinc is a co-factor for a number of enzymes involved in immune response. Zinc deficiency is associated with compromised immune response; zinc replacement therapy normalizes immune response.

Echinacea, goldenseal, pau d'arco, capsicum, elderberry, astragalus, garlic, sheep sorrel, burdock, slippery elm, Turkish rhubarb and calendula are herbs that can be very helpful both as natural antibiotics and as part of an overall infection and mucous prevention program. These herbs boost immunity and help normalize the bacterial flora in the large bowel. They are available, in capsule or tincture form, from most health food stores and have very low toxicity potential.

Mucus, in and of itself, is not a bad thing that should be eliminated from the body at all cost. On the contrary, mucus has many protective properties for both the respiratory and gastrointestinal tract. The trick is to have an optimal, comfortable amount. Look to your nutrition and lifestyle habits to achieve balance. If necessary, you also have the option of using an arsenal of safe, natural supplements from time to time.

Preventing Tumors

Lipomas are benign growths and are usually excised by surgeons as the only form of therapy. Diet and environment do have a role to play in both the prevention and treatment of benign tumors.

Most nutritional authorities advise eliminating all animal protein, dairy products (except yogurt and yogurt products), salt, sugar, white flour products, processed and packaged foods from the diet. These foods are difficult to digest, contain no enzymes and form toxins (oxidants or free radicals) in the large bowel and blood. About half of dietary intake should consist of raw fruits and vegetables.

The remainder may include seeds, nuts, whole grains and cultured dairy products such as yogurt, buttermilk and kefir. Juice fasting should also be considered, as it is a good way to detoxify. For detailed information on how to do this the right way and enjoy yourself at the same time, I suggest you pick up a copy of *The Joy of Juice Fasting* by Klaus Kaufmann.

It is now an accepted fact that benign and malignant (i.e., cancerous) tumors are initiated by what is called free radical pathology. This simply means that toxins from air, water and food enter the body, cause damage to the nuclei of cells and initiate tumor growth. There are thousands of possible toxins, or oxidants as they are also called: chemicals, drugs, tobacco smoke, ionizing radiation, pesticides—the list goes on.

Our bodies usually make ample amounts of antioxidant enzymes and thus prevent tumors from forming. In some people, however, antioxidants get depleted and little remains to prevent tumor growth. These antioxidants include vitamin A, beta-carotene, most of the B-complex vitamins, vitamin E, vitamin C, selenium, zinc, cysteine, glutathione, coenzyme Q10, germanium and all the bioflavonoids, especially pycnogenol and quercetin. There is good evidence to suggest that supplementation of the diet with these antioxidants will help prevent tumors from occurring. A health care practitioner familiar with their use can advise you of appropriate doses.

Scientific and anecdotal studies have shown that many different herbs and food supplements are useful in both prevention and complementary medical treatment of lipomas and other benign tumors. These include garlic, pancreatin, raw thymus extract, lactobacillus acidophilus and herbs such as barberry, dandelion, pau d'arco, burdock, slippery elm, sheep sorrel, Turkish rhubarb, echinacea, horsetail, comfrey, ragwort and wood sage. In her book, *Health Through God's Pharmacy*, Maria Treben describes the use of poultices made with horsetail, Swedish bitters and calendula. A naturopath or medical doctor familiar with herbal remedies can be of help in prescribing an individualized treatment plan.

Practical Cancer Prevention

One in three people living in North America will experience cancer during their lifetime. At least half will seek some form of non-drug, non-invasive natural therapy involving diet, nutritional supplements and holistic activities like visualization. People are seeking alternatives at a rapidly escalating rate because of low confidence in conventional medical treatments or reports of success with a wide range of non-toxic therapies. The principles of alternative or complementary medicine can also be applied to cancer prevention.

The consensus of opinion is that the ideal cancer preventive diet is one that is high in fiber and complex carbohydrates, chosen exclusively from the new four food groups: organic whole grains, legumes, fruits and vegetables.

Special Cancer Preventive Foods

The ideal diet for prevention of cancer spread is vegetarian. Avoid all animal products, including chicken, fish and dairy products. Eat plenty of foods from the new "Four Basic Food Groups": whole grains, legumes, fruits and vegetables. Avoid salt, sugar, coffee, tea and alcohol. The rationale for all this can be found in books like *Diet for a New America* and *May All Be Fed: Diet for a New World*, by John Robbins, and *The McDougall Plan*, by John McDougall.

There are foods with particularly strong anti-cancer effects due to their content of beta-carotene, anti-cancer indoles or other vitamins and trace minerals. These include broccoli, cabbage, cauliflower, Brussel sprouts, seaweeds, figs, beets, beet tops, papaya, mung beans, licorice, cucumbers, carrots, garlic, walnut, lychee fruit, mulberries, asparagus, pumpkin, burdock, dandelion greens, taro roots, pearl barley, steamed carrots, spinach, squash and reishi, shiitake, maitake and Chinese black mushrooms.

Avoid all animal products, including beef, pork, lamb, chicken, fish and dairy products. These foods have the highest concentrations of cancer-causing fats and chemicals. Drink lots of fresh juices high in beta-carotene and vitamin C like celery, spinach, beet and carrot juice. Avoid tobacco, salt, sugar, coffee, tea and alcohol.

Antioxidant vitamin and mineral supplements prevent cancer because of their ability to neutralize free radicals (carcinogens). There is increasingly good evidence that antioxidants are a vital part of any cancer prevention or treatment program. The most important of these are vitamin A, beta-carotene, B-complex vitamins, vitamin C, vitamin E, selenium, zinc, germanium, iodine and glutathione. Other supplements that either fight free radicals or boost immunity are pycnogenol, quercetin, garlic, blue-green algae, N-acetyl-cysteine, coenzyme Q10, pancreatic digestive enzymes and the hormones melatonin, estriol and DHEA. Shark cartilage has received a lot of press lately and is one of the alternative cancer therapies undergoing investigation by the Office of Alternative Medicine in the United States.

Herbs and food supplements are used in cancer therapy to boost immunity. Of importance are pau d'arco (taheebo), panax ginseng, flax seed oil, evening primrose oil, black currant oil, calendula, echinacea, goldenseal, astragalus, red clover, Chinese green tea, chaparral, silymarin, artichoke, tumeric, dandelion, bee pollen, propolis, St. John's wort and lomatium. A healthy bowel flora is also vital for a strong immune system. Supplemental lactobacillus acidophilus in powder or capsule form may be a very important way of optimizing colon health and the elimination of toxins from the body.

Consider using a herbal combination made up of slippery elm, burdock, Turkish rhubarb and sheep sorrel. Sheep sorrel appears to be the most powerful anti-cancer component of this herbal tonic. Researchers report that sheep sorrel is effective in breaking down tumors, soothing ulcers and treating skin diseases. It contains carotenoids, chlorophyll, calcium, iron, magnesium, silicon, copper, iodine, manganese, zinc, vitamin B complex and vitamins C, E and K. It's mode of action may be through chlorophyll to provide more oxygen to tissue cells. Since oxygen in higher amounts counteracts cancer cells, viruses and other infections, this could well be sheep sorrel's mechanism of immune system optimization.

Burdock root has long been recognized by herbalists as a blood purifier. Scientific studies have also demonstrated the anti-tumor activity of burdock in animals. It contains carotenoids, chromium, magnesium, potassium, silicon, zinc, calcium, copper, manganese, selenium, iron, B-complex vitamins and vitamins C and E.

Several scientific studies have demonstrated the anti-tumor activity of burdock in animals. The term, "the burdock factor" was coined by scientists at the Kawasaki School of Medicine in Okayama, Japan. In test tube studies, this "burdock factor" was found to be active against HIV (the AIDS virus). Burdock root contains the essential oil inulin—a very powerful immune modulator. It attaches to the surface of white cells and makes them work better. Burdock also contains benzaldehyde, a substance that has significant anti-cancer effects in humans.

Slippery elm is one of the better known herbal remedies. It has traditionally been used as a treatment for ulcers, burns, cuts, hemorrhages and other wounds. It's active component is a mucilage (soluble fiber) similar to the mucilage in flax seed. Other components of slippery elm are gallic acid, phenols, tannins, starches, carotenoids, B-complex vitamins, vitamin C and K, calcium, magnesium, chromium, selenium, silicon and zinc. Slippery elm is a natural antacid and antibiotic and a regulator of the intestinal flora. It too contains chemical components known to have anti-tumor effects.

Turkish rhubarb has strong bowel detoxification effects. In all forms of cancer, the elimination of toxins from the body is crucial to recovery. Turkish rhubarb's primary use is to help cleanse the blood of various toxins. It has a gentle laxative action, cleanses the liver and supports the secretion of bile into the intestine. It contains carotenoids, B vitamins, vitamin C, calcium, magnesium, copper, iodine, manganese, potassium, silicon, sulphur and zinc. Some of its active components include gallic, malic, oxalic and tannic acids, bioflavonoids, pectin, resin, starch and volatile oils. Turkish rhubarb also contains rhein, a chemical member of the anthraquinone family. Rhein has the ability to inhibit the growth of several pathogenic bacteria, parasites and candida in the intestinal tract. This may help explain its ability to fight a wide range of infections. It has also been shown to have anti-tumor properties.

For a full explanation of how this herbal combination works, as well as testimonials, a history of its development and the controversies surrounding its use, refer to *Calling of an Angel* by Gary Glum and *The Essence of Essiac* by Sheila Snow.

Dosages for all food supplements and herbs discussed here are highly variable and depend on the general health and prevention goals of the given individual. A naturopath or medical doctor familiar with nutritional supplements can help guide and supervise someone on an individualized program.

Finally, developing a positive mental attitude, emotional or spiritual health and better control of stress situations in one's life can go a long way toward preventing cancer, or any other disease for that matter.

Coping with Cancer

If you have just been diagnosed with cancer, the most important thing you can do is involve yourself as much as possible with your proposed treatment. Start by reading two excellent books: *Cancer Therapy: The Independent Consumer's Guide to Non-Toxic Treatment and Prevention*, by Ralph W. Moss, and *Options: The Alternative Cancer Therapy Book*, by Richard Walters. Check out the alternatives before subjecting yourself to the mutilating effects of surgery, radiation or toxic drugs that may be no better than doing nothing at all. Although something can be said for the trust between a doctor and patient, do not just glibly accept medical advice before verifying the validity of the recommended treatments independently. You are dealing with a life-threatening illness, not just a sore throat. Ask lots of questions and insist on thorough answers. Get the facts and figures, the cure rates and the side effects. Compare these to doing nothing and to using one or more of the complementary treatments.

Many very worthwhile cancer therapies like ozone, amygdalin (laetrile) and hydralazine are not easily available in Canada and the United States for political reasons (see *Racketeering In Medicine: The Suppression of Alternatives*, by Dr. James Carter) but are available at various foreign clinics (in the Caribbean, Europe and Mexico, for example). Ralph Moss' book, *Cancer Therapy*, gives names, addresses and phone numbers to contact for more information on alternative treatments in other countries.

Complementary cancer treatments are best used to help conventional approaches work better or to reduce the severity of the side effects of radiation or chemotherapy. None are proven alternatives to orthodox cancer treatments. A doctor familiar with natural therapy should be consulted to both prescribe and monitor treatment.

Chemotherapy and Food Supplement Interactions

Despite the fact that millions now supplement their diets with garlic, essential fatty acids, vitamins C and E and other anti-inflammatory, antioxidant immune enhancers, there have been no reported cases of bleeding or clotting disorders associated with these supplements. There is nothing to worry about. Garlic, evening primrose oil and fish oil in large doses prevent platelets from clumping or sticking together. They prevent abnormal clotting in the blood, but do not stop the clotting that would occur under healthy circumstances. Aspirin does the same thing, but has side effects such as gastrointestinal hemorrhage when taken in large doses.

Antioxidants like beta-carotene, vitamin A, vitamin C and vitamin E protect both healthy and diseased (cancer) cells. So do B vitamins, selenium, zinc, glutathione, germanium, ginkgo biloba extract and bioflavonoids. The main value in supplementation with any or all of these is to prevent or ameliorate the side effects of chemotherapy. Obviously, you want to kill the diseased cells and prevent the healthy cells from getting damaged. For this reason, do not take antioxidant supplements during chemotherapy. Take them up to two days before treatment or starting two days after treatment. This will allow for maximal beneficial effects of chemotherapy. There is growing evidence, however, that vitamin A in massive doses has a chemotherapeutic effect. It is, however, too early to advocate its use as a cancer therapy.

A large number of natural food and herbal supplements help boost immunity and may also minimize some of the side effects of chemotherapy. These include rose hips, red clover, wheat grass, blue-green algae, spirulina, cod liver oil, lactobacillus acidophilus, Siberian ginseng, burdock, slippery elm, sheep sorrel, Turkish rhubarb, capsicum, echinacea, goldenseal, astragalus, ginger, germanium, pau d'arco, yarrow, chaparral, liquid chlorophyll, garlic, licorice root, ganoderm, lycium, peony, polygala, ligustrum, schizandra, atractylodes, St. John's wort, lomatium, chickweed and barley juice. The leukocyte (white cell) and platelet counts can be significantly improved with some or all of these measures.

Dangers of Vaccinations

There is a great deal of speculation about the safety and validity of all vaccinations. Some of the concerns expressed by responsible doctors and scientists include:

- Significant differences between the immunity acquired in the natural course of a disease and the immunity gained from vaccines
- Vaccination-induced immune system dysfunction
- The induction of a transient AIDS-like state in healthy children and adults
- The deleterious effects of vaccination on ill or malnourished children
- The suboptimal and inappropriate induction of immunoglobulins caused by the abnormal route of introduction of vaccines into the human system
- The association of an increased incidence of allergies with an increased use of vaccines

A wide range of neurological and immune system disorders are thought to be linked to vaccinations. These include sudden infant death syndrome and autoimmune diseases like lupus.

The control and prevention of infectious diseases is dependent on garbage and sewage control, healthy lifestyles and the promotion of natural immunity with good nutrition. Boiling food and water is helpful. So are supplements such as betaine or glutamic acid hydrochloride, stomach bitters, pancreatin and lactobacillus acidophilus. These help protect the gastrointestinal tract from infection with organisms such as cholera.

Malaria prevention does not involve vaccines. Prescription drugs are used and for the short term they are reasonably safe. Some people suffer side effects, and the risk-benefit ratio favors the use of antimalarial drugs as opposed to no preventive measures at all. Control of mosquitoes with repellents and netting is a must. Supplementing the diet with brewers yeast, high doses of B-complex vitamins and the herb wormwood helps, but is no guarantee of malaria prevention.

Asthma

There are many natural treatments that would help mild to moderate asthma. Avoid food additives, particularly coloring agents, azo-dyes, tartrazine and other chemicals in processed foods. Sulfites, used as a preservative in many foods and beverages, can precipitate asthma. Learn to become a label reader and avoid all these known asthma triggers. In restaurants, the problem may be much more difficult since sulfites are used liberally in practically all dishes, especially salads. Commonly used sulfites include sodium bisulfite, potassium metabisulfite, potassium bisulfite and sulfur dioxide. Test strips are now available to detect the presence of sulfites in foods.*

Many asthma sufferers have hidden or unsuspected allergies to commonly eaten foods, especially milk and wheat. The most accurate way of determining hidden food allergies is with a blood test called the Elisa/Act test. Elimination of reactive foods usually produces symptom improvement within six weeks.

Many asthmatics are sensitive to aspirin, salicylates and other pain killers. Since salicylates are found naturally in many foods, they should be reduced or eliminated from the diet if the asthmatic is sensitive to salicylates. The following is a list of the most common sources of dietary salicylates:

Fruits: Apples, apricots, avocados, all berries, melons, cherries, currants, grapes, raisins, dates, figs, guavas, grapefruit, lemons, lychees, mandarins, nectarines, peaches, plums, prunes, oranges, passion fruit, pears, persimmons, pineapples, rhubarb.

Vegetables: Alfalfa, asparagus, aubergines, broad and green beans, beetroot, broccoli, carrots, chicory, courgettes, cucumber, endive, marrow, mushrooms, okra, olives, onions, parsnips, peppers, chillis, potatoes, radishes, spinach, corn, sweet potatoes, tomatoes, turnips, watercress.

Condiments: Anise, cayenne, celery seed, cinnamon, cumin, curry, dill, fenugreek, mace, mustard, oregano, paprika, rosemary, sage, tarragon, turmeric, thyme.

Beverages: Colas, coffee, tea, most fruit juices, alcohol.

Seeds and Nuts: Almonds, Brazil nuts, coconut, macadamia nuts, peanuts, pine nuts, pistachio nuts, sesame seeds, walnuts, waterchestnuts.

Miscellaneous: Honey, licorice, yeast-containing foods, processed, canned or packaged foods containing any of the above items.

Irrespective of food or other allergies, asthmatics should avoid sugar and white flour products because of their negative effects on the immune system.

It has been known for over 60 years that most asthmatics produce too little hydrochloric acid in their stomachs. Many also have poor pancreatic function and inadequate secretion of digestive enzymes. As a result, high protein foods may not be digested completely and, when absorbed into the bloodstream, may evoke an allergic reaction such as wheezing.

---

* For information on test strips write to Sulfitest, Center Laboratories, 35 Channel Dr., Port Washington, NY 11050, or call 516-767-1800.

I have seen many asthmatics, particularly children, clear up their asthma simply by supplementing with hydrochloric acid and pancreatic digestive enzymes.

Other supplements of proven benefit in the treatment of asthma include vitamin A, vitamin B6, vitamin C, bioflavonoids (especially quercetin and pycnogenol), bromelain, zinc, flax oil, salmon oil, selenium, magnesium and vitamin E. Herbal remedies that have been used with success by asthmatics include echinacea, horsetail, lobelia, ginkgo biloba, licorice, ma huang, taheebo, propolis and slippery elm. Yoga, meditation, psychotherapy, relaxation exercises and stress reduction techniques have also all been shown to reduce the severity and frequency of asthmatic attacks.

Autism and Nutrition

Some reports link autism to childhood immunizations. It is true that vaccines have been associated with immune system abnormalities, mental retardation, autoimmune disorders, arthritis and even sudden infant death syndrome. However, the evidence for this is scanty and highly controversial; most conventional doctors would dispute the validity of any of these associations.

The cause of autism is unknown, but many published studies indicate that autistic children can be helped by the following:

1. Folic acid supplementation.

2. High doses of supplemental vitamin B6 and magnesium: Numerous studies by Dr. Bernard Rimland, a world-renowned autism expert, indicate this to be the case.

3. Amino acid analysis and balancing: Recent studies indicate that autistic children have high levels of free tryptophan and serotonin in their blood. They may be helped by supplements of glutamine, phenylalanine and tyrosine.

4. Food allergy testing and treatment may significantly help clear up autistic symptoms. The Elisa/Act test may be very helpful in diagnosing hidden food allergies. Several published case reports indicate that nearly 50 percent of autistic cases improve when sugar, milk and wheat are removed from the diet.

5. Testing for heavy metal toxicity (lead, mercury, cadmium, etc.) by blood, urine and hair analysis may reveal a previously unsuspected cause of brain chemistry imbalance.

6. Supplementation of the diet with other nutrients designed to enhance brain function, including DMG (dimethyl glycine), octacosanol, choline, B-complex vitamins, vitamin C, vitamin E and ginkgo biloba extract.

Fighting the Hidden Lead Epidemic

There is a growing awareness by the public, if not by the medical profession, of the importance of toxic heavy metals to health. Many of the seemingly mysterious causes of twentieth century diseases are related to the accumulation in the body of minerals such as mercury, cadmium, lead, aluminum, nickel and arsenic. Recently, there has been great interest in the effects of mercury from dental fillings on the immune and nervous systems. This is based on some alarming studies and subsequent media reports. I believe that the lead problem will gradually come to light in much the same way.

Unlike the mercury amalgam story, there is no argument in the scientific literature on the hazards of even low levels of lead in the body. There is, however, a problem with early detection. Low level lead exposure has been linked to many health problems, especially nervous system disorders such as hyperactivity, learning disabilities and behavioral abnormalities in children. Despite the fact that low IQs and nervous system damage in children have been documented with blood lead levels of 10 to 11 micrograms per deciliter, provincial authorities continue to claim that the "acceptable level" of lead is 25 micrograms per deciliter. As a result, many cases of lead poisoning go undetected. Testing for lead in the blood, by the way, is not the best way to screen for the presence of lead in the body.

Early detection of lead in the body may help in preventing other lead-associated health disasters such as stillbirths, cancer, heart disease, high blood pressure, kidney disease, depression, immune disorders and a host of metabolic diseases. We cannot wait for "authorities" to do the responsible things necessary to rid lead from the environment and from our bodies. So, where do we begin?

Most importantly, what are the sources of lead in our environment? Lead seems to be everywhere, but we can reduce exposure to it. Sources to watch for include leaded petrochemical products, dust and dirt, leaded house paint, drinking water (from old galvanized pipes, pre-1930 construction), canned foods, imported ceramics, glazed pottery and painted glassware, cigarette and other tobacco smoke, hair blackeners (e.g., Grecian Formula), mascara, bonemeal, organ meats, dolomite and the list goes on. In their book, *Trace Elements, Hair Analysis and Nutrition*, Drs.

90

Richard Passwater and Elmer Cranton list over 300 different occupational sources of lead contamination.

We may not be able to avoid lead in our urban food supply. It seems to be present in practically all foods that come from lead contaminated soils. What we can do, however, is detect lead in our drinking water and in cookware, plates, cups, bowls and other kitchen utensils. These are the hidden lead sources most likely to produce problems in our daily environment. What the common dental filling is to the mercury problem, drinking water and dinnerware is to the lead problem. When we cook food, lead can be leached out of the cookware. Thanks to the availability of the Frandon Lead Alert Kit and the Frandon Lead in Water Kit, it is now possible to rapidly detect the presence of lead in ceramicware, metalware, glassware, soldered food cans, painted surfaces, children's toys, pipes and drinking water.* These products are the same as those used by the FDA to detect lead in products at U.S. ports of entry.

Once we have done our best to minimize exposure, the next step is to test our bodies for lead levels. According to Passwater and Cranton, hair analysis is the best method for detecting the presence of lead. Blood lead levels are a second choice, because blood rapidly deposits lead into skeletal tissue and hair. Low blood levels of lead may, therefore, be misleading. Hair analysis provides early detection of lead and other toxic heavy metals, often before serious symptoms are manifested. Many labs provide hair analysis to doctors, chiropractors and naturopaths.** If high levels are found, a nutritional supplement program can be started to chelate (bind) lead and remove it from the system. In more extreme, symptomatic cases, intravenous chelation therapy can be used.

There are several nutritional and chelating factors that are effective for lead and that have low toxicity in therapeutic (not RDA) doses. These include vitamins A, C, and E, zinc, calcium, magnesium, iron, chromium, selenium, garlic, kelp, lecithin, L-cysteine, L-methionine, L-glutathione and N-acetyl-cysteine. Foods high in lead-chelating substances include garlic, onions, eggs, soybeans and other legumes. The fact that these foods are so highly effective in preventing heart disease, cancer and neurological disorders may well be due to their ability to chelate lead and other toxic heavy metals. A regular diet of these foods and supplemental nutrients will offer us some protection while we wait for the authorities to clean up their acts.

---

* These lead-testing kits are available for home use from Pace Environs, 81 Finchdene Square, Scarborough, Ontario, M1X 1B4; phone 1-800-359-9000.
** The best known in Canada is Anamol Laboratories, P.O. Box 96, Concord, Ontario, L4K 1B2; phone 416-660-1225.

Warts

A wart is a small benign growth or tumor of the outer layers of the skin occurring singly or in clusters. Warts may occur at any age, but are most commonly seen in children and teenagers. Though they may persist for many years, most warts clear up spontaneously (without treatment) after two years. Warts pose no health threat, but may cause discomfort, depending on their location. There are three basic types of warts: common warts, plantar warts and filiform warts.

Warts are due primarily to viral infections of the skin by a member of the papovavirus group. They are highly contagious and can be spread from person to person by direct or indirect contact with wart tissue or secretions. Warts may also be spread by touch from one part of the body to another.

Any measures that improve general health—and the immune system in particular—will help prevent warts and other viral infections. Eliminate sugar, refined carbohydrates, red meats and processed foods from the diet. Eating foods laced with chemicals or those that are deficient in vitamins and minerals (e.g., empty calorie junk foods) increases the likelihood of catching viruses of any kind.

Natural remedies for warts include vitamin E, garlic, aloe vera, tea tree oil, calendula and castor oil applied directly to the wart. Also helpful is supplementation with high doses of vitamins A, C and E and B-complex, as well as zinc, lactobacillus acidophilus and the amino acid L-cysteine. I have also found that topical application of hydrogen peroxide to the wart is very effective.

Effective herbal remedies, used topically or taken internally, include dandelion, great celandine, mullein, echinacea, thuja, houseleek, goldenseal, calendula, lomatium, pau d'arco and wintergreen. In *Health through God's Pharmacy*, Maria Treben recommends Swedish bitters as an effective remedy. Most of these herbs are not only effective against viruses, but are also helpful in fighting candida infections.

Although there are dozens of herbs and natural food supplements that help the immune system fight viral infections, allergies and cancer, four stand out for special attention: burdock, Turkish rhubarb, sorrel and slippery elm. This is because they are safe and effective even at massive dosages. They have also been advocated by many herbalists and natural healers as immune system boosters.

Different remedies work for different people—it's all a matter of trial and error. Since all the remedies listed are fairly innocuous, they're worth trying before resorting to more invasive medical alternatives—freezing and destruction of the wart with liquid nitrogen, for example.

Middle Ear Fluid

The most common controllable cause of fluid behind the eardrums in children is hidden food allergies, especially to milk, dairy products, wheat, yeast, citrus fruits and peanuts. Many of the food reactions occur on a delayed basis (up to five days after consumption of the reactive food). If trial and error (elimination-provocation techniques) fail to determine the offending foods, the Elisa/Act test can be of tremendous help. Knowing what the reactive foods are can go a long way toward the prevention and treatment of middle ear problems including hearing loss.

A high sugar intake suppresses immunity and may be at the bottom of many allergy problems. One of the least suspected culprits in this area is a high fruit juice intake. I have often seen children in my practice who consume the equivalent of 50 teaspoons or more of sugar each day in the form of "unsweetened" apple juice. Don't let the label fool you. It takes a lot of apples to make a glass of apple juice (the equivalent of up to 10 teaspoons of sugar for some brands). Other hidden sources of sugar include commercial cereals, soft drinks, gelatin desserts, puddings, cookies, granola bars and flavored yogurt.

A number of natural food supplements may be of help in reducing the fluid accumulation behind the eardrum. These include blue-green algae, bee pollen, barley green and other green drinks, vitamin A, beta-carotene, B-complex vitamins, vitamin C, bioflavonoids, vitamin E, essential fatty acids (evening primrose oil, borage oil, flax seed oil, olive oil, cod liver oil), zinc, silica, selenium, echinacea, calendula, goldenseal, elderberry, camomile, ginger, capsicum, mullein, garlic, pau d'arco, lactobacillus acidophilus and N-acetyl-cysteine. Choosing the appropriate supplements and dosages is a matter of biochemical individuality and should be done with the help of a qualified health care practitioner.

Antihistamine Alternatives

There is some concern about the cancer-promoting effects of some commonly used, non-prescription antihistamines. Recent negative reports in the media have prompted many to seek safer, more natural alternatives to antihistamines, commonly used for hay fever. Antihistamines are certainly no cure for hay fever. What about the natural alternatives?

Runny nose, sinus congestion, headache, postnasal drip and itchy eyes, ears and throat are all symptoms of hay fever. The condition is most common in spring, summer and fall and is most often associated with allergies to grasses, weeds, trees and pollen.

Studies have shown an association between sugar consumption and hay fever symptoms. Sugar cane, wheat and grass pollen are all in the same botanical family of grasses. Their association with hay fever symptoms may not be just coincidental. Many of my hay fever patients were able to go off antihistamines altogether when they eliminated sugar, wheat and milk from their diets.

Observant doctors have noted that the treatment of hidden food allergies, nutritional imbalances and deficiencies produces a significant reduction or disappearance of hay fever symptoms. This may be because one can reduce the hypersensitivity of the airways in the respiratory tract by avoiding allergic foods and correcting nutritional imbalances.

Many nutritional and herbal supplements in high doses may be of help to hay fever sufferers. These include the following antioxidant vitamins, minerals and amino acids: vitamin A, beta-carotene, B-complex vitamins, especially pantothenic acid (vitamin B 5) and vitamin B 6, vitamin C, vitamin E, selenium, zinc, coenzyme Q10, rutin, quercetin, hesperidin, catechin pycnogenol, glutathione and cysteine. Deficiencies in essential fatty acids (GLA and omega-3-EPA) often aggravate hay fever and other allergic conditions.

Studies on vitamin C have shown that in very high doses it has properties very similar to antihistamines. Runny noses and mucous congestion respond fairly quickly with high doses. The only side effect is loose bowel movements or diarrhea if the dose taken is too high for the given individual. The best way to take this supplement is in crystalline powder form mixed with juice. You can start by taking about a quarter teaspoon four times daily and gradually increase it to one full teaspoon four times daily or just to the level tolerated by your bowel.

Bicarbonate powder (calcium, magnesium and potassium bicarbonate mixture) can also be used to neutralize acute allergic reactions. This comes in powdered form and should be available from most health food stores or pharmacies. The usual effective dose for adults is one to two teaspoons in juice three or four times daily.

Herbs such as echinacea, goldenseal, St. John's wort, lomatium, astragalus and calendula are very helpful in stimulating proper functioning of the immune system. The herbal combination of ma huang, white willow and kelp is also effective, especially for the control of postnasal drip and sinus congestion.

Sometimes, treatment of a chronic candida hypersensitivity or infection (yeast syndrome) improves the condition. All these natural strategies have low side effect potential and do not cause the drowsiness, potential heart problems or weight gain seen with antihistamines. Additionally, they are widely available in health food stores and pharmacies without prescription. Appropriate dosages can be determined by biochemical individuality testing through a health care practitioner such as a naturopath or nutritional medical doctor.

Laryngeal / Voice Problems

Laryngeal disease, hoarseness, voice problems and difficulty swallowing may all be symptoms of unsuspected food and chemical allergies. If medical investigations and conventional treatments have been fruitless, it may be very helpful to get some allergy testing done.

Testing for inhalant allergies (pollens, grasses, trees, etc.) is adequately addressed by skin scratch/intradermal tests. Skin testing for food and chemical allergies, however, is inaccurate and unreliable. There are a variety of food and chemical allergy tests that one could use, but I recommend a combination of the IgE RAST and the Elisa/Act test developed by Dr. Russell Jaffe. At present, these are the two most reliable blood tests for immediate (IgE RAST) and delayed hypersensitivity reactions (Elisa/Act) to foods and chemicals. Most doctors should be familiar with the IgE RAST since it has been available for over 15 years. For more information on the Elisa/Act test, you or your doctor can contact Serammune Physicians Laboratories (see the appendix for address and phone number).

Test kits can be ordered from the lab and your doctor can take blood to test as many as 300 different foods and chemicals. Once the allergic substances are known, elimination of the offending foods or chemicals is likely to relieve the symptoms within three to six months. (For in-depth information on Food Allergy Testing, see the section on Food Allergies and Allergy Testing.)

Natural Sore Throat Remedies

The most common cause of a dry mouth and a sore throat is insufficient water intake. Another potential cause is essential fatty acid deficiency. Cut down or eliminate intake of animal products and take a supplement of either flax seed oil or evening primrose oil, along with chewable vitamin C and vitamin B6. Sometimes popping five or six zinc gluconate lozenges (25 mgs) daily for a week or two can provide quick relief.

Diabetics, even those with well controlled blood sugar levels, are prone to candida (yeast) infections. In the mouth, this is often referred to as thrush and can cause a burning sensation. A simple, safe and effective remedy is the use of tea tree oil as a mouth rinse or gargle. Candida is killed on contact upon rinsing with tea tree oil and may also help with sore throats caused by bacteria and viruses. If none of these simple remedies help, see a natural health care practitioner for a professional assessment.

Herpes and Cold Sores

Herpes is an annoying and occasionally serious viral infection easily recognized by most as a cold sore. It can also occur in the genital area where the blisters can be extremely painful and stubborn to heal. Since herpes is a virus, it will respond to all the measures designed to improve or optimize the immune system.

Studies indicate that ultraviolet light can stimulate the reactivation of the herpes simplex virus. Application of a PABA sunscreen before going outdoors will help prevent sunlight-induced lesions. Taking PABA (500 to 1,000 mgs three times daily) may also offer some preventive help. Recent studies suggest that the prescription mineral lithium may be of help to women who cannot tolerate acyclovir. Lithium interferes with the replication of the virus without affecting the host cells. It can be used in a topical ointment (8 percent lithium succinate) or combined with zinc (zinc sulphate solution 0.025 percent).

Nutritional excesses and deficiencies can have a remarkable impact on any viral illness. We know that starvation (particularly protein deprivation) causes a lower production of antibodies and a greater risk of developing infections. In order for the immune system to function optimally, the body requires adequate amounts (at least RDA levels) of zinc, vitamin C, vitamin E, vitamin A, iron, copper, folic acid, vitamin B12 and essential amino acids.

Studies have also shown that refined carbohydrates (glucose, fructose and sucrose) have a depressant effect on the immune system as early as an hour after eating them. So does cigarette smoking and alcohol consumption. Even moderate alcohol consumption can make viral illnesses worse. Complete abstinence is mandatory. A diet high in saturated animal fats (beef, pork, lamb, dairy products, eggs) also impairs immune function. A higher intake of the omega-3-EPA oils (found in halibut, cod, mackerel, salmon, trout, tuna, among others) and gamma linolenic acid (flax seed oil, evening primrose oil, black currant oil, etc.) enhances immune function. A high protein intake is helpful simply because it enhances antibody production.

Additionally, many doctors have noticed that a diet high in the amino acid lysine and low in the amino acid arginine helps with genital herpes outbreaks. Lysine (1,000 to 2,000 mgs three times daily) taken with vitamin C (2,000 mgs three times daily) decreases the frequency and severity of herpes outbreaks, but not necessarily the healing time. Lysine should be taken preventatively at low doses (500 mgs daily) and at higher doses at the first sign of symptoms (6,000 mgs daily). Symptoms correlate with the time of greatest viral replication. The best results are obtained if the lysine supplements are combined with the low arginine diet. High dose lysine is harmless, but may cause higher cholesterol levels in rare individuals. Blood tests can be done for anyone taking lysine for prolonged periods of time.

Foods high in lysine include fish, poultry, lima beans, shrimp, mung bean sprouts and yeast. Foods high in arginine include walnuts, filberts, pecans, peanuts, almonds, cashews, Brazil nuts, sesame and sunflower seeds, coconut, gelatin, oats, corn, buckwheat, barley, cereals, chocolate, dairy products and meats.

Some doctors and authors have advocated the use of megadoses of the synthetic preservative BHT (butylated hydroxytoluene) as a treatment for herpes. They argue that this is a safe and effective treatment for outbreaks as well as being a preventive that can be taken on a more or less permanent basis. Most reputable scientists disagree and point to the carcinogenic effects of BHT. Another problem with high dose BHT is that it can irritate the lining of the stomach, leading to ulcers and perforation.

Natural remedies that enhance immunity or combat herpes are lactobacillus acidophilus, echinacea, goldenseal, burdock, sheep sorrel, Turkish rhubarb, slippery elm, myrrh, red clover, capsicum, calendula, aloe vera, lomatium, St. John's wort, propolis, garlic, olive oil, castor bean oil, thymus extract, astragalus, colloidal silver and tea tree oil.

Topical calendula cream and aloe vera gel may be effective as antiseptics and for relief of the pain of herpes blisters. Alternating direct application of vitamin A cream and vitamin E cream can help speed healing. For individualized dosages, see a naturopath or doctor familiar with these safe, natural remedies.

Recurrent Colds and Flus

Recurrent flus and colds are are often associated with hidden food allergies and/or excessive sugar intake. The general rule observed by most natural health care practitioners is that more than one antibiotic prescription per year equals hidden food allergies. Milk, dairy products, wheat, corn, citrus fruits, chocolates and eggs are the most common culprits. One way of determining which foods are at the root of the problem is to try an elimination diet. This is described in detail in *Detecting Your Hidden Food Allergies*, by Dr. William Crook. Other books along the same lines are *Superimmunity for Kids*, by Dr. Leo Galland, and *Five Day Allergy Relief System*, by Dr. Marshall Mandell. The general idea is to eliminate the most likely allergens from the diet for at least a week and add them back one at a time, noting the reactions. Whether or not you follow the advice in these books, it's a good idea to keep a daily food intake diary, noting the degree of symptoms seen each day. Correlations between symptoms and foods eaten will start to emerge.

If the elimination-provocation approach fails to reveal the hidden allergies, consider an Elisa/Act blood test. In many ways, this blood test is similar to other Elisa tests, which measure antibodies to viruses, bacteria and fungi. Since 90 percent of all food allergies occur on a delayed basis (the flu or cold may occur up to three days after ingestion of the offending food), this blood test can be helpful in uncovering unsuspected food allergies of the delayed type.

There are several nutrient and herbal supplements that can be taken to help both boost immunity and prevent respiratory infections. Cod liver oil is a good place to start. Most people can tolerate one tablespoon daily. To get a proper balance of all the essential fatty acids, add 1 tablespoon daily of flax seed oil. With an increase in fatty acid intake, it is also important to take extra vitamin E. Buy 200 IU natural vitamin E capsules, break open the capsules and add the contents to either the cod liver oil or the flax seed oil with each dose. Next, add 1/4 teaspoon of vitamin C crystals (with bioflavonoids) to papaya or cranberry juice daily. Gradually increase the dose by a 1/4 teaspoon every day until bowel tolerance is reached. Some people tolerate buffered vitamin C powder or ester-C powder better than pure ascorbic acid; it depends on the sensitivity of your stomach to acidity. Bioflavonoids like pycnogenol, quercetin, hesperidin, rutin and catechin help control other symptoms related to allergies. Zinc gluconate lozenges (25 mgs of zinc per tablet) should also be a part of the program. Zinc is a cofactor for a number of enzymes involved in the immune response.

Echinacea, goldenseal, propolis, garlic, astragalus, capsicum, chaparral, red clover, ma huang, white willow, sea kelp, elderberry, pau d'arco (taheebo), calendula and the herbal combination of burdock, slippery elm, sheep sorrel and Turkish rhubarb are herbs that can be very helpful both as natural antibiotics and as part of an overall infection prevention program.

These herbs boost immunity and help normalize the bacterial flora in the large bowel. They are all available in capsule, powder or tincture form and have no toxicity. Aloe vera juice is another natural immune booster that can be had on a daily basis to help prevent infections.

N-acetyl-cysteine is a natural antibiotic capable of dissolving mucous buildup anywhere in the respiratory tract. Other supplements that may be effective for both prevention and treatment include vitamin A, beta-carotene, vitamin B6, blue-green algae and bee pollen.

If you must take prescription antibiotics, it is important to replace the friendly bowel bacteria that have been killed off by the drugs. These bacteria (lactobacillus acidophilus) are important to help prevent yeast (candida) and other infections. Although all these natural remedies are of very low toxicity, it's best to see a natural health care practitioner for an individualized diet and supplement program.

Nasal Polyps and Hay Fever

Nasal polyps are often seen in people allergic to salicylates. This compound is found in pain control medications (aspirin, for example) and naturally in many foods. A three-month trial therapy with a low salicylate diet is worth trying for anyone suffering from hay fever and/or nasal polyps. Not all patients with nasal polyps will respond to this diet because they may have other causes for their condition. These include chronic candida infection, specific food allergies and hypersensitivity to other drugs or chemicals, especially food coloring agents.

The following are high salicylate foods and should be eliminated from the diet for three months:

Fruits: apples, avocados, apricots, all berries, cherries, currants, dates, figs, grapes, guavas, grapefruit, lemons, lychees, mandarins, melons, nectarines, oranges, peaches, plums, prunes, passion fruit, pears, persimmons, pineapples, rhubarb, raisins

Vegetables: alfalfa, asparagus, aubergines, broad and green beans, beetroot, broccoli, carrots, chicory, chillis, courgettes, corn, cucumber, endive, marrow, mushrooms, okra, olives, onions, parsnips, peppers, potatoes, radishes, spinach, sweet potatoes, tomatoes, turnips, watercress

Condiments: anise, cayenne, celery seed, cinnamon, cumin, curry, dill, fenugreek, mace, mustard, oregano, paprika, rosemary, sage, tarragon, turmeric, thyme.

Beverages: alcohol, colas, coffee, tea, most fruit juices

Seeds and Nuts: almonds, Brazil nuts, coconut, macadamia nuts, peanuts, pine nuts, pistachio nuts, sesame seeds, walnuts, waterchestnuts

Miscellaneous: honey, licorice, yeast-containing foods, processed, canned or packaged foods containing any of the above items

If the salicylate-free diet fails to produce significant symptom relief, consider having an Elisa/Act blood test done. This test can determine allergies to as many as 300 foods and chemicals. The most common food allergies associated with the condition include milk, wheat, yeast, corn, chocolate, citrus fruits and eggs.

Besides food hypersensitivity control, several nutritional/herbal supplements may be of help to nasal polyp sufferers. These include all the antioxidant vitamins, minerals and amino acids: vitamin A, beta-carotene, B-complex, especially vitamin B5 (pantothenic acid) and B6, vitamin C, vitamin E, selenium, zinc, silicon, kelp, rutin, quercetin, hesperidin, catechin, glutathione N-acetyl-cysteine and cysteine. Deficiencies in essential fatty acids (GLA and omega-3-EPA) and other trace minerals (e.g., germanium) worsen nasal polyps and other allergic conditions.

Herbs such as echinacea, goldenseal, St. John's wort, capsicum, pau d'arco, burdock, sheep sorrel, slippery elm, Turkish rhubarb, lomatium, ma huang, astragalus and calendula are very helpful in stimulating proper functioning of the immune system. So is lactobacillus acidophilus. Sometimes, treatment of a chronic candida hypersensitivity or parasitic infection improves hay fever symptoms. Appropriate dosages can be determined by biochemical individuality testing through a health care practitioner.

Platelet Problems

Idiopathic thrombocytopenic purpura (ITP) is an immune system disorder characterized primarily by rapid destruction of blood clotting factors called platelets. The cause is unknown and treatment usually involves steroids and removal of the spleen. There are no proven effective alternative therapies. There are, however, complementary nutritional therapies that may help speed recovery.

Elimination of allergic foods from the diet prevents the inflammatory response that manifests as flare-ups of the disease. The most common food allergy associated with ITP is milk. If food allergies are not known, go on a hypoallergenic diet (no animal products, processed foods, sugar, white flour products, coffee, tea, alcohol). At your earliest opportunity, get food allergy testing done.

Some studies indicate that high doses of vitamin C and bioflavonoids are helpful in the treatment of ITP. Bioflavonoids such as rutin, hesperidin, catechin, quercetin, eriodictyol and pycnogenol help strengthen the walls of capillaries, thereby preventing bruising. They stabilize the mast cell membranes and thus block the series of reactions that are associated with almost any allergy. If the condition is associated with any allergy, supplementation with vitamin C and bioflavonoids would be beneficial.

Bioflavonoids are found in many foods, including citrus fruits (the white material just beneath the peel), onions, garlic, peppers, buckwheat and black currants. In supplemental form, they have been successfully used for many years as a treatment for pain, bumps, bruises and more severe athletic injuries. Bioflavonoids work together with vitamin C to protect blood vessels. They are also useful in the treatment of asthma and other allergic conditions.

Side effects of bioflavonoid supplementation are unlikely, even in megadoses, but due to the serious nature of ITP, it is important that even this natural therapy be supervised by a doctor.

Lupus

Systemic lupus erythematosus (SLE) is a disease of the blood vessels and connective tissues that is characterized by periods of remission and exacerbation (i.e., it waxes and wanes). It affects primarily the joints and skin, but can involve other body organs. In some cases the disease becomes severe enough to produce irreversible kidney damage. Women are affected eight times as often as men during non-childbearing years and fifteen times as often in childbearing years. A mild case may require little or no treatment, while severe forms are treated medically with aspirin, cortisone and antimalarial drugs.

The exact cause of SLE is not known, but the theory is that it results from an abnormal body reaction to its own tissues. This autoimmune breakdown leads to the production of antibodies such as ANA (antinuclear antibody) that attack different tissues, resulting in their damage. Complexes of antigens and antibodies deposit in the kidneys and joints, leading to further damage. It's as if the immune system was no longer able to differentiate friend from foe.

Some predisposing factors are thought to make a person susceptible to SLE. These include physical or mental stress, streptococcal or viral infections, exposure to sunlight or ultraviolet light, immunization, pregnancy and genetic disposition. Another theory is that SLE is triggered or aggravated by the use of certain drugs like procaineamide, hydralazine, anticonvulsants, penicillins, sulfa drugs and oral contraceptives.

A diet low in saturated fat and alkaline ash may be helpful. This means that intakes of beef, pork and dairy products should be reduced as much as possible. Most autoimmune diseases benefit from a higher dietary intake of essential fatty acids from primarily vegetable sources. The Swank diet, recommended for treatment of multiple sclerosis, is ideal, but many SLE victims also benefit from food and chemical allergy testing.

Of possible importance to SLE is the role of mercury toxicity or hypersensitivity from dental fillings. Dr. Hal Huggins and several other dentists concerned with heavy metal toxicity have described some cases of lupus that resolved on the removal and replacement of silver mercury dental amalgams.

Supplements that may be helpful as complementary medical treatment for SLE include beta-carotene, bicarbonate mixtures, buffered vitamin C, flax seed oil (or cod or halibut liver oil), evening primrose oil, B-complex vitamins (especially vitamin B5, vitamin B6 and PABA), selenium, silicon, zinc, calcium, potassium, magnesium, vitamin E and bioflavonoids such as hesperidin, rutin, catechin, quercetin and pycnogenol.

Please note that in low doses (under 1,200 IU per day), vitamin E may have little or no effect on SLE. In doses well above 2,000 IU, vitamin E weakens autoimmune disease. I have purposely not recommended any specific doses since there is a great deal of variability of response to all supplements in SLE sufferers. Herbs such as aloe vera, comfrey, licorice root, white willow bark, feverfew, devil's claw, yarrow, yucca and marshmallow may also be helpful. Doses have to be carefully individualized. Supervision by a nutritional medical doctor or naturopath is highly recommended.

Sarcoidosis

Sarcoidosis is a rare (1 in 10,000), systemic inflammatory disorder that may involve almost any organ or tissue in the body. It is most often found in the thoracic lymph nodes and the lungs. The cause of sarcoidosis is unknown, but it is characterized pathologically by the presence of "noncaseating granulomas" (non-infected inflammatory lumps) in all affected tissue. An imbalance in T lymphocytes has been suggested as a mechanism for granuloma formation. The diagnosis is ultimately made by biopsy.

The conventional medical therapy for sarcoidosis is corticosteroids, although not all patients will need this form of treatment. The usual practice is to give from 40 to 60 mg of prednisone a day for one year, with a gradual tapering of the dosage thereafter. The prognosis for survival for patients with sarcoidosis is very good. In large studies, only about four percent of patients die from the disease, and only half of them die from pulmonary sarcoidosis. Patients with extensive systemic manifestations have a less favorable prognosis.

Sarcoidosis is likely to benefit from the use of natural, anti-inflammatory supplements, which may be used as a complement to conventional medical care. Examples of such supplements include cold-pressed flax seed oil, gamma linolenic acid (GLA found in evening primrose oil, black currant seed oil and borage oil) and omega-3-EPA (found in trout, cod, halibut, mackerel, salmon, shark, herring and other seafoods). Increasing these in the diet, or taking them in encapsulated supplement form, while decreasing the intake of saturated animal fats can have a remarkably good anti-inflammatory effect.

Optimizing the body's trace mineral balance may also be crucial to achieving natural, anti-inflammatory effects. Avoid foods known to interfere with mineral absorption such as bran, coffee and tea. Minerals that may be involved include iron, zinc, copper, manganese, calcium, magnesium, boron, silicon and selenium. Excess lead and iron in the body can cause a great deal of damage. If tests indicate that this is a problem, oral or intravenous chelation therapy may be necessary.

Vitamins such as A, B-complex, C, beta-carotene, bioflavonoids, (especially pycnogenol) and vitamin E can be supplemented in higher than RDA doses because of their antioxidant properties that help prevent certain aspects of inflammation. The recommended intake dose for all these nutrients would have to be determined for the individual by a qualified health care practitioner based on appropriate biochemical tests. Tests that would be of particular value include blood, urine and hair mineral analysis.

Many people with sarcoidosis have reported benefits from the use of certain herbs. Alfalfa, for example, which has been extensively studied, contains many important substances including saponins, sterols, flavonoids, coumarins, alkaloids, vitamins, amino acids, minerals, trace elements and other nutrients. Numerous clinical and anecdotal reports support its use as a natural anti-inflammatory. Other herbs with beneficial anti-inflammatory effects include devil's claw, comfrey, sassafras, licorice and ginseng. Like vitamin and mineral supplements, herbs are not without their side effects and are best administered and supervised by an experienced health care practitioner.

There are many ways to stimulate the body's natural production of cortisone. This is done by nutritional support of the adrenal glands with a diet high in protein and low in refined carbohydrates (i.e., no sugar and white flour products) and the following natural supplements: pantothenic acid (vitamin B5), vitamin C, magnesium citrate, potassium citrate, zinc picolinate, raw adrenal concentrate, bioflavonoids and licorice root capsules, tea or tincture. Siberian ginseng, DHEA (an extract of wild yam), astragalus and evening primrose oil also provide adrenal support. Work out an individualized dosage schedule and supplement regime with a naturopath or health care practitioner.

There are a growing number of studies that demonstrate the relationship between food allergies (hypersensitivity) and chronic inflammatory diseases. The purported benefits of juice or water fasting for inflammatory problems may simply be because the fast eliminates the food or foods to which the person is allergic. For those who find the rigors of fasting and food elimination diets too inconvenient or risky, the Elisa/Act or RAST blood tests can pick up hidden allergies to any number of foods. For more information on these tests, please see the section Food Allergies and Allergy Testing.

In some people that react adversely to all foods (pan-allergic), the possibility of an intestinal tract parasitic or fungal (candida) infection needs to be investigated and treated before starting on a food allergy elimination program. Although one cannot say that parasites or candida cause chronic inflammatory diseases, many nutrition oriented physicians have reported successes when either the candida or parasitic infection was cleared first. Look into some of these possibilities with a health care practitioner.

Mercury and the Dental Filling

The subject of mercury toxicity from dental amalgams continues to be in the news. Unfortunately, there is still a great deal of resistance to and denial of the problem by mainstream dentistry. Mercury is a lethal substance that has been associated with hundreds of serious nervous and immune system problems. There is no scientific justification for its use in the human body. In 1991, the use of mercury in dental fillings was banned altogether in Sweden. Other countries will soon follow suit as research data continues to accumulate.

Gloves and masks are not a foolproof protection against mercury vapor in the dental office. Autopsy reports on dentists and dental technicians indicate alarmingly high levels of mercury deposits in the brains of these individuals. Unless the dentist is a member of the Environmental Dental

Association (EDA), it is unlikely that he or she has been properly trained in the safe use of mercury. Why use it anyway? There are plenty of new, safer alternatives to mercury, despite what the dental associations are saying.

The presence of mercury can be reliably detected by an instrument that measures mercury vapor in the mouth. Dentists who are members of the Environmental Dental Association have such a machine in their offices and can do the test for you. The Elisa/Act blood test can also determine whether or not your immune system is reacting adversely to mercury. Other types of blood and urine tests for mercury yield misleading information. Hair analysis can measure mercury excess in the body but is not a reliable test for mercury hypersensitivity (allergy). Skin testing for mercury is also not foolproof.

A decision to replace mercury fillings should depend on objective tests as well as your intuition about dental filling toxicity. It is simply not good enough to listen only to dentists, many of whom have a limited and biased understanding of the dangers of mercury dental fillings.

For concise information on mercury and dental fillings, get a copy of *Eliminating Poison in Your Mouth*, by Klaus Kaufmann. It's available at your local health food store or library. Also, get in touch with Dr. Joyal Taylor and the Environmental Dental Association.* They can provide lots of material on the continuing controversy.

Low White Cell Counts

A low white cell count can be associated with nutritional imbalances, a chronic viral condition, a chronic fungal or candida condition and/or toxic heavy metal excesses, especially of mercury, lead and cadmium. Chemical hypersensitivities, x-rays and other types of radiation can also be suspected as potential causes. Avoid cigarette smoking and frequent consumption of coffee, tea, caffeinated products or alcohol. Nutritional deficiencies are often seen with a low white cell count, particularly deficiencies in protein, essential amino acids, beta-carotene, zinc, copper, iron, vitamin B6 and vitamins A, C, D and E. If you are already taking most of these supplements to no avail, it could be that dosages are not high enough, absorption is inadequate or supplement quality is poor.

The mercury found in the common silver dental filling (amalgam) and the mercury found in ever-increasing amounts in fish and other seafoods may have an immunosuppressive effect, leading to many neurological disorders. These could include anxiety, depression, insomnia, a loss of sex

* Write to: EDA, 9974 Scripps Ranch Blvd., Suite #36, San Diego, CA 92131; phone: 1-800-388-8124 or 619-689-8124.

drive, poor memory, poor concentration, muscle aches and pains, among others. Some authors have associated the mercury amalgam problem with multiple sclerosis, Parkinson's disease and chronic fatigue syndrome.

Visit a naturopath or a nutrition-oriented medical doctor for a more thorough evaluation of your biochemistry, including an Elisa/Act blood test for candida, mercury and other toxic heavy metals. A viral antibody screen, a hair mineral analysis and an amino acid analysis might also be very helpful.

Baldness and the Immune System

It is thought that alopecia areata (patchy baldness) is the result of an immune system malfunction. As in cases of other immune system disorders (e.g., thyroiditis, rheumatoid arthritis, lupus, scleroderma, myasthenia gravis), knowing what food or chemical allergies are associated with the flare-ups is often helpful in symptom control. Most of these are delayed-onset allergies (type II–IV allergies), aggravating the symptoms of the immune disorder up to a week after ingestion or exposure. Type I reactions occur on an immediate basis (e.g., peanut allergy causing an acute asthmatic attack). Type II–IV allergies are not necessarily the cause of immune system disorders. However, avoidance or neutralization of these hidden allergies may go a long way toward controlling or even reversing the signs and symptoms of the disease in question.

Long-term zinc supplementation may be very helpful for baldness. In some cases, however, oral zinc supplements in tablet or capsule form fail to produce changes in the scalp condition. This may be because of selective malabsorption of zinc from the gastrointestinal tract. White spots on the nails or horizontal ridges ("washboard nails") may be signs of zinc deficiency. One way of determining zinc status in the body is to get a hair mineral analysis done. Results that indicate a low level of zinc in the face of a normal to high intake of zinc from the diet may mean zinc malabsorption. Those without body hair obviously cannot get hair analysis done. Finger and toenail samples can be used instead to yield the same kind of information.

In cases where zinc gluconate or amino acid chelated zinc tablets have failed to improve hair growth, I recommend a liquid zinc supplement such as zinc sulphate heptahydrate solution or zinc citrate. Effective dosages are between 150 to 200 mgs per day. The only possible drawback to this might be a zinc-induced copper depletion. To prevent this, take a copper supplement, roughly in a ratio of 8 to 1 (eight parts zinc to one part copper). I also recommend that fiber intake from grain and legume sources be reduced to less than 40 grams per day. Excessive dietary fiber and hidden food allergies may inhibit zinc absorption. Avoid sugar, white flour products and other junk foods.

Pancreatic digestive enzyme supplements may be very important in some cases. These enzymes break down dietary protein, carbohydrate and fat so that zinc, as well as other minerals and vitamins, is better absorbed. Pancreatic enzyme supplements are available at most health food stores. The dosage is two tablets or capsules after each meal (three times daily); this should be sufficient to enhance zinc absorption from the gastrointestinal tract. A better alternative for some people is a completely plant-based digestive enzyme supplement containing proteases, lipases and amylases.

A recent clinical trial using supplements of shark oil concentrate (400 mg capsules of Squalene) found that more than 70 percent of participants had regrowth of hair in previously bald areas. The dosage used was one capsule three times daily after meals. No side effects were reported. It is likely that this supplement works because the biochemical structure of shark oil resembles that of the steroid hormones. Although corticosteroid therapy in the form of injections, cream or pills seems to help some cases, the long-term side effects may be prohibitive. One can boost the body's own production of steroid hormones without significant side effects by using natural supplements such as vitamin C, pantothenic acid, raw adrenal glandular concentrate, DHEA and licorice root extract.

A large number of essential nutrients are involved in healthy hair growth. These include vitamin A, biotin, inositol, vitamin B12, PABA (para amino benzoic acid), other B-complex vitamins, unsaturated essential fatty acids (from primrose, flax seed, rice bran, borage, black currant or fish), vitamin E, coenzyme Q10, dimethyl glycine (DMG), silica, copper, iron, iodine, cysteine and methionine. See a naturopath or a medical doctor familiar with nutritional evaluations to get an individualized diet and supplement program to match your specific needs.

Too little facial and body hair can be hereditary. The other possibility is that it is the result of the long-term effects of stress on adrenal hormones, especially the androgens. Vitamins that might help are biotin, inositol, PABA and other B-complex vitamins. A complete nutritional analysis including blood, urine and hair tests would help determine individual nutrient needs. Adrenal steroid tests (particularly DHEA-S) cortisol and progesterone may also be worth doing. Supplementation of DHEA (available by prescription in Canada and without a prescription in health food stores in the U.S.) or natural progesterone might be of help if the steroid profile is abnormal. Other forms of adrenal support, such as vitamin C, magnesium, zinc and licorice root, could also be considered.

The breakdown product of testosterone, dihydrotestosterone, is thought to cause male pattern baldness, an enlarged prostate and acne. This breakdown product can be inhibited or blocked by zinc, essential fatty acids and the herbs saw palmetto and pygeum. The amounts used depend on the individual. See a naturopath or a medical doctor experienced with nutrition and herbs for a personalized regime of diet and supplements.

Blocked Eustachian Tubes

Undiagnosed or hidden food allergies may be responsible for a blocked eustachian tube—the passageway between the middle ear and the throat. Such allergies are not immediate or Type I food allergies that one could easily recognize, but are Type II, or delayed hypersensitivity reactions (occurring up to five days after consuming the offending food or foods). An allergic reaction can lead to inflammatory swelling of the tube, thus causing blockage. Another mechanism by which the tube can become blocked is through inflammatory swelling of the nose. This occurs when one swallows with the nose and mouth closed, thus forcing air and secretions into the tube.

Another thing to consider is the use of natural decongestants and antihistamines. Vitamin C crystals (with bioflavonoids) in papaya or cranberry juice daily may help a great deal. Start with a 1/4 teaspoon every half hour and gradually increase the dose by a 1/4 teaspoon every day until bowel tolerance is reached.

Allergic reactions of any kind can also be dampened with the use of a bicarbonate powder. There are several good ones on the market, available from health food stores or pharmacies. Look for brands with a mixture of potassium, calcium and magnesium bicarbonate.

N-acetyl-cysteine is a natural antibiotic capable of dissolving mucous buildup anywhere in the respiratory tract. It may be taken in addition to the vitamin C and bioflavonoids with no concern for harmful side effects.

Herbs may also be helpful. Echinacea, goldenseal, propolis, garlic, astragalus, burdock, slippery elm, sheep sorrel, Turkish rhubarb, capsicum, chaparral, red clover, ma huang, white willow, sea kelp, elderberry, pau d'arco (taheebo) and calendula are herbs that can be very helpful as immune system boosters and natural antibiotics. For a personalized natural regime, see a naturopath or medical doctor familiar with herbs, vitamins and other drugless therapies.

Hypothyroidism

The standard blood tests for thyroid disease will tell a doctor whether or not the thyroid gland is diseased, but will not necessarily indicate whether the thyroid hormones are functioning at an optimal level. According to alternative health care doctors, consistent underarm temperatures of 97.6° F or below (or average oral temperatures below 98.6° F) combined with symptoms of low metabolism are likely due to a hidden hypothyroid (low thyroid) condition.

Classic symptoms of a low functioning thyroid include depression, fatigue, cold extremities, fluid retention, trouble losing weight, a higher than average body fat composition, hypoglycemia, gastrointestinal symptoms such as multiple food sensitivities/allergies and poor response to exercise (e.g., getting weaker after months of aerobic exercising).

Checking temperature for indications of low thyroid is best done using the old-fashioned shake down thermometer. Taking daily readings for a few weeks will show an accurate trend. It should be remembered, however, that not all cases of low temperatures are caused by a functionally low thyroid. This and many other aspects of low thyroid are explained in great detail in Broda Barnes' book, *Hypothyroidism: the Unsuspected Illness.*

Hair loss may also be a symptom of hypothyroidism and other hormonal imbalances (e.g., adrenal, gonadal, etc.). Because low temperatures may also be a reflection of suboptimal nutrient levels in the body, nutritional factors must also be considered, particularly deficiencies in protein, zinc, selenium, silicon, iodine, vitamin A, B-complex vitamins (particularly biotin and inositol), essential fatty acids, vitamin C and vitamin E. Routine blood tests for thyroid may be normal in unsuspected (subclinical) hypothyroidism. One may find, however, a higher than normal level of cholesterol, a low level of vitamin A and a high carotene level. This phenomenon occurs because active thyroid hormone is required to convert carotene from the diet into vitamin A (retinol). It is also required to help keep cholesterol blood levels low.

In most cases of hypothyroidism, especially in vegetarians, blood tests will show low levels of vitamin A and high levels of carotene. Evidence of this is a carrot-orange color on the palms and soles. Many people who have normal thyroid function tests with multiple hypothyroid symptoms will occasionally show high levels of anti-thyroid antibodies and anti-microsomal antibodies (Hashimoto's thyroiditis). High doses of the B vitamin PABA, vitamin E and evening primrose oil or other essential fatty acids may then be very helpful to reverse the condition. If not, low doses of prescribed thyroid hormone (i.e., desiccated thyroid), slow-release lio-thyronine (T3), glandular thyroid extract or homeopathic thyroid drops may help relieve symptoms.

In some cases, there may be a goiter (an enlarged thyroid gland) in the neck. A goiter is a definite indication of weak thyroid function. Supplements with thyroid extract and/or iodine eliminate the signs and symptoms within six weeks. Suddenly, a depression caused by abnormal thyroid function—for many years unresponsive to the usual anti-depressant drugs—disappears. The food sensitivities, the inability to lose weight on very low calorie diets, the lack of positive results from exercise and the general malaise all improve dramatically.

Treatment with desiccated thyroid is safe when supervised. An alternative to the use of thyroid hormone is supplementation with zinc, vitamin B6, tyrosine and iodine. This does not always work, however, and thyroid hormone (L-thyroxin) supplementation may be necessary. Some companies make a glandular thyroid extract without the L-thyroxin, although there are trace amounts of this active hormone. In some cases these work as well as the hormone tablet. A homeopathic doctor should assess suitability for this remedy.

Yet another alternative for the treatment of subclinical hypothyroidism is the use of time-released liothyronine (T3). For more information on T3, see Dr. Denis Wilson's book, *Wilson's Syndrome: The Miracle of Feeling Well*. Treatment for Wilson's syndrome can sometimes get complicated: supervision by a medical doctor is required on a regular basis, mainly to decide on dosages and monitor for side effects. Liothyronine has a very low toxicity potential, and side effects can be controlled entirely by drinking much more water and reducing the two daily doses by 7.5 mcgs or more. Make sure you are taking compounded, slow-release liothyronine capsules, not the Cytomel tablets. There is a world of difference between the two prescription forms of T3.

Most endocrinologists object to the use of thyroid medication in a person with normal thyroid blood tests. This is understandable, given the rigidity of medical education, but illogical. For example, in insulin-dependent diabetes with high blood sugar levels, the insulin blood levels are usually either normal or higher than normal. Despite this, doctors give insulin. Diabetes is an endocrine disease where the real problem is not the blood levels of insulin but the tissue receptivity to insulin. To get around this lack of receptivity the person is given more insulin, forcing the tissues to use some of the excess insulin. Megadoses of insulin are used; standard diabetes therapy could therefore be called an orthomolecular therapy.

In the orthomolecular treatment of hypothyroidism, thyroxin is given despite the normal thyroxin levels. If blood levels of insulin or thyroxin alone are used to make a diagnosis of diabetes or hypothyroidism, few would get the proper treatment for either of these conditions. It is unwise to rely only on biochemical tests for deciding on a treatment. These tests are guides and must be used together with the individual's history and physical examination. Check with your natural health care practitioner for a more comprehensive assessment.

Hyperthyroidism

Hyperthyroidism (also known as thyrotoxicosis or Grave's disease) is a condition in which the thyroid gland produces too much hormone. It is most commonly seen in women between the ages of 20 and 40. The cause is unknown, but it is thought to be due to an autoimmune mechanism. This means that for some reason the immune system makes antibodies against the thyroid gland, resulting in a hyper-metabolic state which may be associated with one or more of the following signs and symptoms:

- Goiter (enlargement of the thyroid gland); a goiter may also be associated with iodine deficiency
- Rapid heart rate (tachycardia) and palpitations
- Nail problems, thinning hair and warm, fine, moist skin
- Tremor
- Heart beat irregularities
- Nervousness and hyperactivity
- Increased perspiration, heat intolerance
- Weight loss, increased appetite
- Insomnia, fatigue, weakness
- Increased bowel movements
- Exophthalmos (protruding eyeballs), blurred and double vision
- Myopathy (muscle pain and weakness)
- Pretibial myxedema (red and very itchy skin rashes)

Prognosis with conventional medical treatments is generally very good, but variable from person to person. Conventional treatments include high-dose iodine, anti-thyroid drugs, radioactive iodine and surgery. Some alternative medical doctors have successfully used the mineral lithium in high doses to help suppress thyroid function. Beta-blocker drugs may be required to prevent heart beat irregularities and high blood pressure. Natural treatments can often reduce the need for drugs and surgery; they should be considered as complementary to the conventional approach, not an alternative to it.

Many foods help suppress thyroid function naturally. These include broccoli, Brussel sprouts, cabbage, cauliflower, kale, mustard greens, peaches, pears, rutabagas, soybeans, spinach and turnips. It may be wise to increase these foods in the diet of anyone suffering from a hyperthyroid state. Some doctors have found that unsuspected food allergies may make hyperthyroidism worse. The most common of these are milk, dairy products, wheat, chocolate, caffeinated soft drinks and stimulants like coffee, tea and nicotine gum or patches. These should be avoided completely until comprehensive food and chemical allergy testing can be done to determine the offending foods and chemicals. Mercury hypersensitivity due to dental fillings should also be suspected.

Besides food and chemical allergies, victims of hyperthyroidism may also be suffering from extreme stress, a variety of other hormonal imbalances (pituitary, adrenal, gonadal, etc.), bowel infections and other digestive problems. These may all need to be addressed for a complete recovery to take place.

The hyper-metabolic state seen in hyperthyroidism requires a greater intake of supplemental vitamins and minerals, including vitamin A, B-complex, vitamin C, vitamin E, calcium, magnesium, potassium, silicon, selenium, iodine, zinc, copper and essential fatty acids (e.g., flax seed oil, evening primrose oil). If possible, consult a naturopath or holistic doctor for a nutritional assessment and a personalized supplement program.

3

The Heart and
Circulatory System

A surprising amount of research in the past decade has been done on the natural treatment of heart disease, high blood pressure and circulation problems. Bypass surgery and drugs with horrendous side effects are not always necessary to clear coronary artery disease. A number of popular books by authors such as Nathan Pritikin, John Robbins, Dr. John McDougall and Dr. Dean Ornish have touted the merits of a low fat, high fiber diet for preventing and treating heart disease. In addition, Dr. Joe Goldstrich, at one time chief cardiologist and medical director at the Pritikin Longevity Center in California, has recently published a new book (*The Cardiologist's Painless Prescription for a Healthy Heart and a Longer Life*) on heart disease treatment and prevention containing over 4,000 references to medical literature.

The Goldstrich program for heart disease is the one I recommend most often. His approach is to blend the best of conventional medical treatment (e.g., lifesaving cardiac drugs, ASA, pacemakers, etc.) with the best of nutritional remedies like garlic, coenzyme Q10, magnesium, vitamin C, vitamin E and dozens of others. One treatment philosophy does not replace the other. Diet changes, exercise, antioxidant and herbal supplements are all a part of a regime aimed at both preventing and reversing cardiovascular disease. Many natural approaches can be done with little or no supervision from a health care practitioner. Some must be monitored very closely due to drug interactions or effects on the blood clotting system, digestion, blood pressure and blood sugar. The good news, however, is that using the natural approach pays off in a healthier heart and an improved quality of life.

Reversing Heart Disease the Natural Way

Over 36 percent of all deaths in North America are caused by heart disease. The good news is that even severe cases of atherosclerosis can respond well to changes in diet and lifestyle. The more severe the case, the more strictly one has to adhere to a nutrition program. For the most serious cases, I usually recommend a complete vegetarian diet, the best example of which is written up in the book The McDougall Plan. Do not compromise. There must be complete avoidance of saturated animal fats, sugar, refined carbohydrates, white flour products, cholesterol and sodium in the diet. Also, avoid trans-fatty acids, hydrogenated oils (margarine, vegetable shortenings, imitation butter spreads, most commercial peanut butters) and oxidized fats (deep-fried foods, fast foods, ghee, barbecued or smoked foods). All these may increase the levels of free radicals in the bloodstream and lead to more hardening of the arteries.

Foods that may have a therapeutic effect in the reversal of coronary artery disease include garlic, wheat germ, liquid chlorophyll, alfalfa sprouts, buckwheat, carrots, watercress, rice polishings, apple, celery and cherries. Water soluble fiber sources like flax seed, pectin, guar gum and oat bran can be added to the diet to assist in further lowering blood cholesterol levels and cleansing the body of toxins. Other foods which have therapeutic benefits include onions, beans and other legumes, soy and ginger. A great deal of evidence also indicates that one can prevent heart attacks by increasing the intake of omega-3 and omega-6-EPA oils. I recommend vegetarian sources for these oils: walnuts, flax seed oil, borage oil, evening primrose oil or black currant oil.

Fresh fruit and vegetable juices are also an important part of the nutritional program. The juices recommended by naturopaths include combinations of carrot, liquid chlorophyll, beet, asparagus, lettuce, parsley, alfalfa, spinach and celery. Pineapple with honey is the recommended fruit juice.

Supplemental Nutrients

Note: Dosages for all these supplements will vary from individual to individual; consult a medical doctor or naturopath.

Chromium can decrease both cholesterol and triglycerides while improving glucose tolerance. A good source of chromium is brewer's yeast, but not torula yeast which is chromium-poor. The best supplemental forms are chromium picolinate and polynicotinate.

Copper in optimal doses controls cholesterol and is vital in the prevention of aortic aneurysms. The zinc to copper ratio must be balanced in the body (8 to 1 zinc to copper is ideal) and can be determined through a combination of blood, urine and hair tests.

Magnesium can do virtually anything that prescription heart medications can do. Doctors frequently prescribe "calcium channel blockers" to treat heart problems. Magnesium has been referred to as "nature's calcium channel blocker." The problem is that in order to correct an arrhythmia it usually has to be given at dosages far above those that can safely be tolerated in oral supplement form. In practice, it is always wise to balance magnesium intake with both calcium and potassium. Evaluation of blood and tissue levels can be done with the help of a health care practitioner.

If one takes high amounts of magnesium (2,000 to 5,000 mgs per day), the effect, after a day or so, is diarrhea and loss of magnesium and other minerals from the body. This is known as "magnesium-induced magnesium deficiency." The only way to get around this problem is through intravenous or intramuscular injections. Many people can learn to give themselves intramuscular injections of magnesium and thus help control their heart beat irregularities.

Potassium, like magnesium and calcium, is very important in the control of blood pressure and heart rhythm. It is crucial that potassium be balanced with calcium and magnesium. Food sources include bananas, oranges, cantaloupe, baked potato, spinach, lentils, split peas and all beans.

Omega-3-EPA oils reduce cholesterol and prevent platelet stickiness. Good dietary sources include flax seed oil, rice bran oil, trout, mackerel, salmon, herring, sardines, cod, halibut and shark. There is, however, some controversy about the cholesterol-lowering effects of fish oils, some studies reporting an elevation of blood fats.

Selenium is an antioxidant that works in conjunction with vitamin E to protect vascular tissue from damage by toxins. Low selenium levels are associated with an increased risk of atherosclerosis.

Vitamin E is otherwise known as alpha-tocopherol. Studies indicate that supplementation with as little as 200 IU daily can reduce the risk of a heart attack by 46 percent for men and 26 percent for women. Whether natural source or synthetic source, all forms supply the body with at least some vitamin E activity. The natural forms of vitamin E are d-alpha-tocopherol, d-alpha-tocopheryl acetate, d-alpha-tocopheryl succinate and mixed tocopherols. The synthetic forms are dl-alpha-tocopherol, dl-alpha-tocopheryl acetate or dl-alpha-tocopheryl succinate.

Studies indicate that the most biologically active are the esterified natural forms: d-alpha-tocopheryl acetate and d-alpha-tocopheryl succinate. Both have been found to provide full antioxidant activity in the body and are the ones recommended by the top authorities on vitamin E at the Shute Institute and Medical Clinic in London, Ontario.

Recent studies indicate that high levels of stored iron in the body (ferritin) are associated with a greater risk of heart disease and diabetes. High-dose vitamin E supplements can interfere with iron absorption and iron destroys vitamin E in the body. Thus, if you have been prescribed iron to correct iron deficiency, and if you are also taking vitamin E, make sure you take the supplements about 12 hours apart. Iron absorption is enhanced by sufficient acid in the stomach. A supplement of vitamin C (500 to 1,000 mgs) can increase iron absorption by up to 30 percent. Other good absorption aids include Swedish bitters, betaine or glutamic acid hydrochloride, apple cider vinegar and lemon juice.

Vitamin C lowers high blood cholesterol levels and helps prevent atherosclerosis by directly promoting the breakdown of triglycerides.

It is essential to collagen formation and thus to the regulation of arterial wall integrity.

Beta-carotene is the precursor to vitamin A. It is a fat-soluble antioxidant that protects LDL-cholesterol from oxidation. Supplementation has been shown to raise HDL-cholesterol levels. Beta-carotene has also been shown to protect smokers from coronary artery disease.

Vitamin B6 prevents accumulation of high levels of the amino acid homocysteine, which is implicated as one of the tissue-injuring substances initiating atherosclerosis. Other supplements which lower homocysteine levels include vitamin B12 and folic acid. Vitamin B6 deficiency has been linked to elevated serum cholesterol, atherosclerosis and a greater risk of coronary artery disease. Vitamin B6, B12 and folic acid are best taken together in the form of a B-complex vitamin supplement.

Carnitine is therapeutically effective in the treatment of coronary heart disease because normal cardiac function is dependent on adequate concentrations of carnitine in heart muscle. Carnitine helps increase muscle strength and stamina. In the body, carnitine is manufactured from the amino acids lysine and methionine with the help of vitamins B3, B6 and C. Linus Pauling advocates the use of high doses of L-lysine and vitamin C in patients with angina. His studies indicate a significant improvement, possibly because of greater manufacture of carnitine in the body due to the lysine and vitamin C.

L-carnitine transports fatty acids into cells so that they can be burned as fuel. In fact, some types of metabolic obesity are caused by a deficiency of carnitine. L-carnitine can dramatically lower blood levels of triglycerides. D-carnitine and DL-carnitine can be toxic and should not be used. Use only L-carnitine. Unfortunately, this very special amino acid supplement is only available in the United States

Proline is a nonessential amino acid highly concentrated in many tissues in the body. Proline is important to the health of the skin and to the synthesis of collagen, cartilage, joints and tendons. Proline helps strengthen the heart muscle and is an ingredient found in many natural commercial formulations marketed to the general public for reversing heart disease. Proline is synthesized in the body from other amino acids, namely ornithine and glutamic acid. The metabolism of proline is intimately connected to enzymes using niacin (vitamin B3) and vitamin C as co-factor. Good vegetarian sources of proline include wheat germ, granola, oat flakes and avocadoes. Proline is found in nearly all high protein foods and deficiency of it is rare.

Knowledge of proline supplementation is limited. Excess levels of proline have been linked to convulsions, elevated blood calcium levels and osteoporosis. I hesitate to recommend specific dosages.

N-acetyl-cysteine (NAC) is a sulfur-containing amino acid and is a strong antioxidant. It is a constituent of glutathione peroxidase, one of the most important antioxidants in the body. NAC is very important in the treatment of angina because it can make patients more sensitive to the beneficial effects of nitroglycerine. NAC must be used with caution by diabetics. A physician should supervise its use as a treatment.

Choline lowers blood levels of triglycerides and cholesterol. Lecithin is a source of choline, but some brands of lecithin may have 20 percent or less choline content, the remainder being saturated fat. Unfortunately, no study confirms the benefits of lecithin in lowering cholesterol. Much of the lecithin sold commercially in pill or loose powder form may be nothing more than rancid fat. Look for pure choline capsules.

Chondroitin sulfate, a component of collagen, lowers cholesterol and triglycerides while preventing thrombus (vessel blockage) formation.

DHEA (dehydroepiandrosterone) is a steroid hormone produced in the adrenal gland. It is found in significantly lower levels in men with documented coronary artery disease and men who die of heart attack. DHEA supplementation (a natural source is Mexican wild yam) has benefits not only for heart disease, but for memory, obesity, diabetes, arthritis, cancer, immune system problems and osteoporosis as well.

Niacin has long been known to be a potent agent for lowering cholesterol. Unfortunately, severe side effects (flushing, gastrointestinal distress, ulcers, glucose intolerance and liver irritation) make it an unpopular remedy. Those wishing to take it should be under the care of a physician. There are time-release supplements, as well as forms combining niacin with inositol, that are not associated with any significant flushing reaction. Inositol hexaniacinate is the safest form of niacin and produces virtually no flushing effects. Niacin can lower total cholesterol blood levels by as much as 18 percent, raise HDL-cholesterol by 32 percent and lower triglycerides by 26 percent at dosages ranging from 600 to 1,800 mgs daily.

Coenzyme Q10 (CoQ10) is an antioxidant supplement that has been found to be effective in the prevention and treatment of coronary artery disease. It is particularly effective in the treatment of chest pain and heart beat irregularities. It improves cardiac function in cardiomyopathies (diseases of weak heart muscle), reduces angina attacks and pain and works synergistically with other antioxidants like vitamin E, beta-carotene and vitamin C. CoQ10 can significantly lower high blood pressure as well as lower LDL-cholesterol while raising HDL-cholesterol.

Bioflavonoids are special antioxidant compounds found in many fruits (especially berries), vegetables, green tea and wine. Some better known bioflavonoids include catechin, hesperidin, rutin, quercetin, pycnogenol, pronogenol and polyphenols. Bioflavonoids can lower LDL-cholesterol levels and inhibit platelet stickiness. Together with vitamin C in large doses, bioflavonoids are also very effective in the treatment of allergies.

Ginkgo biloba increases the blood supply to the brain, prevents platelet aggregation and controls angina pectoris (chest pain from coronary heart disease). It is a potent antioxidant much like vitamin E.

Garlic is probably the best known of the herbs that lower cholesterol (by up to 10 percent) and triglycerides (by up to 13 percent) while raising HDL-cholesterol (by up to 31 percent). It also lowers blood pressure and prevents thrombus formation.

Gugulipid is a standardized extract of the mukul myrrh tree native to India. Gugulipid can lower both cholesterol and triglyceride levels by up to 27 percent and 30 percent respectively. It has no side effects and is even considered safe for use during pregnancy.

Onions are effective for lowering blood pressure and cholesterol as well as preventing platelet aggregation.

Alfalfa lowers cholesterol because of its content of saponins.

Ginger has a tonic effect on the heart, lowers cholesterol and inhibits platelet aggregation.

Cayenne also lowers cholesterol and inhibits platelet aggregation and is an excellent natural remedy for the chest pain seen in angina pectoris.

Bromelain, a proteolytic enzyme found in pineapples, can break down atherosclerotic plaques.

Many of these nutrients are sold in combination form at health food stores. It may not be necessary, therefore, to take large numbers of capsules or tablets. A naturopath or medical doctor familiar with herbal remedies can recommend specific dosages. The world's leading medical journals are increasingly reporting that diet and lifestyle changes by themselves can reverse hardening of the arteries and its complications. Drugs and surgery are not always a given when it comes to heart disease.

When one is taking heart medication and wishes to switch to a more natural regimen, it must be done gradually over a long period of time. Additionally, there are bound to be many drug-nutrient interactions. For example, digitalis (Lanoxin) depletes the body of vitamin B1, vitamin B6 and zinc. Deficiencies of these and other nutrients will lead to further complications and, no doubt, more drug prescriptions. Taking a broad-spectrum multiple vitamin and mineral supplement may offer you some protection against drug-induced nutrient deficiencies. A thorough nutritional evaluation from a health care practitioner can help sort out your specific supplement needs.

Coronary artery disease is also often helped by behavior modification, various stress management techniques, relaxation therapy, visualization, biofeedback, yoga, psychotherapy, hypnotherapy and aerobic exercise. Different approaches suit different people. Whatever appeals to the individual should be pursued as a way of enhancing the diet and supplement program. Whatever helps to control stress for the victim is valid.

Discuss all this with a health care practitioner; he or she can then develop an individualized holistic health program aimed at reversing heart disease. Studies prove it can indeed be done the natural way.

Niacin Problems

The purported toxicity of niacin has been exaggerated by both doctors and the mass media. These same mainstream sources say virtually nothing about deaths caused by "safe and effective" drugs. Authors like Thomas J. More have actually gone on record as saying that it's healthier to keep your cholesterol high than take potentially toxic prescription drugs to lower it artificially.

I have been prescribing niacin for over 15 years in high doses (3,000 to 5,000 mgs daily) without one episode of liver toxicity. Niacin lowers blood pressure, improves circulation, helps anxiety and insomnia, controls blood sugar and may relieve certain types of schizophrenia. Although it is true that niacin can raise liver function tests, this is usually mild and does not represent liver damage. In rare cases, especially with the various time-released forms of niacin, liver irritation is more likely but also reversible by lowering the dose or discontinuing the supplement. The problems, in any event, are preventable if regular liver function blood tests are done and if dosages are monitored by a doctor who is not bashful about vitamin therapies.

Additionally, there are now some very safe, non-flush-producing, non-time-release forms of niacin complexed with inositol. These forms of niacin lower cholesterol every bit as well as pure niacin. Brand names include Niasitiol, Nianate, Chol-less and Niachol. Another way of preventing a niacin flush is to take an ASA tablet with each niacin dose. A natural ASA source is white willow bark.

Some stubborn cases of high cholesterol, particularly when combined with fatigue, weight control problems and a subnormal body temperature, are associated with subclinical hypothyroidism (low thyroid function). This clinical entity is written up in the books, *Hypothyroidism: the Unsuspected Illness*, by Dr. Broda Barnes, and *Wilson's Syndrome: The Miracle of Feeling Well*, by Dr. Denis Wilson.

Cholesterol-lowering foods include carrots, oat bran, garlic, onions, apples, apple pectin, alfalfa sprouts, legumes, psyllium seed, lactobacillus acidophilus, plain yogurt, soy beans and soy bean products like tofu and soy milk. Complete elimination of sugar, white flour products, red meats, milk, cheese, coffee and processed foods is necessary. See the section Reversing Heart Disease the Natural Way for cholesterol-lowering supplements.

Buerger's Disease

Buerger's disease (also called thromboangiitis obliterans) is relatively rare and considered to be directly related to smoking. Blockages occur in the small and medium-sized arteries of the arms and legs, much like what occurs with most cases of atherosclerosis (hardening of the arteries). Gangrene and the loss of a limb frequently occur.

Although there are effective medical treatments for many victims, complementary natural remedies aimed at improving the circulation may also be of great value. Narrowing and blockages of arteries are not always irreversible. Studies by Dr. Dean Ornish and others indicate that a large percentage of people who suffer from hardening of the arteries can reverse the disease at any stage by natural means alone.

In order to accomplish this, follow a completely vegetarian diet. Avoid all animal products, including chicken, fish and dairy products. Eat plenty of whole grains, legumes, fruits, vegetables, seeds and nuts. Avoid salt, sugar, coffee, tea, tobacco and alcohol. The rationale for all this can be found in books like *Diet for a New America* by John Robbins and *The McDougall Plan* by Dr. John McDougall. The supplemental nutrients listed as useful in the section Reversing Heart Disease the Natural Way can be very helpful for Buerger's disease as well.

Edema

Ankle swelling (edema) is a common problem with many different causes. In some cases it may cause pain, numbness, tingling or restriction of mobility. It is not a disease in itself, but a symptom of specific disorders.

Before deciding on a treatment for edema it is necessary to identify the underlying causes. Edema in the legs and ankles occurs when the veins fail to maintain pace with the arteries. Lying horizontally allows the fluid pooled in the lower extremities to return to the heart, while standing or sitting for long periods causes fluid to accumulate. There are literally hundreds of predisposing factors that can lead to ankle and leg swelling.

Ankle edema is a common problem for people who stand in one position for too long, who wear restrictive garments, who have weak legs (especially calf muscles) who consume excess salt or who are sensitive to warm weather. Certain high blood pressure medications (beta-adrenergic blockers) can cause edema. So can protein deficiency or imbalance, varicose veins, premenstrual syndrome, obesity, high blood pressure, oral contraceptives, pregnancy, liver disease, thyroid disease, adrenal problems, various forms of heart disease, pancreatitis and kidney disorders. It is therefore very important to investigate all the medical causes for edema before doing anything else.

Once this has been done, look into the possibility of nutritional-biochemical imbalances. For example, some nutrition-oriented doctors have found that a significant number of people suffering from edema of unknown origin have hidden or delayed food allergies. Many women are put on diuretics to control their tendency to retain fluid. Weight fluctuations are very often associated with fluid retention problems and are usually indicators of unsuspected food allergies. Changing the diet to avoid or rotate the allergic foods will quite often result in the elimination of the excess fluid and may significantly help those with chronic weight control problems. Dairy products, wheat and other grains are the most common offenders, but any food can produce fluid retention in susceptible individuals.

Aside from hidden or delayed food hypersensitivities, the diet should be analyzed for excessive sodium or salt intake. Studies have shown that suboptimal intakes of certain nutrients may also be involved. These include bioflavonoids (found in garlic, onions, chives, cherries, peppers and the white covering of citrus fruits), vitamin B1, vitamin B5 (pantothenic acid), vitamin B6, gamma linoleic acid (from evening primrose or flax seed oil), iodine, magnesium (especially from deep green leafy vegetables such as parsley and spinach) and vitamin C. Eating more of the foods containing these nutrients will be of some help.

Frequently, doctors prescribe these nutrients in supplemental form, occasionally in megadoses. Herbalists, on the other hand, may additionally recommend taking horseradish, parsley, nettle or sassafras to help rid the body of fluid excess. Herbal diuretics are safe as long as the recommended doses are not exceeded.

The problem with non-herbal diuretic drugs is that they may cause a loss of potassium, magnesium, zinc and other trace minerals from the body. People on such drugs should be monitored by their doctors for mineral imbalances.

In cases of poor muscle tone from many years of sedentary behavior, some practitioners recommend therapeutic massage or shiatsu treatment. Aerobic exercise or rebounding on a mini-trampoline on a regular basis may also be beneficial to improve lymphatic circulation. None of these natural remedies should be tried without the supervision of a qualified health care practitioner and certainly not before all treatable medical reasons for edema have been ruled out.

Preventive and Therapeutic Oils

Fats and oils are often decreased or eliminated by people concerned about weight control and cholesterol. It is definitely wise to cut down on saturated animal fats and cholesterol in the diet, but there are certain fats that are as essential for the body as vitamins and minerals. These are alpha-linolenic acid (omega-3), linoleic acid (omega-6) and oleic acid (omega-9). They are crucial for healthy skin, cholesterol metabolism, prostaglandin synthesis, prevention of infections, proper growth and development, and proper brain and nervous system function. Supplementing them in the diet will help an obese individual lose weight. Eliminating them from the diet may very well be the cause of obesity that fails to respond to low calorie diets. Not all fats behave the same way.

Your choice of oils in the diet may be more important than you think. All your body cells have membranes which are made up of the essential fatty acids. The body must get these from the diet since it cannot synthesize them from other nutrients. A diet deficient in essential fatty acids will eventually lead to abnormal cell function, dry skin and hormonal imbalances. As many responsible nutritionists have pointed out, we have only just begun to scratch the surface of the diseases attributed to an imbalance of essential fatty acids. For example, studies show that omega-3 oils are vital for the prevention of blood clots and damage to the walls of arteries. Blood clotting factors called platelets become far less sticky and aggregate (get together to form clots) less if aspirin is taken on a daily basis. Much the same thing can occur when one supplements the diet with omega-3 oils. Besides lowering platelet stickiness, omega-3 oils help lower blood pressure, blood cholesterol and triglycerides. All this reduces the risk of heart attack and stroke. With aspirin, there is always the risk of bleeding internally; thus, many modern cardiologists prefer the supplementation of diets with hefty doses of fish oils. Although fish oils are a good source of omega-3 oils, flax oil is superior in several ways: it is better tasting, less expensive and more likely to be toxin-free. It is high in omega-3, omega-6, omega-9, silicon, vitamin E and other essential nutrients. Side effects, even in higher-than-recommended doses, are minimal or non-existent.

Aside from its role in cardiovascular disease, flax oil has been used as an anti-inflammatory agent to lessen the symptoms of migraine headaches, female problems like premenstrual syndrome and endometriosis, rheumatoid arthritis, multiple sclerosis, lupus, scleroderma and other autoimmune conditions. When flax oil is taken with high doses of vitamin E and other antioxidant nutrients, the anti-inflammatory effect may be equal or superior to prescription analgesics and non-steroidal, anti-inflammatory drugs. Some of these drugs have been reported to cause gastrointestinal hemorrhage and unexpected deaths. Side effects of this severity have never been reported with flax oil at any dose.

Recent research also suggests that flax oil can help regulate the immune system; prevent cancer; eliminate constipation; soothe gastritis, colitis and peptic ulcers; and combat bronchial asthma, eczema, psoriasis, kidney disease, mental illness, yeast infections, impotence and other glandular problems. One illness of near epidemic proportion is chronic fatigue syndrome. Studies indicate that virtually all victims have a deficiency of essential fatty acids, and that there is a good therapeutic response to supplementation with evening primrose oil or flax oil.

In purchasing a good flax oil, make sure that it has an expiry date and that it was cold-pressed in an oxygen and light-free environment. Unless these criteria are met by the manufacturer, the composition of the oil may be altered and potentially harmful to health.

Natural Blood Thinners

Although it is theoretically possible to reduce dependence on prescription anticoagulants, this should be done carefully over a long period of time and with the supervision of a medical doctor. Blood tests have to be done weekly until blood clotting ability has stabilized.

Foods that are high in vitamin K increase blood clotting. They do not have to be eliminated, just reduced as much as possible. These foods include all the dark green vegetables like spinach, alfalfa and broccoli, as well as cauliflower, egg yolks, liver and red meats.

There are many nutrients that work like anticoagulants in high doses (i.e., help prevent the blood from becoming too sticky or from clotting less easily). Some of these nutrients work by preventing platelets from sticking together, while others work by decreasing the blood levels of certain clotting factors or proteins. The net effect is referred to by most laymen as "blood thinning."

The best known natural anticoagulants are garlic oil and omega-3-EPA oils (flax seed oil, rice bran oil, cod liver oil, salmon oil, among others). Wheat germ oil, evening primrose oil, black currant oil, olive oil, soybeans, sunflower seeds, vitamin E, ginkgo biloba, butcher's broom and various Chinese herbs also help decrease the blood's ability to clot. Most of these are available from your local health food store or supermarket. Since no two people are alike, the recommended effective amounts are highly variable. Work with a doctor to establish a more natural blood thinning regime.

Nosebleed Prevention

Nosebleeds can be caused by trauma (accidents, nose-picking), sinusitis, rhinitis, vitamin deficiencies, upper respiratory infections or dryness of the mucous membranes. On a systemic level, nosebleeds are often seen with aspirin usage, high blood pressure, atherosclerosis and bleeding disorders (hemophilia, aplastic anemia, leukemia and others).

Prevention of nosebleeds is often possible through dietary changes. Foods high in vitamin C and bioflavonoids, such as garlic, onions, citrus fruits, berries, cherries and peppers, are helpful, as are foods high in vitamin K, like spinach, alfalfa, broccoli and other deep green leafy vegetables, as well as cauliflower. Avoid sugar, white flour products, coffee, tea and alcohol.

For prevention in more serious cases, higher than RDA doses of the following vitamins, minerals, herbs and other supplements should be considered: vitamins A, C, E and K, calcium, zinc, calendula, hawthorn, bioflavonoids (rutin, hesperidin, catechin, pycnogenol, progenol) and chlorophyll-containing "green" foods (chlorella, spirulina, barley green, blue-green algae, green kamut). Dosages for all these supplements can be personalized by a natural health care practitioner.

Treating Capillaries and Veins Naturally

Most doctors tell their patients that superficial varicose veins and broken capillaries are the result of heredity. Women tend to get them more after pregnancy or if they take hormones such as the birth control pill. Jobs that involve a lot of standing increase the likelihood of getting the problem, as does a lack of exercise and being overweight.

It is also known that superficial capillaries and veins are rarely seen in populations where unrefined, fiber-rich carbohydrates comprise a large portion of the diet. These medical conditions are prevalent in societies accustomed to refined, westernized diets. While there is no conclusive evidence that a high fiber diet prevents or improves varicose veins and broken capillaries, such a diet should be followed for its proven effects against diverticulosis, constipation and its possible protection against this unsightly problem.

The integrity and health of capillaries relates to many dietary micronutrients. Supplemental vitamins and minerals may be very helpful. These include bioflavonoids, calcium, copper, magnesium, vitamin C, vitamin E and zinc. Such a regimen may help to prevent broken capillaries.

Pycnogenol, an antioxidant derived from pine tree bark, has an antioxidant activity 50 times stronger than vitamin E. It is safe and effective in the treatment of circulatory problems such as varicose veins, diabetic retinopathy, water retention and other inflammatory conditions. It has useful anti-allergy and anti-arthritic effects.

Some herbalists and homeopaths have claimed both preventive and therapeutic successes with barberry, hawthorn berries, white oak bark, witch hazel and calendula. These herbs can improve circulation and prevent the buildup of toxins in the large bowel.

The most immediately effective treatment for superficial varicose veins and broken capillaries is sclerotherapy. This involves injecting saline (salt solution) into the tiny blood vessels at the surface of the skin. The salt solution destroys the broken capillaries, which are then absorbed into the neighboring connective tissue below the skin. The treatment is safe and yields excellent cosmetic results in most cases. Many dermatologists and other types of doctors offer this natural treatment. Combining it with a high fiber diet and the supplements previously mentioned would give the best chance of resolving this problem.

Cold Hands and Feet

In the absence of other symptoms, cold hands and feet may indicate an inherited problem or indicate a greater need for certain nutrients. It is important, however, to rule out various medical conditions that are associated with this problem. These include Raynaud's disease, hypothyroidism, adrenal insufficiency, reactive hypoglycemia (low blood sugar attacks) and circulatory abnormalities of other kinds. Check with a doctor to make sure such medical problems have been excluded as potential causes of the problem.

Cigarette smoking and drugs that constrict blood vessels (e.g., birth control pills, migraine medications, blood pressure drugs, caffeine) are also common causes of cold hands and feet. If possible, avoid tobacco smoke and use natural alternatives to drugs.

A variety of nutritional supplements may be of help. Coenzyme Q10 is a natural supplement that improves oxygen supply to tissues. Vitamin E does the same and improves circulation because of its effects as an anti-clotting agent. Vitamin C supplementation in high doses often improves cold hands and feet. The B-complex vitamins, particularly vitamin B3 (niacin), are extremely important for the heart and vascular system. Anyone who has ever taken niacin (over 100 mgs on an empty stomach) will attest to the feelings of warmth and even flushing that it produces. This is because niacin dilates small arteries throughout the body.

Herbal remedies that improve circulation and warm up hands and feet include ginseng, cayenne, garlic, ginkgo biloba extract and pau d'arco. Doses depend on your individual needs and tolerance for the supplement concerned. See a naturopath or a doctor experienced in using these remedies.

Controlling High Blood Pressure Naturally

Many people who suffer from high blood pressure (also called essential hypertension) can benefit from a natural approach. I must caution, however, that treating high blood pressure with natural remedies can get complicated, even with the help of a practitioner who is familiar with both drug and natural remedies. It's not just a matter of taking a few supplements as an alternative to a prescription. The ideal approach would be to continue the prescribed medical treatment, then start whatever natural therapy is appropriate. As the blood pressure goes lower, one can gradually be weaned off the prescription drug(s). Several diseases are associated with high blood pressure. These include diabetes mellitus, kidney disease, obesity, high blood cholesterol, hyperthyroidism, adrenal glandular diseases and other metabolic disorders. Most people taking anti-hypertensive drugs have already had these treatable conditions ruled out by their doctors.

Scientific literature reports that high blood pressure responds very well to the following diet and lifestyle changes:
- Periodic juice fasting
- Vegetarian (high fiber) diet
- Stress reduction techniques (biofeedback, meditation, relaxation response, etc.)
- Aerobic exercise
- Weight loss
- Food allergy detection and elimination
- Quitting smoking and chewing tobacco
- Balancing blood levels of amino acids
- Balancing trace minerals (especially calcium, magnesium and potassium)
- Avoidance of salt, sugar, caffeine and alcohol
- Oral and intravenous chelation therapy

High blood pressure may be the result of excessive amounts of cadmium and lead in the body. These heavy metal pollutants are often found in cigarette smoke and, hence, are elevated in smokers. This may be one of the reasons why cigarette smoking causes high blood pressure. Since zinc is antagonistic to cadmium, it can be used as a supplement to help rid the body of excess cadmium. Oral and intravenous chelation therapy programs are often very effective when toxic heavy metals are the source of the blood pressure problem.

Mercury hypersensitivity or toxicity affects primarily the nervous system. Through a nervous system mechanism, high blood pressure can, theoretically, occur as a result of mercury exposure. There are indeed anecdotal reports of a relationship between high blood pressure and mercury from dental amalgams. The scientific literature, however, does not support this association. As more researchers study the effects of mercury dental amalgams on health, new information will, no doubt, come to light. Hair mineral analysis can be used to determine body levels of many toxic heavy metals including aluminum, arsenic, lead, mercury, cadmium, copper, silver and nickel. If any of these are elevated, appropriate detoxification/cleansing programs can be implemented.

There are a large number of nutritional supplements that have been reported to help control blood pressure naturally. These include calcium, magnesium, potassium, coenzyme Q10, garlic, vitamin C, flax seed oil, fish oils, evening primrose oil and tryptophan. Herbs that are helpful include cayenne, camomile, valerian, fennel, hawthorn, parsley and rosemary. Watch out for licorice root. It contains glycyrrhetinic acid, which, in excess, can produce high blood pressure in susceptible individuals.

Phenylalanine should be avoided as a supplement since high amounts can elevate blood pressure. Phenylalanine is found in large amounts in aspartame, the ubiquitous artificial sweetener. If you drink a lot of diet pop or chew a lot of sugar-free gum you may be consuming large amounts of phenylalanine. Avoid it and any other chemical sweeteners, many of which are high in sodium. Work with a natural health care practitioner to help lower blood pressure naturally.

Low Blood Pressure (Orthostatic Hypotension)

Orthostatic hypotension is a low blood pressure condition that causes lightheadedness, blurred vision, weakness and, in severe cases, fainting or seizures. In most victims, there is a diminished ability of the body to respond to the pressure changes in the vascular system when rising to a standing position. Orthostatic hypotension is often caused by interference (by drugs or disease) with the autonomic nervous system or a lack of blood volume (due to anemia or blood loss). There are many causes of low blood pressure that are often ignored by patient and doctor, but should not be, as they may be warning signs of underlying problems like diabetes, kidney disease, pernicious anemia, porphyria and Guillain-Barre syndrome. Orthostatic hypotension may be one of the signs of Parkinson's disease. Medical treatment depends on the cause of the hypotension.

There are many metabolic imbalances that can cause orthostatic hypotension, including weak thyroid or adrenal glandular function. Vitamin and trace mineral deficiencies may also be involved. If no specific cause can be found that could explain the symptoms (e.g., idiopathic orthostatic hypotension), consider trial therapy with the following supplements:

Bioflavonoids	Potassium citrate
Licorice root capsules or tincture	Raw adrenal concentrate
Magnesium citrate	Vitamin C
Pantothenic acid (vitamin B5)	Zinc citrate

Siberian ginseng and DHEA (an extract of wild yam), astragalus and evening primrose oil (or borage or black currant oil) also provide adrenal support. Consult a naturopath or medical doctor before undertaking any supplement program. Working together, an individualized dosage schedule and supplement regime can be developed.

Vasculitis

Vasculitis is an inflammation of a blood vessel. There are many different causes of vasculitis, including infection, drug toxicity, allergy and auto-immune disease. Vasculitis can lead to severe pain, rashes and other circulation problems. It can sometimes be life threatening. Prednisone (synthetic cortisone) is often prescribed on a long-term basis as a treatment for the type of vasculitis associated with auto-immune diseases like lupus, rheumatoid arthritis and polyarteritis nodasa. Prednisone is also used for vasculitis of unknown cause.

Research indicates that vasculitis may be associated with hidden food and chemical allergies. A diet low in saturated fat and alkaline ash (mainly vegan) may be helpful. This means that intake of beef, pork and dairy products should be reduced as much as possible. Also of benefit is a high dietary intake of essential fatty acids from primarily vegetable sources (e.g., flax seed oil).

Of possible importance is the role of mercury toxicity or hypersensitivity from dental fillings. Dr. Hal Huggins and several other dentists concerned with heavy metal toxicity have described some cases in which vasculitis was resolved upon the removal and replacement of silver mercury dental amalgams. The best immunological test for determining hidden food and chemical allergies as well as a potential mercury problem is the Elisa/Act test developed by Dr. Russell Jaffe. I strongly recommend this test for anyone suffering from auto-immune diseases.

Supplements that may be helpful as complementary medical treatments for vasculitis include beta-carotene, bicarbonate mixtures, buffered vitamin C, flax seed oil, cod liver oil, shark oil, halibut liver oil, evening primrose oil, oil of borage, B-complex vitamins (especially vitamin B5, vitamin B6 and PABA), selenium, silicon, zinc, calcium, potassium, magnesium, vitamin E and bioflavonoids such as hesperidin, rutin, catechin, quercetin and pycnogenol.

Please note that in low doses (under 1,200 IU per day), vitamin E may have little or no effect on vasculitis. In doses well above 2,000 IU, vitamin E weakens autoimmune disease. I have purposely not recommended any specific doses since there is a great deal of variability of response to all supplements in vasculitis sufferers. Herbs such as aloe vera, comfrey, licorice root, white willow bark, feverfew, devil's claw, yarrow, yucca and marshmallow may also be helpful. Doses have to be carefully individualized. Supervision by a nutritional medical doctor or naturopath is highly desirable.

Hemangiomas

Hemangiomas are benign tumors of arteries or veins. They can occur anywhere in the body and their cause is unknown. Natural therapies designed to help arrest or reverse these usually benign tumors of blood vessels are harmless and worth trying in conjunction with routine medical care. Ultrasounds can be ordered at time intervals recommended by a conventional doctor to help assess changes in the size of the hemangiomas.

The basic principles that apply to the prevention and treatment of any benign tumor also apply to hemangiomas. Most nutritional authorities advise eliminating all animal protein, dairy products, salt, sugar, white flour products, processed foods, coffee, tea and alcohol. The reasoning behind this is that these foods are difficult to digest, contain no enzymes and accumulate toxins (oxidants or free radicals) in the liver, large bowel and blood. Approximately half of dietary intake should consist of raw fruits and vegetables. The remainder may include seeds, nuts, legumes (starchy beans) and whole grains. Soy products like tofu, miso, tempeh, soymilk, soy burgers and soya nuts may be good initial replacements for animal proteins and dairy products. For some tasty vegan recipes, see the book *Vegan Delights* by Jeanne Marie Martin.

It is now an accepted fact that benign and malignant (i.e., cancerous) tumors are initiated by what is called free radical pathology. This simply means that toxins (oxidants) from air, water and food enter the body, cause damage to the nuclei of cells and initiate tumor growth. Our bodies usually make ample amounts of antioxidant enzymes and prevent tumors from forming. In some people, however, antioxidants get depleted and little remains to prevent tumor growth. There is good evidence that supplementation with antioxidants will help prevent tumors from occurring.

Scientific and anecdotal studies have shown that many different herbs and food supplements are useful in both prevention and complementary medical treatment of benign tumors. These include deodorized garlic, pancreatin, raw thymus extract, lactobacillus acidophilus and herbs such as barberry, dandelion, pau d'arco, chaparral, echinacea, horsetail, comfrey, ragwort, wood sage and the mixture of burdock, slippery elm, Turkish rhubarb and sheep sorrel. A naturopath or medical doctor familiar with herbal remedies can be of help in prescribing an individualized treatment plan.

Reversing Macular Degeneration

Macular degeneration is the leading cause of visual loss in Europe and North America. It is thought to be the direct result of free radical damage to the macula, a small area located at the center of the retina that is responsible for fine vision. Free radical damage occurs with excessive exposure to UV light and may lead to both cataracts and macular degeneration. With the accelerated depletion of the ozone layer, free radical damage from sunlight may become a more common occurrence in the next decade. There are at least 70,000 chemicals that have been introduced into our environment since the 1940s: there is little doubt that some of these are initiators of free radical damage to the eyes. Aging, hardening of the arteries and high blood pressure are other risk factors associated with macular degeneration.

There is a very good chance that the problem of macular degeneration can be reversed with dietary changes and antioxidant supplementation. All animal products, including fish and organic meats and chicken, must be eliminated from the diet. Follow a completely vegetarian diet. This minimizes exposure to free radicals originating from rancid animal fats and chemicals found in their fat cells. As John Robbins correctly points out in *Diet For A New America*, even "organic" animal products contain harmful chemicals.

This is unavoidable in our polluted world, as "free range" animals eat, drink and breathe chemically contaminated air, water and food. Eating lower on the food chain does not guarantee chemical-free foods, but it sure reduces the concentration of free radicals in the diet (by a factor of 20 or more).

Eat more legumes; they have a cleansing effect due to their high content of sulphur-containing amino acids. Eat more fresh fruits and vegetables, especially yellow vegetables, berries (particularly blueberries because of a high content of bioflavonoids) and cherries because of their content of carotenes, flavonoids, vitamin E and vitamin C. In addition, take the following antioxidant supplemental vitamins and minerals:

Beta-carotene	Vitamin C
Coenzyme Q10	Vitamin E
Pycnogenol	Zinc chelate, picolinate or citrate
Selenium	

Studies have also indicated that ginkgo biloba and blueberry extract show impressive results with macular degeneration.

None of these natural supplements have any serious side effects, but it's always best to get supervision from a naturopath or medical doctor familiar with nutrition.

Hemochromatosis

Iron overdosing may lead to hemosiderosis (generalized or focal iron deposition) and hemochromatosis, damage to heart, spleen, liver, and pancreas. Hereditary hemochromatosis occurs in approximately 1 out of 20,000 individuals. There is no general agreement on the cause of hemochromatosis, but it is believed to be the end result of an inborn error of metabolism. Some of the signs and symptoms include greyish skin, headache, shortness of breath, fatigue, dizziness, weight loss, bronzing of the skin, cirrhosis, diabetes mellitus, cardiomyopathies, congestive heart failure and heart beat irregularities. The conventional medical treatment is via phlebotomy (blood letting).

It may be helpful to avoid high sources of iron in the diet. The foods with the highest sources of iron are meats, poultry, fish, seafood, grain products, kelp, brewer's yeast, blackstrap molasses, wheat bran, pumpkin seeds, squash seeds, wheat germ, sunflower seeds and millet. Avoid cooking foods in iron pots and pans, and use distilled water or filtered water with a low or absent iron content for drinking and cooking purposes. Vitamin C increases iron absorption; thus, those with hemochromatosis are advised not to supplement with high doses of vitamin C.

Published research supports the use of many natural remedies for liver diseases of all types. For example, low sugar (sucrose) consumption is beneficial. So is the avoidance of all fats, animal protein, raw fish, shellfish, alcohol and highly processed foods. Great benefits may be derived from following a raw vegetable and fruit diet for several weeks. Short-term juice fasting is also helpful (see the *Joy of Juice Fasting*, by Klaus Kaufmann). Therapeutic juices include radish and pineapple, black cherry concentrate mixed with liquid chlorophyll and a combination of carrot, beet, green pepper, spinach, papaya and cucumber juices.

Milk thistle extract (silymarin) helps most liver disorders. So does coenzyme Q10, black radish, red clover, dandelion, B-complex vitamins and the amino acids methionine and cysteine. Injections of folic acid, vitamin B12 and other B-complex vitamins may be dramatically effective in cases where energy levels have been severely impaired. Many patients can learn to give themselves regular injections until the liver has had a chance to repair and rebuild itself.

The herbal tea combination of slippery elm, burdock, Turkish rhubarb, cress and sheep sorrel may be of great help in cleansing the liver (three to six months). Periodic liver function blood tests, as well as supervision by a natural health care practitioner, are strongly recommended.

Intravenous chelation therapy or oral chelation therapy using antioxidant vitamins and minerals (N-acetyl-cysteine, beta-carotene, B-complex vitamins, vitamin E, selenium, zinc, manganese, magnesium, glutathione, choline, cysteine, methionine and others) may help keep iron levels under control. For more information on chelation therapy contact the EDTA Chelation Lobby Association of B.C. or the American College of Advancement in Medicine. See the resource section in the appendix for addresses and phone numbers.

Raynaud's Disease

Raynaud's disease is a condition that involves spasms of the arterioles, especially in the hands and feet, which turn white, blue and then red. Cold or emotional upset often stimulates the spasms, which may last from minutes to hours. The pain may be excruciating, with sensations of tingling, numbness and burning. It is most often seen in young women and rarely leads to any serious consequences (skin ulcers or gangrene, for example). When the signs and symptoms occur secondary to another disease, the term "phenomenon" is used. When they are seen unassociated with other diseases (i.e., idiopathic, of unknown source), it is referred to as "Raynaud's disease."

Primary conditions associated with Raynaud's include connective tissue disorders like scleroderma, rheumatoid arthritis, lupus, thyroiditis, trauma, primary pulmonary hypertension, and thoracic outlet syndrome. Conventional treatment is with drugs and, in severe cases, surgery (sympathectomy) may be required. Chiropractic treatments may be of some help in selected cases. Not much can be done for the condition medically. Birth control pills, female hormone prescriptions and cigarette smoking make Raynaud's symptoms worse. Calcium channel blockers are currently the drug therapy of choice. There are a great number of things you can do to relieve the problem with natural therapies.

From the dietary viewpoint, naturopaths have noted that eating more liver-cleansing foods (such as beets, carrots, artichokes, lemons, parsnips, dandelion greens, watercress and burdock root) helps to normalize circulation. Ideal fresh juices include carrot, spinach, beet, cucumber and lemon. Citrus peel, figs, honey and magnesium-rich foods (spinach, parsley, alfalfa and other greens rich in chlorophyll) are also helpful. Avoid beef, pork, alcohol, hot sauces, spicy foods, fried foods, processed foods and cold or cooling foods. Some cases of Raynaud's are triggered by certain food sensitivities. Food allergy testing may be worth while, especially in severe, intractable cases.

Vitamin and mineral supplements that have been reported to be effective are:

Coenzyme Q10	Phosphatidyl choline (lecithin)
DMG (dimethylglycine)	Pycnogenol
Evening primrose oil	Quercetin
Liquid chlorophyll	Trial of vitamin B12 injections
Magnesium (Magnesium is nature's calcium channel blocker; some do better when magnesium is given as an injection.)	Vitamin B3 (niacin)
	Vitamin E

Note: Niacin may cause some liver irritation, skin flushing, redness and itching at almost any dose. These side effects may be blunted by taking one or two 500 mgs capsules of white willow bark along with the niacin. Alternatively, use a complex form of niacin like niasitol (e.g., niacin plus inositol combination), which produces neither skin reactions nor liver irritation. Always take niacin and any single B vitamin together with a high potency B-complex to prevent other B vitamin deficiencies from developing.

Additionally, there are herbal remedies that have been noted to be helpful. These include ginkgo biloba extract, butcher's broom, capsicum (cayenne), garlic, ginger root, bee propolis, pau d'arco, oat, St. John's wort, passiflora, valerian, licorice root and alfalfa. Most Raynaud's victims find that one or more of these natural remedies relieves their symptoms. Supervision by a health care practitioner is recommended.

Diabetes

I gave a lecture on the hazards of milk and sugar to a group of diabetics in November 1993. At the time, a dietitian representing the local chapter of the Diabetes Association stated that their policy is that "sugar in moderation" is an acceptable part of a diabetic's diet. I strongly disagree. Sugar in any amount is an appetite stimulant. The more sugar you eat, the more you are likely to eat in general. Sugar increases the body's loss of chromium through the urine and leads directly to glucose intolerance (i.e., diabetes and hypoglycemia). Sugar in moderation for any diabetic is unrealistic, hazardous and perpetuates the disease.

Evidence is continuing to mount that one of the triggers of insulin-dependent diabetes mellitus (IDDM) is an allergy to cow's milk albumin and possibly to wheat gliadin. Diabetes mellitus affects nearly two million children and young adults in North America. It is responsible for over 25,000 amputations and at least 37,000 deaths each year. Aside from eliminating simple sugars from the diet, a wise preventive action might be to test children for antibodies in their blood against cow's milk and wheat. Doctors like Benjamin Spock have argued that milk is an inappropriate food for children, regardless of individual sensitivity. According to Dr. H. C. Gerstein, it is estimated that up to 30 percent of cases of IDDM could be prevented by removing cow's milk from the diet of 90 percent of the population in the first three months of life.

Natural Treatment of Diabetes

There is effective complementary medical therapy for both insulin dependent diabetes mellitus (IDDM) and non-IDDM. Although many of the self-help nutritional and herbal supplements are without significant side effects, drug interactions are possible in those on oral hypoglycemic prescriptions and/or insulin injections. Ideally, work with a sympathetic medical doctor to supervise progress. If on any amount of insulin or hypoglycemic drugs, make sure blood sugar levels are monitored with a glucometer at least twice a day, or as directed by a health care practitioner.

Eating Plan:
1. **Eat a high complex carbohydrate, high fiber (HFC) diet:** Seventy percent of calories should come from complex carbohydrates, 15 percent from protein and 15 percent from fat. Eat one to four servings of fruit daily, depending on blood sugar response. Caloric intake should be based on age, sex, height, weight and activity level.

2. **Eat five or six small meals throughout the day** instead of large meals; the closer the diet is to vegetarian principles, the better.

3. **A hypoallergenic/rotation diet is optimal,** if at all possible, get food allergy testing done by your doctor using the Elisa/Act blood test. Eliminate the reactive foods and place everything else on a four-day rotation diet. This is especially important to the overweight diabetic.

4. **Eat More of the Following:**

   Sugar-Controlling Foods (provided no allergies exist to them): Cucumber, string beans, garlic, Jerusalem artichokes, parsley.

   Chromium-Rich Foods: Brewer's yeast, mushrooms, beets, grapes, raisins and whole grains.

137

Note: Chromium is an essential mineral, and is an active ingredient of a substance called glucose tolerance factor (GTF), along with vitamin B3 (niacin) and amino acids. In supplemental form, chromium picoli nate is best absorbed and utilized by the body.

Zinc-Rich Foods: Sunflower and squash seeds, peanuts, meats, wheat germ, soymeal, hard wheat berries, wheat bran, buckwheat, rice bran, millet, whole wheat flour, oatmeal, brown rice, cornmeal, black-eyed peas, green beans, chickpeas, lima beans, spinach, green onion, green leafy vegetables, sprouted grains.

Foods High in Water-Soluble Fiber: Psyllium, flax seed, pectin, guar gum and oat bran.

Complex, Whole Grain and Legume Carbohydrates: Whole rice, millet, yams, pumpkin, squash, celery, onion, spinach, peas, cabbage, radish, mung beans, blueberry, peach.

Foods Rich in Other Trace Minerals Like Iodine and Silicon: Kelp, dulse, Swiss chard, liquid chlorophyll, turnip greens, watercress, celery, alfalfa sprouts, alfalfa, buckwheat, wheat germ, rice polishings, sesame seeds, other seeds and nuts, onions, beans, legumes, cherries, garlic, brewer's yeast, ginger, soy, yogurt and raw goat milk.

Foods Rich in Omega-3 and Omega-6 Fatty Acids: Salmon, herring, mackerel, sardines, walnuts, flax seed oil, evening primrose oil, black currant oil, vegetable, nut and seed oils.

Spices: Cinnamon, turmeric, bay leaf, cloves.

5. **Drink Therapeutic Fresh Juices and Teas:** String bean, cucumber and celery. Raw sauerkraut and lemon. Raw sauerkraut and tomato. String bean, brussel sprout, carrot and lettuce. Watermelon and tomato. Parsley tea. Huckleberry leaf tea.

6. **Avoid:** Any foods that cause allergic/intolerant reactions.

   Sugars (glucose, fructose, lactose, malt, maltose, dextrose, corn syrup), candy, honey, molasses, dried fruits, concentrated sweets, concentrated juices, fried foods, caffeine, spicy foods, processed foods.

   Trans-fatty acids, hydrogenated oils (margarine, vegetable shortenings, imitation butter spreads, most commercial peanut butters), oxidized fats (deep-fried foods, fast food, ghee, barbecued meats).

Iron (diabetes has been found with increasing frequency in those with high blood levels of ferritin, or stored iron).

7. Supplements:

Please note that doses are dependent on biochemical tests, individual needs and practitioner supervision. Several companies make combination supplements in tablets or capsules, thus significantly reducing the number of pills to be taken. As improvement occurs, doses are reduced and many of the supplements can be stopped.

Beta-carotene

Bioflavonoids (pycnogenol, rutin, hesperidin and quercetin)

Biotin

Burdock root (a plant source of insulin)

Cedar berries (a plant source of insulin)

Chromium picolinate

Coenzyme Q10

Copper citrate

Folic acid

Myoinositol (especially helpful in cases of neuropathy)

Ginkgo biloba extract (helps prevent diabetic retinopathy and peripheral vascular disease)

Goldenseal root

L-carnitine

Licorice root

Magnesium

Manganese

Omega-3 fatty acids and omega-6 fatty acids (flax seed oil, cod liver oil, evening primrose oil)

Potassium citrate

Selenium

Silica (horsetail)

Time-released niacin (vitamin B3)

Trace minerals[1]

Uva ursi

Vanadyl sulphate (produces an insulin-like reaction when taken with meals)

Vitamin B6

Vitamin B1

Vitamin B12

Vitamin C[2]

Vitamin E

Zinc picolinate

[1]Alfalfa, aloe vera, garlic, onions, fenugreek, capsicum, ginger, kelp, liquid chlorophyll, blue-green algae, psyllium, ginseng and lactobacillus acidophilus may all be used to provide other trace minerals and to promote tissue healing, digestion and elimination.

[2]If ferritin or blood iron levels are high, vitamin C should not be supplemented until levels return to normal. Vitamin C increases iron absorption and may create iron toxicity problems. Also of concern is a relationship between diabetes incidence and high blood iron or ferritin levels.

At first glance, all of this might seem overwhelming for someone educated in the conventional medical school of nutrition. The good news is that the implementation of only a few of the suggested changes can dramatically lower the requirements for insulin and hypoglycemic drugs. For example, several studies indicate that just increasing the fiber content of the diet to a total daily intake of 40 grams while eliminating refined (simple) sugars lowers insulin requirements by as much as 30 percent. A little effort goes a long way toward both the prevention and treatment of diabetes—this is a most promising area of complementary medicine.

Aplastic Anemia

Aplastic anemia is characterized by bone marrow failure—the bone marrow simply doesn't develop any new blood cells. Total suppression (aplasia) of the bone marrow may be the result of a toxic reaction to radiation, certain drugs or chemicals. In rare cases, the cause may be a tumor in the thymus gland. In about half the cases, the cause is unknown (idiopathic).

In some cases, aplastic anemia strikes suddenly. In most cases, however, the onset is insidious, occurring weeks or months after exposure to the offending toxin. Symptoms may include weakness, fatigue, lassitude, headache and breathing difficulties. Infections may be more frequent and severe than would normally be expected. In chronic cases, the skin has a waxy pallor with some brown pigmentation. Due to a decrease or absence of platelets, internal bleeding may occur. Other manifestations include ulcerations, heart murmurs, rapid heart rates, fever and enlarged spleen and lymph nodes.

Acquired (as opposed to hereditary) aplastic anemia is a result of exposure to radiation, chemical agents and solvents (e.g., benzene, urethane, arsenic), drugs (e.g., phenylbutazone, chloramphenicol) and insecticides. Some antibiotic drugs, anti-inflammatory drugs and anticonvulsants have also been implicated. The exact mechanism for the development of acquired aplastic anemia is not clear. It may be related to a genetic hypersensitivity to certain drugs, chemicals or radiation. Bone marrow failure may also be the result of kidney failure, liver disease, various glandular (endocrine) disorders, some hereditary diseases and chronic infections. Advanced cancers, particularly those that spread to the bone marrow, may also produce the condition.

Standard medical therapies start with the elimination of the source when the cause is related to chemicals, drugs or radiation. Bone marrow transplants are still considered to be the most effective therapy for aplastic anemia. Blood transfusions are also done, but only if absolutely necessary. In patients older than 30 years of age, the treatment of choice may be antilymphocyte globulin. Some anabolic steroids (androgens) may also be effective in stimulating the bone marrow. If the condition stems from an immunologic basis, immunosuppressive drugs such as prednisone and cyclophosphamide may be useful. The prognosis for aplastic anemia is unpredictable. Scientists are studying a new biotechnology product called GM-CSF (Recombinant Human Granulocyte-Macrophage Colony Stimulating Factor) and using it as experimental treatment for severe cases that are unresponsive to other therapies.

Nutritional (complementary) therapy may have a place in the management of acquired aplastic anemia. Although highly controversial as a treatment for hardening of the arteries, EDTA chelation therapy is an accepted treatment for toxic heavy metal poisoning. Hair mineral analysis and specialized blood and urine tests can help determine the presence of various toxic heavy metals, drugs and chemicals.

Since the 1940s, our bodies have been exposed to over 70,000 new chemicals. These include not only drugs, but many substances that have found their way into our food, water and atmosphere. The problem is not so much that they are there, but that our bodies have no efficient way of deactivating them. The human race has not had enough time to evolve protective mechanisms. Consequently, many of these chemicals are stored permanently in our muscle and fat cells. This fact has been verified by human tissue biopsy studies on chemical levels (DDT, PCBs, drugs, pesticides, dyes, etc.).

The real danger is that these stored chemicals (also known as xenobiotics) can cause cellular changes leading to tissue damage in any part of the body. Some scientists hold to the theory that cancer, heart disease and immunodeficiency diseases have their origin thanks to these toxins. All agree that tissue damage (oxidizing effects) is possible. This concept is also referred to as the free radical theory of aging. Free radicals are highly reactive molecules that are formed in the body both from internal and external pollution. They are capable of damaging any weak cells not adequately protected by antioxidants (enzymes, amino acids, vitamins and minerals that inactivate free radicals).

The most powerful antioxidants are beta-carotene, vitamin A, vitamin C, bioflavonoids, vitamin E, selenium, zinc, B-complex vitamins, cysteine and methionine. A proper balance of these nutrients in the food we eat will offset the free radical effects of xenobiotics, helping to prevent disease and slow down the aging process. But, if our food is contaminated with chemicals and is of poor quality, a balanced diet alone will do little to help prevent toxin accumulation. Countless authors, myself included, have used this argument to justify the daily supplementation of our diets with antioxidants in pill, powder or liquid form. Dosages, of course, depend on the individual and the degree of toxemia. Even so, daily supplementation of the previously mentioned antioxidants does little, if anything, for the up to five grams of stored toxins in the average adult.

So, what can one do to rid the body of chemicals stored in muscle and fat tissues? Some have advocated colonic irrigation, fasting, chelation therapy and proper food combining. Although testimonials abound for the sense of well being these methods bring, they have little effect on the stored xenobiotics.

Over the past decade, some studies have hinted at the effectiveness of a combination of supplemental antioxidants, daily exercise and sauna. The exercise and supplemental antioxidants help stimulate the circulation and mobilize the stored chemicals, while the sauna allows the individual to expel toxins through the skin. Crucial to the release of toxins from fat cells are high doses of vitamin B3 (niacin). Most authors recommend a hypoallergenic diet (primarily vegetarian) free of as many chemicals as possible along with heavy intake of distilled or uncontaminated spring water. Some authors recommend the use of herbal diuretics, laxatives or enemas to round out the therapy. Still others recommend tissue oxygenation with supplements such as organic germanium, pycnogenol and dimethyglycine (DMG). The length of time it takes to rid the body of toxic stores varies with each individual, but the average adult requires three months of a healthy diet and daily exercise, saunas and nutritional supplements. This approach has been used by some clinical ecologists over the past decade as a last resort therapy for patients suffering from total allergy syndrome (twentieth century disease). Many claim that the sauna, exercise and megavitamin program is the only effective method of detoxification of stored pesticides.

Unfortunately, scientific studies on the validity of these techniques are scanty. Many individuals and groups have made claims about the effectiveness of detoxification programs of this nature. However, the fact remains that this approach is still experimental and unrecognized as a legitimate therapy for any specific disease or set of symptoms. At this stage, all that can be confidently asserted is that we should do our best to prevent toxin accumulation through a healthier diet, exercise and antioxidant supplements. See the appendix for the names of organizations that can provide more information on aplastic anemia.

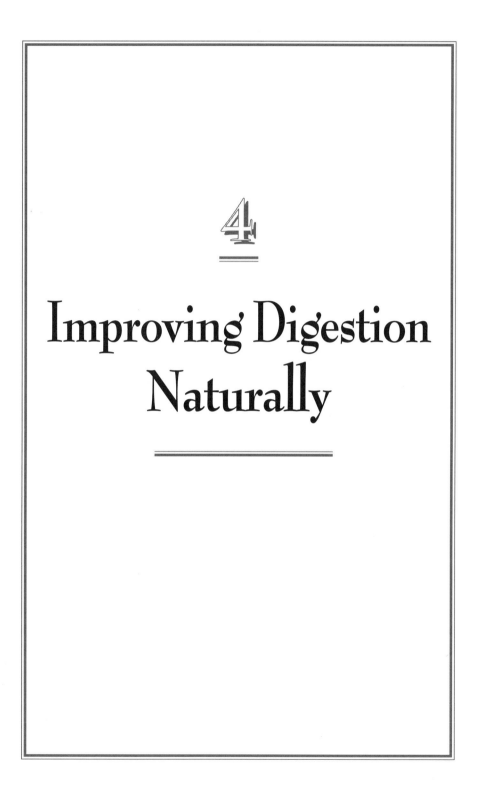

4

Improving Digestion
Naturally

The mouth, esophagus, stomach, duodenum, small intestine and large intestine make up the tube known as the gastrointestinal tract. The pancreas, liver and gall bladder manufacture various secretions, which empty into it on a continual basis. Problems associated with the function of these organ systems account for the second most common reason to seek medical attention (fatigue being the first). Drug sales in North America for antacids, antispasmodics, acid suppressors, motility modifiers, laxative and anti-diarrhea agents continue to escalate, despite the fact that they only suppress symptoms and never treat the true source of the problem.

The real source of problems such as irritable bowel syndrome, chronic constipation, bloating, gas, cramps, ulcers, indigestion, malabsorption and many other conditions can usually be found in nutritional medicine. Food allergies, bacterial flora imbalances, parasitic infections, fungal infections and digestive enzyme insufficiencies are just some of the real causes of chronic gut illnesses suppressed by commonly prescribed drugs.

In this chapter, you will learn that there are safe and effective alternatives that deal with the source of almost all gastrointestinal problems. These natural remedies reduce and often eliminate the need for prescription drugs.

Constipation

A healthy colon eliminates waste in 12 to 18 hours. The most common cause of constipation in North America is a lack of fiber and water in the diet. Other less common causes include the use of drugs that effect motility (opiates, iron tablets, antidepressants). Antacid and laxative abuse can also lead to a chronic constipation problem. Constipation may be a feature of irritable bowel syndrome, food allergy, diverticulosis, abdominal infection, dehydration, bowel obstruction, long periods of immobility, stress and depression.

The first thing to do about constipation is to increase water intake to at least eight large glasses of spring water per day. Avoid coffee and regular tea. Diluted fruit juices are fine. Increase consumption of high fiber foods such as whole grain breads, pastas and cereals, vegetables, legumes, fruits, seeds and nuts.

It is also very important to eliminate intake of refined carbohydrate foods such as sweets, chocolates, cakes, white flour products, white rice and other processed foods. Sugar and other junk foods are constipating.

High fiber supplements such as unsweetened wheat bran, oat bran and psyllium seed husks may not only help move the bowels better but will also decrease cravings for sweets. Some people may not be able to tolerate these grain fibers due to hypersensitivity; in such cases, fruit, vegetable or herbal alternatives may be substituted. Children of all ages can follow this advice as well as adults.

One of the common causes of chronic constipation, especially in children, is heavy milk consumption. Another is magnesium deficiency. Magnesium is the central element of chlorophyll and is found in all greens. Folic acid deficiency may also lead to chronic constipation. It too is found in green leafy vegetables. Lack of physical activity also plays a role. Physical fitness optimizes circulation to the bowel as well as other vital organs. If possible, take regular exercise, preferably aerobic.

Other natural remedies that have been effective for more stubborn cases of constipation include aloe vera juice, digestive enzyme supplements, B-complex vitamins, (especially vitamin B5, pantothenic acid), vitamin C, magnesium citrate or chelate, liquid chlorophyll, flax seed oil, lactobacillus acidophilus, Swedish bitters, cascara sagrada, comfrey, goldenseal, buckthorn, senna leaf and barley juice.

As a word of caution, please remember that each case has to be assessed on an individual basis and special medical or nutritional tests may be necessary to decide on the optimal treatment. One such test is the comprehensive digestive and stool analysis (CDSA). This is done on a sample of your stool by one of many different laboratories in the United States. A health care practitioner can provide you with the collection kit and send the stool sample to the U.S. by courier.

The CDSA is a battery of 24 screening tests of gastrointestinal status. Although some components of this test are available in Canada, the quality of the test is superior in the U.S., where some labs specialize in detailed stool analysis. The test has its main value in the assessment of how well a person digests and assimilates his or her food, whether or not there is a bacterial bowel flora imbalance, hidden infections with yeast or parasites, possible food allergies or digestive enzyme insufficiencies. Once the specific functional problem is determined by the CDSA, further investigations and treatment can be carried out as indicated by the results of the test.

According to Dr. Leo Galland, "every patient with disorders of immune function, including multiple allergies, patients with unexplained fatigue, or with chronic bowel symptoms, should be evaluated for the presence of intestinal parasites." In a study reported in the *Journal of Nutritional Medicine* in 1990, Dr. Galland found that one of the symptoms of hidden giardia infection may be constipation. In the U.S., it is estimated that about 50 percent of the water supplied to communities is contaminated with the parasite giardia lamblia. This parasite and several others (particularly blastocystis hominis and entamoeba histolytica) have been implicated in a large number of physical and emotional illnesses. People can easily pick up these infestations from salad bars, day care centers and household pets. Fortunately, natural herbal remedies are available to treat the growing epidemic of these parasites in the North American population. These include wormwood, grapefruit seed extract, black walnut, pumpkin seeds, chinchona and garlic.

The Family Herbal, an excellent book by Barbara and Peter Theiss, has an entire chapter devoted to Swedish bitters. Although most people know of the beneficial effects of Swedish bitters on digestion, few realize that this combination product has a myriad of other uses. Rather than go into a lot of detail, I suggest you get a copy of the book.

Swedish bitters can be safely taken on a long-term basis, provided the user does not suffer from ulcer or hyperacidity problems. This is because this herbal digestive aid increases stomach acidity. Also, if you have diarrhea, bitters may be detrimental because of its laxative effect. As its name suggests, it does taste very bitter and that's just about the only complaint I've heard about the product.

Stomach acid is absolutely essential for digesting protein and for the absorption of vitamins and trace minerals. Most people who benefit from bitters have a problem with low stomach acid (hypochlorhydria). Some authorities claim that about half the population of North America is hypochlorhydric. Betaine and pepsin HCL, glutamic acid HCL and Swedish bitters all help to increase stomach acidity. There is no toxicity and no dependence developed, even if taken for long periods of time. The stomach, in fact, will learn to secrete higher amounts of acid on its own thanks to the supplement.

Low stomach acidity has been associated with a very long list of maladies, including anemia; asthma; auto-immune diseases like vitiligo; spider veins on the face; vitamin B 12 deficiency; deficiencies in iron, copper, zinc, manganese and calcium; food allergies; the yeast syndrome; parasites; other gastrointestinal conditions—the list goes on. This is the reason for the many testimonials on the benefits of bitters for a wide range of conditions seemingly remote from the digestive system. By increasing stomach acidity you are getting at the physical root cause of many diseases.

Irritable Bowel Syndrome

Irritable Bowel Syndrome (IBS) is a common condition characterized by abdominal pain, constipation or diarrhea, increased colonic mucous secretion, flatulence, nausea, anorexia, along with varying degrees of anxiety or depression. It has also been referred to as nervous indigestion, spastic colitis, mucous colitis and intestinal neurosis. It is the most common gastrointestinal condition seen by doctors in general practice and represents up to 50 percent of all referrals to gastroenterologists. Some have estimated that up to 15 percent of the population suffers from some of the symptoms of IBS.

In the classic scenario, sufferers make the rounds of general practitioners, internists and gastroenterologists, are subjected to multiple investigations, including x-rays and internal scoping procedures, and are usually prescribed either tranquilizers, antispasmodics or other symptom-suppressive drugs. In many cases, patients seem satisfied with a partial resolution of their IBS symptoms. Unfortunately, more than half the cases fail to respond to this conventional medical approach; consequently, many seek natural alternatives.

Intractable cases may respond to food allergy detection and treatment, supplemental gastric and pancreatic digestive aids, bowel flora normalization and the treatment of any underlying large bowel infections caused by parasites, yeast, fungi or bacteria. An ideal test for IBS sufferers is the CDSA (comprehensive digestive and stool analysis).

Parasites do not always have to be treated by repeated courses of potentially toxic drugs. In my experience, the use of natural anti-parasitic supplements are effective and unlikely to produce side effects. These include wormwood, grapefruit seed extract, berberine, garlic, black walnut and dairy-free acidophilus. Goldenseal, ginger root, vitamin B6, Swedish bitters, plant enzymes and pancreatic digestive enzymes (pancreatin) may also be helpful and free of side effects. Another natural treatment to consider is a supplement of N-acetyl glucosamine. The usual therapeutic dosage for cases of irritable bowel syndrome is 2,000 to 3,000 mgs daily. For maximum beneficial results, a natural anti-parasitic program should be followed for at least three months, sometimes longer.

Numerous published studies in British medical journals have shown that peppermint oil may provide effective treatment for many of the symptoms of irritable bowel syndrome not complicated by infection. The oil inhibits gut muscle cramps or spasms and excessive gas. It is important to use enteric coated capsules. They allow the oil to arrive intact in the colon where the therapeutic effect is needed. Ordinary peppermint oil is broken down in the stomach and does not reach the large bowel. Double-blind studies do indeed prove that enteric coated capsules of peppermint oil are safe and effective treatment for IBS. Additionally, they are potent anti-candida (yeast) agents and may be of considerable benefit in the treatment of intestinal candida overgrowth.

The successful treatment of IBS can be complex and slightly different for each sufferer. Work with a natural health care practitioner for an individualized natural program.

Colitis and Crohn's Disease

The general term "inflammatory bowel disease" includes two major gastrointestinal diseases: Crohn's disease and ulcerative colitis. Both involve large bowel inflammation and tissues outside the colon. There is some degree of overlap with respect to signs and symptoms in both conditions, but the cause is poorly understood.

Crohn's disease is primarily a disease of white adults between the ages of twenty and forty, although it can occur in both children and the elderly. Its main signs and symptoms include abdominal pain, diarrhea, weight loss, rectal bleeding, anal fissures, abscesses and arthritis. In a minority of cases there may be inflammation of the liver, kidney and skin. The disease process involves the small bowel in 30 percent of patients, the colon in 15 percent and both the small bowel and colon in 55 percent of cases.

Ulcerative colitis is a chronic inflammatory disease that deteriorates the lining of the large bowel. It shows up primarily in the twenty to forty age group and affects predominantly females. Most often, the inflammation begins at the rectum and extends up through the colon. The inflammation can progress until ulcerations and abscesses develop. The disease can be mild and localized or excruciatingly painful with perforations of the colon. There is usually diarrhea with blood and mucus in the stool. Sudden attacks followed by periods of remission are typical.

Ulcerative colitis tends to occur in families and is associated with a high incidence of eczema, hay fever, arthritis and ankylosing spondylitis. There is a school of thought that believes that inflammatory bowel disease, especially ulcerative colitis, is the result of an allergy or a hypersensitive reaction to food by the colon. Salicylate (e.g., aspirin) sensitivity is found in some patients with ulcerative colitis. Some researchers have shown the existence of circulating antibodies against cow's milk and other foods.

Conventional medical treatment for Crohn's and ulcerative colitis often ignore the value of diet despite a large amount of published medical literature that stresses its importance. Studies and research information are well documented in the book *Food and the Gut Reaction*, by Elaine Gottschall. Many victims of inflammatory bowel disease can control their symptoms simply by eliminating lactose (milk sugar), starches, grains and refined carbohydrates from the diet. Gottschall's book contains menus, recipes and other self-help information for anyone suffering from inflammatory bowel disease. The salicylate-free diet and the Gottschall Specific Carbohydrate Diet have a high success rate with both Crohn's disease and ulcerative colitis. Some patients need only follow these diets for six months, while others must follow them for years before being able to eat the disallowed foods without symptoms.

More difficult cases require help from a natural health care practitioner for treatment of hidden food allergies, candida (yeast) infections, bacterial flora imbalances and parasite infestations. The best currently available immunological test for determining hidden food or chemical hypersensitivities (allergies) is the Elisa/Act test. This special blood test, developed by Dr. Russell Jaffe, measures circulating antibody levels to as many as 300 foods and chemicals. Candidiasis can also be determined by the Elisa/Act test, while parasitic infections can be diagnosed by comprehensive parasitology stool analysis. Diet therapy can then be more specifically tailored to account for the individual food allergies or infections.

Nutritional imbalances and deficiencies arise in sufferers of Crohn's disease because of malabsorption. Zinc deficiency is common, as are deficiencies in B vitamins (especially vitamin B12), vitamin A and vitamin D. Most cases require periodic vitamin B12 injections.

Herbs that can help inflammatory bowel disease include camomile, ginger, comfrey and a combination of slippery elm, Turkish rhubarb, burdock, sheep sorrel and cress. This same combination of herbs can be used in the complementary treatment of hemorrhoids, constipation, ulcers, diverticulitis, obesity, adult onset diabetes and hypoglycemia. Side effects are negligible.

Grains are a problem for Crohn's and colitis sufferers. Aloe vera juice is soothing for practically all gastrointestinal inflammations. Garlic and acidophilus (dairy- and grain-free) may be helpful too. None of the natural treatments interfere with conventional medical treatments. In fact, it's quite possible that diet change alone will help make any medical therapy work better.

Halitosis

Halitosis (bad breath) is a very common problem and can be a sign of many different conditions. The most common causes include dental and gum disease, upper or lower respiratory tract infections (nose, sinuses, throat, lungs), improper diet (too much refined food and red meat), constipation and cigarette smoking. Other fairly common causes of halitosis are food allergy, sugar diabetes and hypochlorhydria (low stomach acid).

Low or absent stomach acid causes poor digestion of foods leading to excessive bacterial fermentation. This can be alleviated by natural supplements like Swedish bitters, glutamic acid and betaine and pepsin hydrochloride. A heavy intake of onions, garlic, alcoholic beverages and other highly odoriferous foods can also be a factor in some cases. Fasting causes bad breath due to the production of ketones. This is easily relieved when the fast is broken.

If you have already ruled out these potential causes of halitosis, and conventional treatment has been unsuccessful, there are a number of effective measures you can take. First, brush your teeth and tongue after every meal. To prevent bacteria build-up, change toothbrushes every month. Use dental floss and a chlorophyll mouthwash daily (two tablespoons to one glass of water). A dentist can take a scraping of dental plaque and examine it under a microscope for the presence of parasites and candida infections.

Green drinks such as liquid chlorophyll, wheatgrass or barley juice are very effective against bad breath. Drink these liberally. Herbal toothpastes made from myrrh, peppermint, spearmint, rosemary and sage should be used. Gargling and rinsing the oral cavity with tea tree oil two or three times daily may help eliminate a low-grade chronic infection of parasites, fungi or bacteria. Another effective remedy for gum and pharyngeal infections is hydrogen peroxide. A diluted three percent solution can be used as an oral gargle and rinse.

Nutritional supplements that are helpful in most cases of halitosis include vitamin A, beta-carotene, B-complex vitamins, vitamin C, zinc, selenium, silicon and bee propolis. These are important for healing of mouth and gum disease and control of infection. An overgrowth of harmful bacteria in the large bowel can cause bad breath. So can hidden candida or parasitic infections. Lactobacillus acidophilus supplements are very important in order to offset these bugs with friendly bacteria in the large intestine.

If all these self-help measures fail to eliminate halitosis, see a naturopath or nutritional medical doctor so that more detailed investigations and specific treatments can be undertaken.

Spring Cleansing

We are all aware of the many toxic chemicals that find their way into our bodies from the air we breathe, the food we eat and the water we drink. Research indicates that these toxins are stored in our bodies for years and are at the root of chronic degenerative diseases like cancer, heart disease, diabetes and arthritis. As spring approaches, people concerned about health and prevention take it upon themselves to do something about ridding their bodies of these toxins. Many go on one of the internal cleansing programs available from health food stores.

The most popular and safest of these is the Sambu Elderberry Cleanse. When taken as directed, body toxins are eliminated and energy levels are increased. Over 90 percent of overweight subjects report an average of ten pounds of weight loss that does not return once the program is terminated. Individuals who are of normal weight or underweight may lose a pound or two but will rapidly regain this weight once the program is stopped.

The Sambu Elderberry Cleanse was popularized by Swiss naturopathic physician Brunhild Zechelius. His book, *Elderberry Internal Cleansing Program*, and Dr. Morton Walker's book, *Elderberry Internal Cleansing*, will provide anyone with a good understanding of the mechanisms by which detoxification takes place with this comprehensive program—consisting of elderberry juice and tablets, flax seed, psyllium seed powder, a herbal diuretic (containing uva ursi, juniper berries, corn silk and parsley) and a herbal laxative (containing senna, cascara sagrada or buckthorn).

The Sambu Elderberry Cleanse is a ten-day program that involves one day of preparing the body for a juice fast, seven days of exclusively liquid nourishment and two days of coming off the fast and getting the body used to eating solid foods again. A detailed booklet explaining the step-by-step procedure is included in the Sambu kit, which is available at most health food stores.

Elderberry has long been used in naturopathic medicine as an effective remedy for fevers, colds, influenza, hay fever, allergies, sinusitis, rheumatism and mucous congestion. These all happen to be the ailments most frequently experienced as the season changes to spring. Elderberry contains many biologically active compounds, including essential oils, terpenes, beta-carotene, B-complex vitamins, vitamin C, bioflavonoids (rutin, quercetin), calcium, potassium, mucilage and tannin. Most of these have been advocated, either alone or in combination, by naturopaths as treatments for various immune system problems such as allergies, viruses and flu-like illnesses. It is therefore not surprising that taking the elderberry cleanse leads to greater vitality and resistance to disease.

Flax seed, another major component of the Sambu program, is high in silicon, vitamin E and omega-3, omega-6 and omega-9 essential fatty acids. The most recent research suggests that essential fatty acid deficiency can lead to obesity, immune system problems (especially chronic viral illnesses like chronic fatigue syndrome) and many other chronic inflammatory and autoimmune diseases. Flax seed not only plays a role in the prevention of the major degenerative diseases, but may also play a vital role in their successful treatment.

Any good detoxification program involves a thorough cleansing of the bowel. This can be accomplished quite readily with soluble fiber products like psyllium seed powder or the mild purgatives and diuretics that come in the Sambu Elderberry Cleanse program. A healthy colon eliminates waste in 12 to 18 hours. Unfortunately, the majority of North Americans do not eliminate this efficiently. The most common cause of poor elimination is a lack of water and fiber in the diet. Other common causes of constipation include a diet of very refined, high sugar, high protein and high fat foods and the use of drugs that affect motility (opiates, iron tablets and antidepressants). Antacid and laxative abuse can also lead to a chronic constipation problem. So can excessive intake of milk and other dairy products.

Although most healthy people can undertake the Sambu Elderberry Cleanse program without supervision, those with health problems are best supervised by a natural health care practitioner. For more detailed information on the benefits of juice fasting, I highly recommend the *The Joy of Juice Fasting* by Klaus Kaufmann.

Ulcers, Gastritis and Helicobacter Infection

Helicobacter pylori infection is a type of bacterial infection that occurs in the stomach and duodenum and is thought to be the cause of stomach and duodenal ulcers. The infection has all the signs and symptoms of a peptic ulcer (pain, burning, gas, bleeding, etc.). There are some natural, common sense measures to both prevent and treat these infections. These include dietary elimination of fried foods, salt, strong spices, animal fats, alcohol, black tea, coffee, chocolate, cola, other carbonated soft drinks and peppers of all kinds. Quitting cigarettes and avoiding aspirin, steroids and other drugs is desirable. Non-steroidal anti-inflammatory drugs used in the treatment of arthritis or other types of inflammation have recently been implicated as potential sources of severe stomach problems. Also, studies done in England by John Yudkin strongly suggest that sucrose (table sugar) is involved in the development of ulcers and other digestive problems.

A very effective natural remedy is freshly made cabbage or potato juice (drink immediately after juicing; do not store). Cabbage or potato juice dilutes stomach acid and flushes it through the duodenum. Both reduce pain and lead to faster healing.

Do not drink milk. Although milk neutralizes stomach acid, the calcium and protein in milk stimulates the production of more acid. Cow's milk has a rebound effect and makes acidity worse in the long run. Almond milk, raw goat's milk or soy milk are good substitutes, provided there are no allergies to these foods. Over the past two decades, researchers have also found that a significant number of gastritis and ulcer sufferers have an allergy or hypersensitivity to cow's milk. These people may be perpetuating their stomach problem simply because they drink milk on a regular basis. Most people who have food allergies crave the foods to which they are allergic. If you crave milk, you are probably allergic to it.

Get food allergy testing done, eliminate the reactive foods from your diet and discuss some of the natural remedies outlined below with a naturopath or doctor. For more information on the impact of food allergies on health, how to test for them and how to treat them, see the section Food Allergies and Allergy Testing.

Eat small and frequent meals. Foods that are well tolerated by most sensitive stomachs include well-cooked millet, cooked rice, avocados, bananas, potatoes, squash, yams, broccoli, carrots, raw goat's milk and soured (cultured) dairy products such as yogurt, cottage cheese and kefir. Those with bleeding stomach problems may have to resort to baby foods and non-irritating fiber such as psyllium seed, pectin and guar gum to help promote healing.

L-glutamine is an amino acid that is important in the healing of hyperacidity. Vitamin E, chelated zinc, vitamins A, B6 and K, unsaturated fatty acids (evening primrose oil, flax seed oil, omega-3-EPA oil) and sodium ascorbate have all been shown to promote faster healing. Iron supplementation may be required to prevent anemia and other complications resulting from blood loss.

Herbal remedies that have traditionally enjoyed success in healing sensitive stomachs include aloe vera, slippery elm, bentonite, comfrey, camomile, goldenseal, peppermint, angelica, fennel, yarrow, St. John's wort and deglycyrrhizinated licorice (DGL). The latter is licorice minus the portion that can affect the adrenal hormones and raise blood pressure.

The herbal combination of slippery elm, burdock, Turkish rhubarb and sheep sorrel can help reduce stomach acidity, pain and bleeding. It may also significantly improve hemorrhoids, tumors and liver disorders. Work with a naturopath or nutrition-oriented doctor for a personalized treatment program that complements conventional medical therapy.

Hiatus Hernia Help

A hiatus hernia occurs when a portion of the stomach moves into the thoracic cavity through an enlarged esophageal hiatus (opening) in the diaphragm. Hiatus hernias are common and may be seen in up to 60 percent of the population over 50 years old. Although often asymptomatic, many sufferers complain of chest pain or heartburn with esophageal reflux. These symptoms can be aggravated by alcohol, smoking, coffee and highly acidic foods. Discomfort is worse lying down after eating and the diagnosis is often made by special x-rays (barium swallow).

Although most conventional doctors still treat hiatus hernia with a variety of drugs, there are quite a few effective natural alternatives for those willing to change their diets and lifestyles. Many hiatus hernia victims are surprised by the relief they experience from chiropractic treatments, shiatsu or massage therapy. A good chiropractor, osteopath or massage therapist can sometimes work wonders with a series of hands-on treatments.

Hiatus hernia symptoms can be prevented by eating frequent small meals throughout the day. Therapeutic vegetable juices include carrot, spinach, beet, cucumber, parsley, celery, cabbage and potato. These should be used liberally throughout the day (two quarts daily). Raw potato juice just before breakfast can help with acid regurgitation. Avoid meat, alcohol, hot sauces, spicy and fried foods, added salt, caffeine products, sugar and refined carbohydrate products. If you use aspirin, replace it with white willow bark capsules. At least this will not further aggravate the discomfort.

Supplements that have a healing effect include essential fatty acids (flax seed oil, cod liver oil, evening primrose oil, borage oil, black currant oil), licorice root tincture or herbal tea, choline, lecithin, PABA, bismuth, bentonite, goldenseal, slippery elm, burdock, aloe vera and lactobacillus acidophilus.

The herbal tea combination of burdock, slippery elm, Turkish rhubarb, sheep sorrel and cress has been successfully used for a wide range of gut problems, including hiatus hernia, duodenal ulcers, colitis, Crohn's disease, non-specific indigestion, irritable bowel syndrome, hemorrhoids and bowel infections. It's well worth using until symptoms clear up.

Leaky Gut Syndrome

People who treat candida endlessly, or continue to have auto intoxication symptoms despite multiple attempts at bowel cleansing, are wasting their time unless they also do something to repair the lining of their gastrointestinal tract.

The ecology of the gastrointestinal tract is intimately connected to the health of the immune system. The intestine is involved with nutrient uptake, but it also serves as a barrier to toxic substances. Nutrition-oriented doctors and naturopaths have noticed that a large number of people suffering from varying degrees of environmental illness and autoimmune diseases (e.g., rheumatoid arthritis, lupus, thyroiditis, scleroderma) have "leaky gut" syndrome. In this syndrome, the intestinal barrier is porous or more permeable to various microbial toxins, food allergens, polysaccharides and polypeptides. When these materials penetrate the intestinal mucosa they induce inflammation and stimulate the immune system to manufacture antibodies that cross-react with the body's own tissues. Systemic immune complexes are formed and lead to many of the symptoms of autoimmune disorders or environmental illnesses (e.g., total allergy syndrome, twentieth century disease, chronic fatigue syndrome, etc.).

What causes this condition? The list of potential etiologies is a long one, but the most common are undiagnosed infections with parasites, fungi, candida albicans and pathogenic bacteria. Leaky gut can also be caused by a deficiency of pancreatic digestive enzymes, inadequate stomach acidity, a highly refined diet, food allergies and excessive use of alcohol, NSAIDS (non-steroidal anti-inflammatory drugs like aspirin and ibuprofen), steroids and broad-spectrum antibiotics.

The gut becomes leaky in the sense that substances (undigested proteins, toxins, etc.) that are normally not absorbed will pass through a damaged or "leaky" gut. This in itself may cause fatigue and many other symptoms indistinguishable from hypoglycemia. Pathogenic microorganisms can secrete various toxins that not only damage the intestinal mucosa, but the various organ systems and the joints as well. Intractable arthritis cases, for example, have been documented to respond to therapy aimed at clearing a chronic, unsuspected bowel infection with parasites or pathogenic bacteria. Herbs, antioxidant vitamins and minerals, glutamine, N-acetylglucosamine, essential fatty acids, soluble fiber like psyllium and fruit pectin, digestive enzyme supplements and lactobacillus acidophilus might all be considered as part of the leaky bowel healing program. There is also an excellent 12-week program involving diet and a predigested protein/multi-nutrient powdered formulation called Ultra Clear Sustain (Ultra Clear GI in Canada). The formula contains fructo-oligosaccharides, which encourage the growth of a normal bacterial flora. Ultra Clear GI also contains dozens of other vital nutrients designed to repair the damaged lining of the GI tract. It is suitable for even the most "hopeless" cases of irritable bowel syndrome, candidiasis and food allergies.*

Burning Tongue Relief

A burning tongue can be associated with low stomach acidity. Studies also indicate that a burning tongue may occur as a result of deficiencies of iron, vitamin B12, folic acid, vitamin B2, vitamin B6 and zinc. Yeast (candida) infections, dental plaque, ill fitting dentures, mercury leakage from dental amalgams and excessive mouthwash use may also be involved.

Stomach acid is required in adequate amounts to help absorb vitamin B12, iron, manganese, zinc, copper, calcium and many other nutrients. Stomach acid secretion tends to slowly decline with age. Some doctors have reported that over half the population suffers from some degree of low stomach acidity. Heredity, food allergies, stress, prescribed drugs and over-the-counter drugs (e.g., antacids) may all play a role in suppressing stomach acidity.

A burning tongue is not caused by taking too many vitamin or mineral supplements. It often responds to stomach acidifiers like betaine and pepsin hydrochloride, glutaminc acid, apple cider vinegar or stomach bitters. If no improvement is made by trying some of the natural remedies over a period of a few weeks, see a health care practitioner knowledgeable in nutrition so that a nutritional evaluation can be done to help isolate the source of the problem.

---

* If your doctors are not familiar with leaky gut syndrome or how to treat it, have them contact Great Smokies Diagnostic Laboratory, 18A Regent Park Blvd., Asheville, NC, 28806; phone 704-253-0621/800-522-4762. Information on Ultra Clear GI can be had by calling Professional Health Products at 1-800-661-1366 (4307-49 St., Innisfail, AB, T4G 1P3).

Gas Relief

A product called "Beano drops" is often used as a natural remedy for gas problems caused by beans and other gas-forming vegetables. The potential for a negative reaction to the product exists if one is allergic to yeast, fungi or molds. Since everyone has some yeast in their bowel, this is not likely to be a problem unless the yeast population gets very high. Yeast tends to grow rapidly after taking antibiotics, the birth control pill or cortisone derivatives.

The literature from the distributor of Beano warns of potential problems for diabetics or those with a rare carbohydrate disease called galactosemia. This is only a theoretical concern. Those who suffer from carbohydrate problems may want to get their blood sugar tested every few months to see what impact, if any, this enzyme supplement has on their sugar tolerance. The product sounds like a good idea for symptom relief. Unfortunately, it does not do anything to cure the problem.

Many people are not genetically programmed to tolerate certain foods, based on blood types, food allergies, enzyme deficiencies and other hereditary factors. Until we find "cures" for all the causes of intestinal gas problems, this is one product that can provide symptomatic relief naturally. Beano is available in health food stores or from Jan Distributing. For information on how to cook beans to avoid gas, see the section Healing Foods for Healing Diets.

Parasites and Natural Therapies

Parasites do not always have to be treated by repeated courses of potentially toxic drugs. In my experience, the use of natural anti-parasitic supplements are effective and unlikely to produce side effects. These include garlic, wormwood, grapefruit seed extract, berberine, black walnut, cloves, Swedish bitters, pumpkin seeds, bentonite, aloe vera, psyllium seed husks or powder and dairy-free acidophilus.

Blastocystis hominis can be a very stubborn parasite and it may take six months or longer to completely eliminate it from the system. Regular use of Swedish bitters or stomach acidifiers (betaine or glutamic acid HCL) along with pancreatic digestive enzymes, plant enzymes and an acidophilus supplement may be necessary on a long-term basis.

A test called the CDSA (comprehensive digestive and stool analysis) and a comprehensive parasitology test will often detect parasites in people suffering from chronic digestive symptoms.

Diverticulitis Treatment

A diverticulum is a small, pouch-like area in the large intestine. The appendix can be considered to be a particularly large diverticulum: when stool gets stuck in it, inflammation develops (appendicitis). Diverticula (more than one diverticulum) come about as a result of increased pressure needed to force hard, dry stool through the bowel when constipated. They do not cause symptoms unless waste matter becomes trapped in them. The diverticula can then get infected and inflamed (diverticulitis). Conventional doctors usually prescribe antibiotics for diverticulitis attacks in addition to pharmaceutical brands of psyllium seed products. This approach works for the majority of cases.

Diverticulitis is a completely preventable problem through natural means alone. It is the end result of a poor diet, the overuse of alcohol and drugs (antibiotics, codeine, etc.) and stress. Avoid sugar, white flour products, all animal products (including milk and cheese), fried foods, coffee, tea, alcohol and processed foods. Get tested for food allergies to see which foods specifically cause problems. Tests to consider include the CDSA (Comprehensive Stool and Digestive Analysis) and the Elisa/Act blood test for food allergies.

If grains, seeds and nuts are well tolerated, leave them in the diet. If these give problems in any way (bloating, gas, constipation, cramps, etc.), stay with only well cooked brown rice, fruits, vegetables, legumes and juices. Oat bran, psyllium seed powder, glucomannan, guar gum, prune juice, aloe vera juice and green drinks such as Barley Green, Green Magma or cabbage juice are good things to take on a regular basis. Periodic juice fasting is a very good idea, particularly when attacks occur. Follow the guidelines discussed in Klaus Kaufmann's excellent book, *The Joy of Juice Fasting*, available from *alive* Books.

Herbal remedies that may be very effective for diverticulitis include alfalfa, cayenne, camomile, echinacea, pau d'arco, goldenseal, garlic, red clover and yarrow. Swedish bitters, a combination herbal digestive supplement, has remarkable soothing effects. Dairy-free acidophilus supplements should be taken on a daily basis to prevent bacterial or yeast (candida) infections of the large bowel. Trapped gas and symptoms related to it can be absorbed/eliminated by charcoal tablets. Have these on hand to prevent and treat embarrassing gas attacks if you are forced to follow a less than optimal diet at various social functions.

Reversing diverticulitis requires an unshakable commitment to healthy eating and lifestyle habits. Aside from a vegetarian, high complex carbohydrate, high fiber diet, supplements that promote healing include digestive enzymes (pancreatin, etc.), vitamin A, B-complex vitamins, buffered vitamin C (Ester C is best), vitamin E and essential fatty acids (flax seed oil, oil of borage, evening primrose oil). A naturopath or doctor familiar with nutritional remedies can help with a personalized program.

Bloating

In an otherwise healthy person, bloating after meals is the result of gas manufactured in the large bowel by intestinal bacteria. Incompletely digested protein due to insufficient stomach acid, weak pancreatic digestion and an imbalance between friendly and potentially pathogenic bacteria all may have something to do with bloating after meals. It may also be the end result of a fermentation process carried out by yeast (candida) on carbohydrates. Unsuspected food allergies may be yet another source of the problem.

A number of things may be needed to reestablish balance, including a bowel detoxification program (juice fasting, psyllium seed husks or powder, flax seed oil, bentonite, etc.). Proper food combining or a candida control diet may also help resolve the bloating.

Also helpful to those suffering from abdominal bloating is supplementation with betaine or glutamic acid hydrochloride, Swedish bitters, pancreatic digestive enzymes, lactobacillus acidophilus, activated charcoal capsules, N-acetyl glucosamine (NAG), peppermint oil capsules and the herbal combination of slippery elm, sheep sorrel, burdock and Turkish rhubarb. Most people arrive at a resolution of their symptoms by trial and error, but the problem can often be determined by doing a CDSA (comprehensive stool and digestive analysis). Ask a naturopath or health care practitioner to order this test for you.

Hepatitis C

Hepatitis C is the virus that is the major cause of post-transfusion and community-acquired, non-A, non-B hepatitis. About 60 percent of cases are thought to be contracted through intravenous drug use, blood transfusion, sexual contact or by accidental perforation of the skin with a needle in the presence of contaminated blood. In 40 percent of cases the source of the infection is unknown. The majority of chronic hepatitis C sufferers have no symptoms, although approximately 50 percent have abnormal biochemical lab tests. About 10 to 25 percent of the cases ultimately develop chronic liver disease (cirrhosis). Rare cases progress to cancer of the liver. Until quite recently there was no proven medical therapy for hepatitis C. Studies now indicate that hepatitis C can be helped by injections of interferon.

Published research supports the use of many natural remedies for hepatitis. For example, low sugar consumption is beneficial. So is the avoidance of all fats, animal protein, raw fish, shellfish, alcohol and highly processed foods. Great benefits may be derived from following a raw vegetable and fruit diet for several weeks. Short-term juice fasting is also beneficial.

Since the 1950s there have been several reports on the benefits of supplementation or infusion of vitamin B12, folic acid and vitamin C. The basic effect of these nutrients is to reduce the mean duration of hepatitis. Supplementation with the bioflavonoid cianidanol (catechin) is also effective in reducing the damage seen with hepatitis.

Milk thistle extract (silymarin) helps most liver disorders. So does coenzyme Q10, black radish, red clover, dandelion, burdock, cascara sagrada, gentian, goldenseal, liquid chlorophyll, licorice, pau d'arco, B-complex vitamins and the amino acids L-methionine and L-cysteine. Blue-green algae stimulates the body to manufacture its own interferon and may help speed recovery. Injections of raw liver extract and vitamin B12 may be dramatically effective in some cases. Many patients can learn to give themselves regular injections until the liver has had a chance to repair and rebuild itself. Dosages for all these remedies depend on individual patient tolerance and disease severity. Supervision by a health care practitioner (medical doctor or naturopath) is strongly recommended.

Kidney Stone Prevention and Treatment

The incidence of kidney stones is steadily increasing. In fact, it is ten times more common now than at the turn of the century. It parallels the dramatic increase in the consumption of animal proteins. It also parallels the rise in other diseases (heart disease, gallstones, high blood pressure and diabetes) associated with the standard North American diet. Over ten percent of all males and five percent of all females experience a kidney stone during their lifetime. Most victims are over 30 years of age.

Kidney stones·are usually composed of calcium and oxalic acid. Less commonly, stones are made of uric acid (in people suffering from gout) and other mixed minerals and amino acids (especially cystine). It is important to determine the type of stone and its cause because this leads to a better designed prevention program. If a stone is passed and caught in the urine with the help of a stainer an analysis can be done by a lab to measure its mineral content. If this cannot be done the alternative is to evaluate a number of criteria. These include diet; any underlying metabolic problems or diseases; blood and urine tests for calcium, uric acid, creatinine and electrolyte levels; 24-hour urinalysis for minerals; urine culture and hair mineral analysis. A combination of these things will usually determine the composition of the stone. Any physician can help in this respect.

The majority of kidney stones are completely preventable. Once you have a stone, no diet or supplement can reverse the problem: you need medical attention. However, you can certainly do a lot to prevent the problem from getting worse. Studies indicate that acute attacks of kidney stone pain that lead to hospital admission can be significantly reduced or eliminated by diet and nutritional supplement therapy alone.

Occasionally, kidney stones may be the result of the following metabolic diseases: hyperparathyroidism (overactive glands located near the thyroid gland that control calcium metabolism), hyperthyroidism (overactive thyroid gland causing bone demineralization and calcium deposits), cystinuria (an inherited metabolic disease causing large amounts of cystine to be manufactured in the body leading to cystine stones), vitamin D excess (caused by over-supplementation), the milk-alkali syndrome (stones caused by excessive use of dairy products or antacids), destructive bone diseases (inherited or caused by benign or malignant tumors), primary oxaluria (an inherited condition causing large amounts of oxalates to be formed in the urinary tract), Cushing's syndrome (a condition whereby large amounts of adrenal hormones lead to bone loss and calcium buildup in the urinary tract) and sarcoidosis (a rare inflammatory disease associated with a disorder in calcium metabolism).

Those prone to forming gallstones should drink enough water to produce two to three quarts of urine daily. A recent study by O. M. Embon et al., published in the *British Journal of Urology*, found that approximately 19 percent of those diagnosed with kidney stones were suffering from chronic dehydration. A 1989 study done on tap water concluded that the higher the magnesium-to-calcium ratio in the water, the lower the incidence of kidney stones. Have an analysis done on water used for daily drinking. (See appendix for testing labs.) It just so happens that most patients suffering from kidney stones benefit from magnesium citrate supplementation (300 to 400 mgs daily). Magnesium increases the solubility of calcium oxalate and prevents precipitation in the urine. A large number of studies support its routine use as a stone preventive supplement.

Avoid sugar and refined carbohydrates; sugar, including the lactose found in milk, stimulates the release of insulin which, in turn, causes a higher calcium excretion by the kidney. Sugar increases the absorption of calcium from the intestines. Those prone to kidney stones benefit from a high fiber, vegetarian (vegan) diet. This is because the metabolic breakdown products of animal proteins are uric acid and oxalic acid, both of which are involved in kidney stone formation. Red meat in particular is very high in phosphorus, which causes the body to excrete more calcium into the urine. It is therefore not surprising that vegans are 40 to 60 percent less likely to form kidney stones than the average population.

Kidney stone victims who have a high calcium excretion in the urine should limit their intake of calcium, sodium, vitamin D and caffeine. A high intake of milk, cheese, calcium supplements and antacids for the treatment of peptic ulcers may raise blood calcium levels and increase the predisposition to stones. Urologists have often joked that if every adult suddenly decided to quit dairy products they would quickly be put out of the kidney stone business.

In some individuals, a high salt intake results in increased losses of calcium from the urine, leading to stone formation. Vitamin D increases calcium absorption from the gastrointestinal tract and releases calcium from bone, leading to stone formation in susceptible individuals. Since milk is fortified with vitamin D, this becomes another potential reason for the high association between dairy product consumption and kidney stone incidence. Caffeine may also increase urinary calcium.

Those who form oxalate stones should limit their intake of high oxalate foods, but only if they are also consumers of animal proteins. High oxalate foods include beans, cocoa, coffee, parsley, rhubarb, spinach, tea, beet tops, carrots, celery, chocolate, grapefruit, kale, peanut, pepper and sweet potato. A supplement of pyridoxine (vitamin B6) of not less than 150 mgs daily should be taken to avoid deficiency of this vitamin, which is more common than we may think. Vitamin B6 deficiency prevents oxalic acid from being degraded in the body. Dietary avoidance of high oxalate foods however, will make only a slight difference with respect to urinary oxalate excretion. Vitamin B6 supplementation may be far more crucial in the overall prevention of oxalate stones.

Vitamin A and vitamin K deficiency may help promote the formation of kidney stones. This is because both vitamins are required by the body to make a common protein found in urine that inhibits calcium oxalate crystalline growth. Low levels of glutamic acid also increase calcium oxalate precipitation. Supplementation with glutamic acid (300 mgs daily) may be important as a preventive in some cases. Aloe vera juice may also be a good kidney stone preventive.

Those who form uric acid stones are helped by a vegetarian diet and supplementation with folic acid and potassium citrate. Citrate is an inhibitor of stone formation and is usually recommended as a supplement by most kidney specialists treating stones. Low levels of citrate are found in 20 to 60 percent of all patients with kidney stones. Avoidance of alcohol is important because alcohol increases the excretion of uric acid, calcium and phosphate and has adverse effects on vitamin B6 and magnesium, both of which help in stone prevention.

Megadoses of vitamin C (more than 6,000 mgs daily) increase urinary oxalate excretion and may be a factor precipitating stones in a minority of cases. There is no study, however, that proves that megadoses of vitamin C lead to a greater incidence of kidney stones. In nearly 15 years of practice, I have never been able to document a single case of kidney stones stemming from vitamin C supplementation. Neither has anyone else. In fact, several published studies claim that the opposite is true: that vitamin C supplementation prevents kidney stones. If vitamin C intake is combined with supplementation with magnesium citrate and vitamin B6, one can be even more confident about prevention.

High body burdens of cadmium have also been associated with an increased incidence of kidney stones. Cadmium excess can be reliably determined by hair mineral analysis. Excesses can be removed from the body by supplementation with zinc, vitamin B6, magnesium and vitamin C. Intravenous chelation therapy can also be done in severe cases. Finally, if there is a history of kidney stones, avoid supplementation with the amino acid L-cystine, a build-up of which can lead to stone formation in genetically susceptible individuals. A prevention program against kidney stones must be individualized as much as possible and followed for life. Work with a doctor to determine the best possible course of action.

Kidney Pain Relief

Kidney stones, cysts and benign tumors can be helped by low protein (low phosphorus), low fat vegetarian diets. Even cases of advanced kidney failure can be helped.

If kidney function is normal, safe and effective pain relief is available from a variety of modalities, including physiotherapy, acupuncture, chiropractic manipulation, hypnosis, behavior modification, muscle strengthening exercises, therapeutic massage, meditation, biofeedback, TENS (transcutaneous electrical nerve stimulation) and natural analgesics. Avoidance of animal fats and coffee reduces the severity of pain from any source.

Most people are not aware of natural pain controllers like DLPA (DL-phenylalanine), magnesium, niacinamide, L-tryptophan, vitamin B1, niacin, vitamin B6, vitamin B12, vitamin C, vitamin E and essential fatty acids (flax seed oil, evening primrose oil, rice bran oil). Megadoses far above the RDA are usually required to produce an analgesic effect when any of these are taken orally.

In more resistant cases, intravenous or intramuscular magnesium sulphate injections are necessary to get a result. Herbs such as alfalfa, capsicum, camomile, clove oil, wintergreen, valerian, burdock, yarrow and feverfew are also effective for chronic pain control. Trial and error may be necessary to decide specific doses and combinations. A natural health care practitioner can be very helpful in prescribing and supervising a personalized pain control program.

Hyperparathyroidism

Hyperparathyroidism is a disease of unknown cause resulting from excessive secretion of parathyroid hormone (PTH). Sometimes the problem is caused by kidney disease or by tumors that secrete PTH. It is usually characterized by high blood levels of calcium, low phosphorus levels and abnormal bone metabolism. Kidney stones and loss of bone mass may occur.

Hyperparathyroidism is usually asymptomatic, but in severe cases there may be ulcers, irritability, memory loss, headaches, muscle weakness and constipation. In advanced cases, large cysts (where bone is replaced by fibrous tissue) can be seen on x-rays. This is called osteitis fibrosis cystica (von Recklinghausen's disease).

There is no specific, recognized alternative therapy for hyperparathyroidism. Kidney stones can be prevented by following a vegetarian diet, high in fiber and complex carbohydrates. Green leafy vegetables (with the exception of spinach) should be increased, while intake of simple carbohydrates and high purines (meat, fish, poultry and yeast) should be kept as low as possible. Avoid high oxalate foods like tea, cocoa, spinach, beets, rhubarb, parsley, cranberry and nuts. Avoid dairy products. Supplements of magnesium, potassium, glutamic acid, vitamin K and vitamin B6 may be of help to offset some of the side effects of excessive calcium.

Bladder Infections

Recurrent infections with repeated antibiotic prescriptions are usually the result of a high simple carbohydrate (sugar) intake or unsuspected food allergies. The most common allergens are milk, wheat, citrus, corn, eggs and chocolate. Whether lactose-free or not, I suggest that milk and all dairy products, including yogurt, be kept out of the diet for at least six weeks. A high sugar intake from fruit juices (except fresh, unsweetened cranberry juice) should also be avoided because sugar feeds the bacteria in the gastrointestinal tract responsible for most bladder infections. The only fluid to push is lots of spring water. A variety of lab tests can help determine hidden food allergies, the best of which is the Elisa/Act test.

Studies have also shown that simple carbohydrates (glucose, fructose and sucrose) have a depressant effect on the immune system as early as an hour after eating them. Removing sugar and white flour products from the diet is often very helpful. A diet high in saturated animal fats impairs immune function. A higher intake of the omega-3-EPA oils (found in halibut, cod, mackerel, salmon, trout, tuna) and gamma linolenic acid (flax seed oil, evening primrose oil, borage oil, black currant oil) enhances immune function. There are many natural supplements that have been documented to help with bladder infections. These include vitamin A (from cod or halibut liver oil), beta-carotene, vitamin B complex, vitamin C, the very potent bioflavonoid pycnogenol, pau d'arco, garlic, astragalus, blue-green algae, bee pollen, propolis, St. John's wort, echinacea, lomatium and common herbs such as calendula, goldenseal, elderberry, capsicum, horehound and camomile.

Most prescription antibiotics wipe out all the friendly bacteria in the bowel. These bacteria aid digestion, boost immune function, help manufacture several vitamins (e.g., vitamin B12, biotin and vitamin K) and synthesize short-chain fatty acids that help prevent bowel cancer. Taking a supplement of lactobacillus acidophilus after antibiotic prescriptions or whenever there is an infection is a good idea. For specific doses and an individualized diet and supplement program, see a natural health care practitioner.

Nephrotic Syndrome and Diet

Nephrotic syndrome is characterized by excess protein in the urine, low albumin in the blood, high blood fats and edema (fluid retention). There are many different health conditions associated with nephrotic syndrome. Each case must be treated somewhat differently.

In serious medical conditions, homeopathic/naturopathic medicine can only be considered to be complementary to conventional medical treatment. In many cases, there are no alternatives to the medical approach, which involves the use of cortisone-like drugs. For some, the natural approach is effective in reducing or eliminating the need for cortisone. Optimizing nutritional intake to match biochemical individuality is desirable. If possible, get a nutritional evaluation done to determine vitamin, mineral and amino acid deficiencies.

Food allergy or intolerance may be the cause of some cases of nephrotic syndrome. One study reports that two out of two cases recovered from this condition when food allergens were removed from the diet, while a second study reports that six out of twenty-six recovered. Food allergy testing done by the Elisa/Act blood test is worth doing. It may open the doors for a recovery without drugs. Unfortunately, this blood test is not accurate if you are taking cortisone, certain analgesics or anti-inflammatory drugs. In other words, you must be off such drugs for several days before having the test done.

Studies indicate that victims of nephrotic syndrome develop deficiencies in zinc. This is probably because of increased urinary zinc loss from the body. If you start taking cortisone, one of the minerals that may need to be supplemented is zinc. Cortisone, and many other drugs, tend to make the body lose zinc in greater amounts than can easily be obtained from the diet. Have your doctor order a 24-hour urine test for minerals such as calcium, magnesium and zinc. Also, get a hair mineral analysis done to find out about toxic heavy metals such as cadmium, lead, mercury, aluminum, nickel, copper and arsenic. Some of these metals can be stored in the body for long periods of time and can lead to kidney damage.

Prostate Problems

The prostate, a male sexual organ, is a solid, chestnut-shaped gland situated around the urethra, under the urinary bladder just in front of the rectum. It provides some secretions that make up semen. It enlarges at puberty due to the influence of androgens and usually ceases growth at about age 20. Studies indicate that nearly every man over age 45 has some abnormal prostate enlargement. Symptoms of an enlarged prostate (benign prostatic hypertrophy or BPH) include pain, burning sensation, sexual dysfunction, difficulty starting and stopping urination and the need to urinate frequently, especially at night (nocturia). Some men with enlarged prostates have no symptoms and are only alerted to the problem during an annual physical examination.

Chronic inflammation of the prostate (prostatitis) can be caused by infection with candida and bacteria. It can be associated with a recurring bladder infection (cystitis), reduced sperm quality, infertility, pain and difficult urination. Conventional treatment includes advice about avoidance of spices, alcohol and sexual activities. Medical treatment may involve the use of sitz baths, antibiotics, anticholinergic drugs, prostate massage, bedrest and analgesics. Treatment often depends on the causative organism isolated by laboratory testing. If no infective organism is found, one should be suspicious of chronic candidiasis or food intolerances/allergies.

Some natural measures can be taken to both prevent and treat prostate problems. Studies have shown that supplemental GLA (gamma linolenic acid), cold-pressed flax seed oil, zinc picolinate or chelate, vitamin C and vitamin E may all be helpful for both BPH and prostatitis.

Vitamin and mineral supplements do not interfere with any medications generally prescribed for prostate problems. Zinc can cause some sensitive individuals to experience nausea. If this happens, take zinc after food or switch to a different brand. If suffering from a hiatus hernia, eat frequent small meals and nothing after 6 p.m. so as to avoid symptoms during sleep. Always take supplements in divided doses after meals.

It is important to take in adequate fluids (at least 64 fluid ounces per day), follow a high fiber diet and use natural stool softeners such as aloe vera, prunes or prune juice. Herbs such as senna, buckthorn, rhubarb, cascara sagrada, slippery elm, burdock, cress, pau d'arco and liquid chlorophyll can certainly enhance elimination. The herbal combination of burdock, Turkish rhubarb, slippery elm and sheep sorrel is not only known for its bowel cleansing effects, but also for its blood purifying properties. All these herbs are effective at optimizing toxin elimination. Regular exercise will also promote good bowel function.

As a general nutritional guide, and if otherwise healthy, have on a daily basis at least five servings of whole grains, three of fruits, three of starchy and non-starchy vegetables and at least two servings of legumes (starchy beans). This prevents strain and discomfort during bowel movements. Psyllium seed and lactobacillus acidophilus supplements may be helpful in the control of the large bowel flora. The use of bee pollen (one to six teaspoons daily) can prevent the frequent urination and poor urine flow that occurs with prostate enlargement.

Recent research has shown that an extract of the saw palmetto berry can reverse benign prostatic hypertrophy (prostate enlargement with aging). The effect of this extract is to inhibit the male hormone breakdown product dihydrotestosterone, which causes the enlargement. Saw palmetto not only shrinks swollen prostate glands, but may also help to increase hair growth in prematurely balding men and to prevent male and female pattern balding, seen as "inevitable" with age. It can also reduce or eliminate hirsuitism (excessive body hair) and virilism in females if taken for several months on a consistent basis. Pumpkin seed oil also inhibits the enzyme that converts testosterone to dihydrotestosterone, and has been demonstrated to reverse benign prostatic hypertrophy. Like flax seed oil, it is rich in essential fatty acids and has a natural anti-inflammatory effect.

Pygeum, another herbal remedy, has been shown to significantly improve the symptoms of benign prostatic hypertrophy in at least 75 percent of patients within 60 days. Pygeum contains sterols, terpenoids and plant alcohols. These substances have an anti-inflammatory effect by inhibiting the production of certain prostaglandins associated with pain and swelling. The special plant alcohols found in pygeum reduce the accumulation of cholesterol by-products in the prostate. Pygeum improves sexual and reproductive functions and is also effective for several male genital infections. Other herbs reported to help prostate enlargement and inflammation are ginger, parsley, juniper, capsicum, uva ursi, ginseng and echinacea.

Although this natural approach has a high success rate, stubborn cases may require food allergy and/or candida detection and treatment. The most common food allergies associated with prostate problems include milk, wheat, yeast, corn, chocolate, citrus fruits and eggs. The treatment of chronic candida infection may involve the use of a special diet, antifungal supplements or prescription drugs.

Penicillin and Bowel Toxemia

The long-term use of penicillin may lead to an overgrowth of candida and other harmful bacteria or fungi in the large bowel. Supplementation with lactobacillus acidophilus and the herb goldenseal is usually helpful in the prevention of such bowel toxemia problems associated with long-term antibiotic use.

The Joy of Juice Fasting, by Klaus Kaufmann, and *Elderberry Internal Cleansing Therapy*, by Dr. Brunhild Zechelius, give information on how one can safely do bowel detoxification and internal cleansing over a period of ten days. The Sambu cleansing program discussed in the Zechelius book is available in health food stores. So is another alternative—the very popular bowel detoxification program developed by Dr. Robert Gray. I believe all these approaches are equally effective. Your choice will depend primarily on lifestyle and on individual likes and dislikes. Before deciding on any detoxification program, check with a doctor or naturopath in case there are any potential health problems that need to be addressed.

Healing Hemorrhoids Naturally

Hemorrhoids (piles) are distended or ruptured veins located within or just outside the anus. They are varicose veins that result from several factors, including heredity, pregnancy, prostate enlargement, obesity, straining at stool, constipation, improper or heavy lifting, sedentary lifestyle, standing for long periods of time, sitting on cold, hard surfaces, liver disease (cirrhosis), food allergies, alcohol or drug abuse and anal intercourse. Hemorrhoids may itch, bleed, tear and cause pain. They can usually be treated naturally, but severe cases may require surgery.

From a dietary standpoint, it is very important to increase fluids. A diet high in fiber and complex carbohydrates is also recommended. Avoid animal products as much as possible as well as coffee, spicy foods, fried foods, alcohol, hot sauces, fatty foods, rich foods, salty foods, sugar and refined carbohydrates. Eat more cranberries, water chestnuts, buckwheat, tangerines, figs, plums, prunes, guavas, bamboo shoots, mung beans, melons, black sesame seeds, persimmons, bananas, squash, cucumbers, tofu, blueberries, blackberries and cherries. Avoid cigarette smoking and a lack of exercise; both habits make hemorrhoids worse.

Fresh juices that may be therapeutic include carrot, spinach, potato, turnip, watercress, celery, and parsley. Topical, soothing herbal remedies are aloe vera and calendula. Herbs that may be helpful in oral supplement form are aloe vera juice, psyllium seed husks or powder, camomile, buckthorn, collinsonia root and elderberry. Flax seed oil (one to two tablespoons daily) creates a natural lubricating effect by softening stools. A garlic clove or raw potato can be made into a rectal suppository for relief of rectal itching. Homeopathic rectal suppositories can also be quite effective. Mineral (sitz) baths are also helpful. Different things will work better for given individuals. Supplemental nutrients that are often prescribed to help shrink hemorrhoidal tissue and promote healing are beta-carotene, bioflavonoids (rutin, hesperidin, catechin, quercetin, pycnogenol) coenzyme Q10 and vitamins A, B-complex, C and E.

For bleeding hemorrhoids, supplementation with vitamin K may be necessary. To get adequate amounts of vitamin K from the diet, eat more dark green leafy vegetables such as spinach, alfalfa, kale and lettuce. Dosages for all supplements would, of course, have to be individualized. Supervision by a naturopath or medical doctor familiar with vitamins, minerals and herbs is ideal.

Pinworms

Pinworms are very common, seldom harmful and treatment is usually not mandatory. Most people who get them, however, are alarmed by the sight of the worms and find the anal itching unacceptable. The drug pyrantel pamoate is well tolerated and there are no adverse effects on the liver or any other organ. Infrequent side effects include vomiting and diarrhea. This drug will eradicate pinworms in close to 100 percent of cases. It is given as a single oral dose based on body weight. In rare conditions, the dosage may have to be repeated.

When treating pinworms, it is very important to treat all other family members regardless of symptoms. Rigorous cleaning of living quarters and clothing will help prevent reinfection. Personal hygiene (i.e., do not scratch the anus) is also very important to prevent spread.

Natural treatment involves following a diet high in fiber and complex carbohydrates and avoiding red meat, sugar and refined foods. Herbal supplements that may be used as alternatives to drugs include high doses of garlic, pumpkin seeds, sesame seeds, pink root, wormseed, worm-wood, black walnut extract and chaparral. Lactobacillus acidophilus supplements are also a good idea. Several manufacturers make supplements containing combinations of these herbs in a single capsule. Please remember that the natural remedies are not without their side effects (nausea, vomiting, diarrhea). A natural health care practitioner or naturopath can help supervise the therapy.

Celiac Disease and Alcoholism

Celiac disease is caused by an intolerance to gluten. Gluten is the name of the protein found in wheat, barley, rye and oats. These same foods can be found to varying degrees in practically all alcoholic products. If one is sensitive or allergic to any of these grains, then one would also be sensitive and allergic to any foods or beverages that contain the same food substances.

Doctors specializing in the treatment of allergic disorders have noticed that many patients found to be allergic to common foods like wheat, also craved or were addicted to the same foods. Alcohol addiction is similar since the alcoholic craves a food that is known to cause damage to his or her system. When an alcoholic is able to give up alcohol, the cravings and addictions are often shifted to foods high in simple carbohydrates, like wheat, sugar, yeast – that is, foods found in alcoholic beverages.

The link between these seemingly different conditions (alcoholism and wheat allergy) may be that both produce varying degrees of hypoglycemia (low blood sugar) temporarily relieved by eating the same foods. This may also help explain why so many ex-alcoholics crave or transfer their addictive behavior to foods high in sugar. Drinking large amounts of alcohol leads to hypoglycemia; so does the consumption of allergic foods. An alcoholic experiences withdrawal symptoms during the first week that he or she abstains from alcohol. These may include insomnia, acute anxiety, rapid pulse rate, extreme perspiration and even seizures. Severe hypoglycemia can produce identical symptoms.

Sclerosing Cholangitis

The passages in the body that connect the liver to the gall bladder are called the bile ducts. When the bile ducts become inflamed and gradually filled with fibrous tissue, a rare, chronic disease called sclerosing cholangitis develops. The fibrous tissue leads to obstruction in the bile ducts and eventually causes deposition of bile salts in the skin. The most common symptoms of this disease are jaundice and itching. Other symptoms may include loss of appetite, general malaise, indigestion and pain in the upper abdomen.

More than half of the victims of sclerosing cholangitis also have ulcerative colitis, a severe inflammatory bowel disease. The cause of sclerosing cholangitis is unknown. The inflammation may spread to the liver, causing the release of various substances that can be measured in the blood. Diagnosis can be made by special x-rays (percutaneous transhepatic cholangiography).

The conventional medical treatment is to use the drug cholestyramine to reduce itching. In some cases of obstruction, balloon dilatation may be done for relief. Sometimes obstruction can be corrected by surgery and, in severe cases, a liver transplant may have to be performed. There is no specific, proven natural treatment for sclerosing cholangitis. There are, however, a number of basic principles that could be considered for complementary medical treatment.

Published research supports the use of many natural remedies for liver disease of all types. For example, low sugar consumption is beneficial. So is the avoidance of all fats, animal protein, raw fish, shellfish, alcohol and highly processed foods. Great benefits may be derived from following a raw vegetable and fruit diet for several weeks. Short-term juice fasting for detoxification is also helpful (see the *Joy of Juice Fasting*, by Klaus Kaufmann). Therapeutic juices include radish and pineapple, black cherry concentrate mixed with liquid chlorophyll and a combination of carrot, beet, green pepper, spinach, papaya and cucumber juices.

Milk thistle extract (silymarin) helps most liver disorders. So does coenzyme Q10, black radish, artichoke, tumeric, red clover, dandelion, B-complex vitamins, Liv 52, lactobacillus acidophilus and the amino acids methionine and cysteine. Injections of folic acid, vitamin B12 and other B-complex vitamins may be dramatically effective in cases where energy levels have been severely impaired. Many patients can learn to give themselves regular injections until the liver has had a chance to repair and rebuild itself.

The herbal tea combination of slippery elm, burdock, Turkish rhubarb, cress and sheep sorrel may be of great help in cleansing the liver. With almost all these natural remedies, the healing process may be slow, requiring a period of months or years. The important thing is to stick to it, get regular lab tests done for liver function and maintain a positive mental attitude. Supervision by a natural health care practitioner is strongly recommended.

Cystic Fibrosis

Cystic fibrosis (CF), an inherited disease of the perspiration and exocrine glands, causes chronic respiratory infections, abnormally thick mucous secretions, pancreatic insufficiency and poor heat tolerance. The sweat, salivary and parotid glands secrete excessive amounts of sodium and chloride and this forms the basis of the "sweat chloride test" used to make the diagnosis. Approximately one in 1,800 people suffer from CF: the incidence is slightly higher in whites than in blacks and is rare among orientals. About 90 percent of cases are discovered during infancy, while 10 percent with milder symptoms are detected in adolescence or young adulthood.

Cystic fibrosis is a serious disorder. The average survival for CF patients is approximately 20 years, but many patients survive into their twenties and thirties. Early diagnosis improves prognosis. Cystic fibrosis affects the lungs, leading to bronchitis, pneumonia, bronchiectasis, lung abscesses, sinusitis, nasal polyps, cardiac complications and even respiratory failure. A long list of digestive problems result from pancreatic insufficiency—the inability of the pancreas to secrete digestive enzymes. Some of these gastrointestinal complications include diabetes mellitus, liver problems, hemorrhoids, constipation and nutritional deficiencies and malnutrition caused by poor absorption. In males, there may be sterility due to defective or absent organs (vas, epididymis, seminal vesicles) in the genital tract.

In females, decreased fertility results from the increased viscosity of the vaginal secretions. Bone development may be retarded and bone itself may be demineralized (osteoporosis).

With respect to diet, it is advisable to avoid animal products, processed foods, cooked foods, coffee, tea, alcohol and caffeinated beverages (colas, chocolate milk), sugar, candies, alcohol, spicy foods, fried and salty foods. Beware of caffeine in various herbs, cocoa-flavored soy or rice beverages and analgesics, as these may aggravate symptoms. The diet recommended for CF is 60 to 75 percent complex carbohydrates (raw fruits, vegetables, nuts, seeds and legumes), 15 to 30 percent protein and 10 to 15 percent fat, mostly from medium-chain triglycerides (MCT). Pancreatin (pancreatic digestive enzymes) must be taken with each meal. It should be noted that in some cases whole grains and dairy products may aggravate the mucous secretion problem. Each case is unique, and food allergy testing may help personalize the diet.

Supplements that may be used and monitored by lab tests to determine optimal dosages are evening primrose oil, zinc, selenium and vitamins A, B-complex, C, D, E and K. Blood, urine and hair mineral analysis are all worth doing to get a good idea of vitamin, mineral and enzyme levels. Digestion can also be improved by regularly drinking aloe vera juice and supplementing with lactobacillus acidophilus. Free-form amino acid supplements ensure adequate protein intake, needed for tissue repair and growth.

Immune system stimulants like raw thymus extract, coenzyme Q10, blue-green algae and other green supplements may help reduce the infection rate. Herbal antibiotics, which may be used either alone or in combination, are echinacea, goldenseal, propolis, garlic, astragalus, burdock, slippery elm, sheep sorrel, Turkish rhubarb, capsicum, chaparral, red clover, ma huang, white willow bark, sea kelp, elderberry, pau d'arco and calendula.

Ginger root and yarrow tea are very soothing for almost any gastrointestinal ailment. The amino acid N-acetyl-cysteine (NAC) is another natural antibiotic. It can dissolve mucous buildup anywhere in the respiratory tract and is particularly effective with sinusitis and bronchitis. If antibiotics have been prescribed, it is important to supplement with lactobacillus acidophilus. These friendly bowel bacteria, which are killed off by prescription antibiotics, are important to help prevent yeast (candida) and other infections.

5

The Brain, Nerves and Mind

D isorders of the brain and the nervous system are traditionally thought to be the domain of the neurologist and psychiatrist. These branches of medicine use drugs primarily to effect changes in brain biochemistry. The "chemical imbalance" of depression, schizophrenia, Parkinson's disease and other nervous system problems can often be improved and even eliminated by the use of modern pharmaceuticals. So, why this chapter?

The answer lies in the fact that most brain and nervous system disorders respond favorably to a natural approach. Multiple sclerosis, insomnia, migraine headaches, dizziness, tinnitus and other ailments can all improve through the use of natural remedies alone or in combination with prescription drugs. This is possible because the chemical imbalance may be the direct result of mercury or lead toxicity, amino acid deficiencies, vitamin B12 deficiency, food and chemical allergies or many other previously unsuspected factors. Correcting the imbalance usually clears up the symptoms. For each condition that a drug is used to treat, there is a natural substance or combination of natural remedies that will work equally well, if not better.

Intelligence, memory, reaction time, vision, hearing, taste and other perceptions can all be optimized through the use of vitamins, minerals, herbs and amino acids. Natural substances like ginkgo biloba (the single most widely used herb in the world) and DHEA have been proven to retard aging, enhance intelligence and memory and improve the health of all the senses. You will find references to ginkgo biloba, DHEA and other natural compounds throughout this chapter. Making good use of them might well be the key to a longer and healthier life.

Migraine Headaches

Most sufferers describe a migraine headache as severe pain on one side of the head accompanied by nausea, vomiting and hypersensitivity to light. Migraines are frequently preceded by a number of warning symptoms, including fluid retention, mood swings, food cravings, fatigue and visual disturbances. They may last from a few hours to several days. Standard medical drug therapy is helpful, but migraines can often be prevented and treated naturally.

Common Triggers:

Airplane travel

Emotional upsets

Excessive smoking

Food and chemical allergies

Menstruation

Missing a meal

Over sleeping

Sleep deprivation

Strong odors (perfumes, tobacco)

Weather changes

Whiplash

The most common foods that should be avoided by migraine sufferers include those that contain tyramine: chocolate, yeast and yeast products (e.g., Marmite), liver, sausages, beans, pickled herring and cheese. Foods that contain histamine, such as sauerkraut, salami and cold cuts, may also be culprits. Other common foods documented to trigger migraines include oranges, bananas, wheat and milk products. Food additives such as tartrazine, benzoate, BHT, BHA and MSG can also trigger migraines. The birth control pill, a high salt intake, caffeine-containing foods (coffee, tea, cola drinks and chocolates), alcohol (especially red wine) and sugar may all act as triggers for sensitive individuals.

Less common and controversial migraine triggers include spinal misalignments (often correctable by osteopathic or chiropractic adjustment), tempero-mandibular joint dysfunction (jaw misalignment; sometimes correctable with dental treatment) and toxic heavy metal hypersensitivity (especially from mercury dental fillings).

Non-Drug Treatments

Natural food supplements that help prevent migraine attacks include vitamin B complex, vitamin C, bioflavonoids (rutin, hesperidin, catechin, pycnogenol or quercetin), vitamin E and essential fatty acids (flax seed oil, evening primrose oil and fish oils). The herbs ginger, white willow bark, ginkgo biloba extract, peppermint, rosemary, wormwood and feverfew reduce pain and nausea. The amino acid DL-phenylalanine is an effective natural pain killer for pain of any source. It is available in health food stores in the United States without a prescription. In Canada, it is generally not available except through the offices of some natural health care practitioners. Supervision by a naturopath, chiropractor or medical doctor familiar with natural therapies is recommended.

Migraine Headaches and Hormones

Some women get migraine headaches either premenstrually or during their periods because of a strong sensitivity to the hormonal changes that occur with each menstrual cycle. These types of migraine are benefited by high-dose vitamin E supplementation. Vitamin E increases the body's synthesis of prostaglandin E-1 (PGE-1), which antagonizes the hormone prolactin. Prolactin has been reported in some studies to be associated with premenstrual pain. Vitamin E is effective in controlling breast tenderness and other PMS symptoms, including mood swings, anxiety, confusion and headaches. Caffeine in coffee, tea, soft drinks and drugs may aggravate the problem and should be avoided at all times.

Hormonal types of migraine often respond favorably to candida therapy. This is because candida manufactures various steroid substances that contribute to hormone imbalance problems. A three-month trial therapy with a candida treatment program may help some victims prevent migraines. Such therapy may include the use of psyllium seed powder, digestive enzymes, glutamic acid, olive oil, garlic, lactobacillus acidophilus, pau d'arco, caprylic acid, fish oil concentrates, flax seed oil or other natural remedies. In rare cases, mercury and other heavy metal toxicities should be suspected as possible contributing factors to a chronic candida overgrowth situation.

Many cases of subclinical hypothyroidism are behind chronic, intractable PMS symptoms like migraine headaches. Although conventional lab tests for thyroid problems may be entirely normal, these cases respond well to natural desiccated thyroid hormone prescriptions. Typically, people with subclinical hypothyroidism have low body temperatures on average. Temperatures normalize, however, once thyroid hormone is taken.

Some cases of subclinical hypothyroidism do better with time-released Liothyronine (T3) prescriptions. There are also those who benefit from L-thyroxine (T4) or a combination of T3 and T4. It's a matter of biochemical individuality, current drug usage, level of stress and current nutritional status. Nutrients like iodine, zinc, copper, selenium, tyrosine, vitamin B6 and other antioxidants are all important for healthy thyroid function.

Many doctors have reported excellent pain relief of menstrual cramps and migraine headaches using natural progesterone cream derived from an extract of wild yam. Applying 1/2 teaspoon to the skin daily for the three weeks prior to menses, then stopping once the period commences, will usually be enough to prevent migraines. In more severe cases, apply the cream every 15 minutes until the pain disappears. This is in addition to the three-week premenstrual use. In rare cases that fail to respond after three months, a trial of higher dose progesterone suppositories may be the only recourse.

Alzheimer's Nutrition Connection

Alzheimer's disease is a devastating disorder in which certain brain cells die prematurely, producing progressive memory loss and generalized intellectual deterioration. The course of the disease is variable, running anywhere from two to twenty years. In North America, about 15 percent of those over age 65 have Alzheimer's. In early cases, there may be loss of orientation to time and place and to persons known only casually. There may be impairment of memory for recent events and of the ability to carry out sequences of events. In early cases, there may also be a loss of spatial orientation. As the disease progresses, memory for remote events becomes impaired, there is a loss of orientation to well-known persons, a loss of vocabulary (i.e., word-finding difficulty) and a loss of self-care capacity (dressing, bathing, eating, toileting). Finally, in the late stages of the disease, there is a loss of physiologic function, including the ability to swallow, control urination or defecation and to regulate breathing and blood pressure.

Although the cause of Alzheimer's is unknown, there is much speculation about aluminum, as researchers have found high concentrations of this metal in the dead neurons of victims. Aluminum is very abundant in our environment, and some theorize that overexposure to it—from pots and pans, antacids, food additives, buffered aspirin, antidiarrheal preparations, shampoos and contaminated water—leads to the disease. High body burdens of aluminum can be determined by blood and hair mineral analysis. It is believed by some scientists that a combination of magnesium insufficiency in conjunction with abnormally high levels of aluminum in the brain cells can inhibit the activity of many magnesium-dependent enzymes, resulting in the progression of Alzheimer's disease. Another theory is that Alzheimer's is caused by a slow virus. A third possibility is that there may be a genetic component. However, a clear pattern of inheritance has not been established.

Alzheimer's must be distinguished from the generalized decline in function we call aging. It is also not the type of dementia that results from hardening of the arteries. Alzheimer's involves a specific degeneration in primarily one system of brain cells located at the base of the forebrain—the uppermost and largest component of the brain. This part of the brain sends information to broad regions of the cerebral cortex and to an area called the hippocampus, which is vital for memory. The cells involved use the chemical messenger (neurotransmitter) acetylcholine: it is this chemical that is lost by cells affected by Alzheimer's. Over a variable period of time, the cells degenerate and die. At that point it is thought that nothing can then be done to revive or replace them. However, if their function can be supported during the period of degeneration by increasing the production of or delaying the destruction of brain supplies of acetylcholine, then the inevitable might at least be delayed.

The raw material used by the brain to make acetylcholine is choline. Choline can be obtained from the diet (soybeans, eggs) or taken as a supplement called lecithin (phosphatidyl choline). Studies indicate that a minimum six-month trial of 10 to 20 grams of 95 percent phosphatidyl choline may be beneficial in retarding the rate of disease progression. Phosphatidyl choline is available at most health food stores without a prescription. Side effects are negligible.

Research in France and Germany indicates that the herb ginkgo biloba may be effective against Alzheimer's. Ginkgo biloba extract has a remarkable effect on different parts of the circulatory and nervous system. Some of its actions include enhancement of energy production, an increase in cellular glucose uptake, an increase in blood flow to the brain and an improvement of the transmission of nerve signals. Coenzyme Q10 has also been shown to be effective because this natural substance carries oxygen to cells. It is available as a supplement at most health food stores. Both ginkgo biloba extract and coenzyme Q10 have negligible side effects.

Many studies and clinical observations indicate that patients with dementia are likely to be nutritionally deficient. Commonly reported deficiencies include folic acid, tryptophan, boron, potassium, selenium, zinc, magnesium, beta-carotene and vitamins B1, B2, B6, B12, C, D and E. Excess body levels of copper, cadmium and manganese have been associated with an increased risk of dementia. Hair mineral analysis may be valuable here. A thorough nutritional evaluation that includes diet intake history, blood, urine and hair mineral analysis can help guide health care practitioners in their prescription of appropriate nutritional supplements.

Finally, in the book *Beating Alzheimer's*, Tom Warren describes his dramatic recovery from the disease. Crucial to his success was the isolation and treatment of food and chemical allergies as well as mercury toxicity emanating from dental fillings. His theory is that Alzheimer's is really an autoimmune response or a type of cerebral allergy. Although this area is still controversial, exploring the possibility of hidden food allergies, chemical hypersensitivities and mercury toxicity from dental fillings may open the doors to recovery for at least some sufferers of the disease.

Anorexia

No one seems to know the cause of anorexia nervosa. It is generally assumed to be the result of social stresses, causing adolescent girls (only five percent of anorexics are boys) to avoid food almost entirely. It is both a psychological and a physiological disorder in which the teenage girl seems to have abdicated all responsibility for the nourishment of her body. There is an intense fear of becoming obese. It is estimated that about one to two percent of the female population between twelve and eighteen is afflicted.

Since the mortality rate has been reported as high as twenty percent, anorexia nervosa is a very serious condition necessitating a multidisciplinary treatment approach which may include hospitalization. Death results from starvation, infections, heart rhythm disorders or suicide. All forms of treatment are normally resisted, and no amount of common sense or persuasion will change the behavior.

There is no specific personality type that is predisposed to anorexia nervosa. The average case may be depressed, anxious, weepy, agitated, hostile, underweight, constipated, amenorrheic (loss of periods) and suffer from a lowered self-esteem. An anorexic is typically preoccupied with avoiding food, has a decreased interest in sex, a disturbed body image and a distorted hunger awareness. Even though sufferers appear emaciated, they are obsessed with the idea that they are fat.

One double-blind, placebo controlled study suggests that zinc deficiency may play a role in causing anorexia nervosa. Most extreme weight reduction diets are low in zinc and, in the long run, lead to overt zinc deficiency. The birth control pill and certain steroid drugs cause the body to increase the excretion of zinc, so these too may be a factor in the development of a zinc deficiency. Additionally, the body's need for zinc is dramatically increased during the rapid growth phase of adolescence. Since zinc deficiency can cause a loss of appetite, researchers have postulated that what is happening is a vicious circle of zinc deficiency leading to appetite loss, leading to more severe zinc deficiency and finally to anorexia nervosa. The implications for prevention are obvious. A zinc supplement in the RDA dosage range (15 mgs daily) should certainly be considered for adolescent girls, especially if they are on the birth control pill, smoking cigarettes or dieting on a regular basis. The best, most bioavailable form of zinc is zinc picolinate.

Natural appetite stimulants that may have a beneficial effect include ginger root, ginseng, gotu cola, catnip, fennel, saw palmetto and peppermint.

Other products that could be helpful (provided the patient is cooperative to some extent) include lactobacillus acidophilus, brewer's yeast, iron citrate, kelp, protein supplements with free-form amino acids and a broad-spectrum multivitamin and mineral supplement. In very resistive cases, daily injections of crude liver extract and vitamin B12 can also be beneficial. Some homeopathic remedies may be helpful in dealing with disturbances in the hormonal (endocrine) system.

Bulimia

Adolescent girls who diet to extremes but do not progress to the full clinical picture of anorexia nervosa may develop a pattern of compulsive binge eating followed by self-induced vomiting or the use of laxatives to expel food quickly from the body (bulimia nervosa). Outward signs of bulimia are not nearly as obvious as those seen in anorexia nervosa, but the condition is just as life-threatening. One of the problems with the frequent use of laxatives is the depletion of potassium from the body. This can cause an irregular heart beat and heart failure.

Periods of extreme low-calorie, low-micronutrient dieting or anorexia may lead to bulimia. As in anorexia nervosa, the condition is usually seen in girls. Patients are often depressed, anxious and have a disturbed body image with a lowered self-esteem. The bulimic behavior (the binge/purge cycles) may become compulsive and uncontrollable. Although long-term psychotherapy is the only effective method of treatment, food addictions or allergies should also be considered.

According to many holistic doctors and nutritionists, some food addictions that lead to binging are really food allergies in disguise. When a food allergy elimination approach is applied to a balanced weight loss program, the binging cycles can be curtailed, in some cases within three to four weeks. In more severe cases, a three-week hypoallergenic fast clears the system long enough to break the cycle of binging and purging. Juice fasting combined with enemas (as described by Paavo Airola in many of his books) may be very effective in clearing food antibodies out of the system. Fasting is best done under the supervision of a health care practitioner.

It is vital, however, that the patient receive either individual or group psychotherapy concurrent with any nutritional therapy. Extreme cases may require medication, but I must point out that no drug therapies have ever been proven to cure eating disorders. The best approach is preventive, which requires a good basic knowledge of nutrition and personal responsibility. For information on anorexia and bulimia associations, see the appendix.

Society and Eating Disorders

The problems associated with eating disorders stem from a sick society. The same is ultimately true for any disease. There are no easy answers to the myriad social problems that lead people to abuse their bodies with food or the lack of it. Alcoholism, drug abuse, cigarette addiction and other forms of self destruction are in the same category. You should be aware, however, that all these conditions can be helped by complementary nutritional therapies. Nutritional status is intimately related to mental health. The nutritional approach discussed will hopefully help many addicted and abused individuals get on the path to better physical health. Improved physical health leads to better mental health and vice versa.

As a physician who sees both men and women for treatment of obesity and other eating disorders, I assure you that the messages in our society that cause women to compromise their good health in an attempt to become skinny are also directed at men in different ways. Why do you think so many men work out at gyms with the attitude of "no pain, no gain" and take anabolic steroids to "tone the body"? It's not just women that suffer from "the famine within." Men are just as much in need of psychotherapy for self destructive behaviors as women.

Eating disorders are not caused by deficiencies. Nutrition is by no means the only factor involved in eating disorders. It is, however, a scientific fact that people who suffer from these disorders have an altered biochemistry that requires nutritional intervention. The specific etiologies are unknown, but the nutritional correlates may nevertheless be of help to many sufferers. Psychotherapy is mandatory for those suffering from anorexia or bulimia, and nutritional therapy is complementary to that. As with all diseases, a holistic approach that incorporates conventional medical care, optimal nutrition and psychotherapy will lead to the best possible outcome for victims of eating disorders.

Attention Deficit Disorder

Attention deficit disorder in children is characterized by hyperactivity, impulsive behavior and the inability to concentrate for extended periods of time. In some cases, the hyperactivity can be so severe that the child is forced into special education classes. Conventional medical treatment involves the use of amphetamine-like stimulants like Ritalin.

In my review of the biochemical and nutritional literature on learning disabilities and attention deficit disorder, three things stand out. First, many reports have claimed that hidden (masked, delayed hypersensitivity) allergies to foods and chemicals may be involved. The most common allergies reported are to corn (present in almost all sweetened foods), milk, wheat, eggs, yeast, chocolate and citrus fruits. Clinically, I have found that the best way to diagnose hidden allergies to foods or chemicals is with the Elisa/Act blood test. It can reveal the immune system's reaction to over 300 foods and chemicals. Second, based on the work of Dr. Russell Jaffe and other nutritional doctors, serum amino acid analysis is another test that should be considered. Since amino acids are the precursors to the neurotransmitters, low levels can lead to neurotransmitter deficiency. Higher than accepted levels may lead to neurotransmitter excess. Once the amino acid levels are determined, treatment can be aimed at balancing brain chemicals more accurately.

Third, it's important to look for micronutrient deficiencies or dependencies. For example, zinc deficiency can have deleterious effects on both short- and long-term memory. White spots on the nails can be a sign of zinc deficiency, even when blood tests for zinc are normal. The expression "no zinc, no think" is not without merit. Many studies have shown that zinc supplementation is helpful for memory, thinking and IQ. The best way of getting zinc is to optimize the diet. The most recently published RDA (Recommended Dietary Allowance) for adults is 15 mgs per day. The richest sources of zinc are generally the high protein foods: organ meats, seafood (especially shellfish), oysters, whole grains and legumes (beans and peas). Beyond ensuring zinc adequacy in the diet, see a health care practitioner to decide whether supplementation is worth trying.

Cognitive impairment may also be associated with a deficiency in iron. Studies show that cognitive development can be impaired when there are low iron blood levels. Deficiencies in B vitamins, particularly vitamin B1 and choline, may also be involved. Toxic heavy metals such as cadmium and lead can accumulate in the body and cause both hyperactive behavior and learning disabilities in some susceptible children. A hair mineral analysis can reveal whether or not these toxic heavy metals are building up in the body. The good news is that with a natural program of vitamins and minerals, accumulations of lead and cadmium can be removed from the system.

Many scientific studies show that ginkgo biloba extract has a remarkable effect on different parts of the circulatory and nervous system. Some of its actions include enhancement of energy production, an increase in cellular glucose uptake, an increase in blood flow to the brain and an improvement of the transmission of nerve signals. Theoretically, one might assume that ginkgo biloba extract could have a beneficial effect on learning disabilities.

Unfortunately, no one has studied its effects in this area. Studies on ginkgo biloba extract support its use for conditions like cerebral vascular insufficiency (short-term memory loss, vertigo, headache, tinnitus, lack of vigilance and depression), senility, Alzheimer's disease, peripheral vascular disorders, Raynaud's disease and postphlebitis syndrome.

Ginkgo biloba extract is a safe herbal compound; thus, for those with learning disabilities, a trial therapy using the extract (if undertaken with the supervision of a naturopath, herbalist or holistic doctor) couldn't do any harm. There is no guarantee that it will be effective, however. More studies and documented clinical experience would have to be done before I could recommend it as a treatment for learning disabilities. Ginkgo biloba extract and the nutrients mentioned here are available from most health food stores and some pharmacies. Work with a doctor to put together a comprehensive nutritional program designed to rebalance the system.

Concussion

Although there are no specific nutritional programs outlined anywhere as a natural treatment for concussion, there are a number of natural supplements that can be taken to speed healing from any type of physical trauma. These supplements come under the broad category known as antioxidants. Antioxidants help stimulate the healing process and prevent oxidative damage from a variety of physical and chemical insults. They include vitamins A, C and E, beta-carotene, all the B-complex vitamins, zinc, selenium, silicon, glutathione and bioflavonoids (e.g., pycnogenol).

In addition to antioxidants, there are a variety of natural supplements that have been proven to be effective in enhancing both short- and long-term memory. Choline, for example, can be obtained from the diet (soybeans, eggs) or taken as a supplement called lecithin (phosphatidyl choline). Studies indicate that a minimum six-month trial of ten to twenty grams of 95 percent phosphatidyl choline may be beneficial in memory enhancement. Phosphatidyl choline is available at most health food stores without a prescription. Side effects are negligible.

Research in France and Germany indicates that ginkgo biloba may be effective in helping many aspects of brain function. Some of its actions include improvement of energy production, an increase in cellular glucose uptake, an increase in blood flow to the brain and an enhancement of the transmission of nerve signals. Coenzyme Q10, has been shown to be effective because this natural substance carries oxygen to cells. Both ginkgo biloba and coenzyme Q10 have negligible side effects.

Homeopathic remedies that speed healing from almost any injury include aconite, arnica and calendula. Dosages of all these natural remedies depend upon the general health situation of the individual and the extent of the injury. Have a natural health care practitioner help supervise a supplement program.

Epilepsy

The cause of epilepsy is often unknown. In some cases, seizure disorders can be linked to infection, meningitis, malaria, cerebral palsy, mental retardation, brain tumors and cysts, head injuries, drugs, lack of oxygen, spasm in the blood vessels or hereditary factors. Some drugs can cause or aggravate epilepsy (e.g., amphetamines, antihistamines, oral contraceptives, antidepressants).

Nutrition does play a role, since seizures may also be associated with malnutrition, food allergies and hypoglycemia (low blood sugar). Avoid all processed foods, sugar, white flour products, caffeine, alcohol, fried foods and tobacco. Recent research has associated epilepsy with consumption of aspartame, an artificial sweetener. Aluminum, mercury and lead toxicity may also contribute to the problem. Hair mineral analysis can determine whether or not these toxic heavy metals are elevated in the body. Other tests should be considered to determine nutritional deficiencies and food allergies.

There are many reports on the benefits of certain nutritional supplements in the control of seizure disorders. These include the amino acids L-taurine, L-tryptophan and L-tyrosine. Also important are magnesium, folic acid, calcium, selenium, silicon, zinc, chromium, manganese, essential fatty acids (evening primrose oil, flax seed oil) vitamins A, C , E and the B-complex vitamins.

Herbs that have a value as part of complementary medical treatment are black walnut, wormwood and grapefruit seed extract (if parasites are involved with epilepsy), burdock, capsicum, pau d'arco, liquid chlorophyll, red clover, propolis, goldenseal, lomatium, St. John's wort, echinacea (for circulation cleansing, infection control or detoxification), hawthorn, hops, lady's slipper, skullcap, valerian, passion flower and ginkgo biloba (for nerves).

Since all cases tend to be different in terms of nutritional needs, it is advisable to see a naturopath or doctor familiar with nutritional medicine for an assessment. Complementary natural treatment may go a long way towards reducing the need for prescription drugs.

Neuropathy

A neuropathy is a disorder of the peripheral nervous system most often producing symptoms in the hands and feet. Signs and symptoms of neuropathy may include weakness, sensory loss, pain, numbness, tingling and other abnormal sensations.

Most serious versions of this problem are seen in those suffering from diabetes and chronic alcoholism. If you are neither a diabetic nor an alcoholic then the source of symptoms may be in various nutritional deficiencies. Heavy metal toxicity, Lyme disease and advanced kidney disease are also associated with neuropathy.

Neuropathy may be caused by deficiencies in zinc and B vitamins, particularly B1, B2, B3, B5, B6, biotin, folic acid, choline, inositol and B12. These are the nutrients most important in nerve health and maintenance. Food sources of these include brewer's yeast, organ meats, whole grains, blue-green algae, sea vegetables, spirulina, berries, nuts and legumes. Oral supplementation with a good B-complex vitamin can help reverse the symptoms in three to five months in many cases. Evening primrose oil and other sources of essential fatty acids are also beneficial in the treatment of neuropathy.

Bioflavonoids such as quercetin, pycnogenol, hesperidin, catechin and rutin inhibit the enzyme aldose reductase. The overactivity of this enzyme is thought to lead to nerve damage in some diabetics. Bioflavonoids are natural aldose reductase inhibitors and may be quite safe and effective in the treatment of diabetic peripheral neuropathy.

In those over age 65, vitamin B12 may become deficient despite an excellent diet. As one ages, a number of imbalances might develop. These include a low or absent secretion of stomach hydrochloric acid, a deficiency of intrinsic factor, a bacterial flora overgrowth in the small intestine or a malabsorption due to excess antacids or previous stomach surgery. In these cases, oral supplementation with vitamin B12 and lactobacillus acidophilus may not be enough. Supplementation with Swedish bitters, apple cider vinegar, lemon juice, betaine or glutamic acid hydrochloride and pepsin may or may not be effective. Regular B12 injections are required in most cases to reverse the deficiency and the symptoms of neuropathy.

Other possible causes of peripheral neuropathy include toxic heavy metals such as mercury, cadmium, lead, aluminum, copper and arsenic. Few people realize that some of these metals are present in dental amalgams and other types of dental work (root canals, crowns, etc.). If you have a mouthful of dental hardware, suspect it as a potential source of your symptoms. A hair mineral analysis as well as other lab tests may be helpful in revealing the problem.

There is a long list of prescription drugs that can cause neuropathy as one of the side effects. Check with a pharmacist or medical doctor.

Schizophrenia

Schizophrenia is a serious mental illness that affects one in one hundred people. Symptoms usually develop in adolescence or early adulthood; men and women are equally affected. There are many different types of schizophrenia, the major ones being simple, catatonic, hebephrenic, paranoid, schizo-affective, borderline and pseudoneurotic. Some of the signs and symptoms include hallucinations, bizarre or inappropriate behavior, withdrawal, depression, agitation, illogical thoughts and ideas, vague speech or disconnected remarks, ambivalence, perceptual disorders and impulsive actions. In paranoid schizophrenics, there may be a constant suspicion and resentment accompanied by fear that people are plotting to destroy or harm them. The hearing of hostile voices not perceived by healthy people is common.

Many researchers believe that the cause of schizophrenia is a chemical imbalance in the brain triggered by extreme mental stress. The exact mechanisms are unknown. Studies on twins indicate that there is a hereditary predisposition for the disease. Psychiatric treatments focus on the use of major tranquilizer drugs, psychotherapy, group therapy and, at times, electroconvulsive shock therapy.

There is a growing body of evidence supporting the use of nutritional intervention as a complementary treatment for schizophrenia. It is by no means an alternative to psychiatry. Conventional psychiatric treatment is of primary importance and patients already on medications such as haloperidol must continue until significant improvements have occurred as a result of any nutritional programs. Withdrawal from psychiatric drugs should be done very carefully and slowly under the supervision of a medical doctor. Beware of self-help nutritional treatment of schizophrenia. The response of a schizophrenic to nutritional intervention is sometimes unpredictable and, for this and other reasons, do not self-prescribe or treat with megavitamins or other supplements.

Two pioneers in the nutritional or orthomolecular treatment of schizophrenia are Dr. Abram Hoffer and the late Dr. Carl Pfeiffer. Their books are well worth reading and are available from the Canadian Schizophrenia Foundation (see the appendix for its address). The CSF puts on an annual conference and provides information and support to the families of schizophrenics.

The Princeton Bio Center (see appendix), founded by the late Dr. Carl Pfeiffer, offers state-of-the-art nutritional assessment and treatment of schizophrenia and other chronic diseases. Some of the nutritional imbalances that could lead to the neurochemical disturbances of schizophrenia include food allergies (particularly to wheat), amino acid imbalances, mineral excesses (especially copper) and vitamin dependencies (especially to niacin, vitamin B6 and vitamin C).

Aside from hypoallergenic diets based on food allergy test results (i.e., Elisa/Act test), many schizophrenics are helped by high-dose supplementation with ginkgo biloba extract, zinc, selenium, manganese, freeform amino acid supplements (based on amino acid analysis), vitamin B12 injections, vitamin B complex, vitamin E, coenzyme Q10, essential fatty acids (e.g., evening primrose oil, flax seed oil, cod liver oil and others), lecithin, choline, and occasionally lithium and thyroid extract. Treatments must be individualized, based on detailed biochemical tests, and supervised by doctors knowledgeable in both allopathic (conventional) and naturopathic medicine.

Stress and Nerves

Stress is a major factor in an irritated nervous system. Counselling and stress reduction techniques such as meditation, aerobic exercise and relaxation can be helpful. A change of lifestyle or environment may be necessary. There are also some nutritional factors to consider.

Stress, anxiety, headaches and other nervous disorders are made worse by excessive caffeine or sugar intake. Common sources of caffeine include coffee, tea, chocolate, carbonated soft drinks and over-the-counter medications for flu, colds, headaches and weight loss. Sugar causes a variety of biochemical changes leading to many nervous system abnormalities commonly referred to as reactive hypoglycemia. Make sure your diet is free of both simple sugars and caffeine.

Nervous symptoms can also be caused by mercury excess in the body. Sources may include contaminated seafood and the erosion of the common silver (mercury) dental filling. High doses of selenium, vitamin C, vitamin E, garlic and N-acetyl-cysteine can help rid the body of toxic heavy metals such as mercury, cadmium, lead, aluminum, arsenic and copper. Getting a hair mineral analysis is a good way of determining whether or not toxic heavy metals are present in the body above acceptable levels.

An overactive nervous system can often be helped by a trial therapy with high doses of vitamin B complex, especially vitamin B3 (niacinamide). Other supplemental nutrients that can control nervousness include calcium, magnesium, potassium, zinc, brewer's yeast, lecithin, octacosanol and vitamin E. In people with low or absent stomach acid secretion, injections of B vitamins, especially vitamin B12, may dramatically improve nervous system function. Often, magnesium sulphate injections will stop spasms, palpitations, headaches or irritability when oral supplementation fails.

Herbal or homeopathic remedies (in tea, capsule or tincture form) such as camomile, hops, lady's slipper, passion flower, skullcap, wood betony, St. John's wort and valerian may also be of help in some cases.

It may take several months to see changes for the better with nutritional, homeopathic or herbal supplement programs. If there is no progress after about three months, see a naturopath or nutrition-oriented doctor for assessment.

Parkinson's Disease

Parkinson's disease involves the deterioration of specific nerve centers in the brain. This deterioration changes the chemical balance of acetylcholine and dopamine. These two chemicals are both essential for transmission of nerve signals. When the balance between these two neurotransmitters is altered, the ultimate result is a lack of control of physical movements.

The main symptom of Parkinson's is a tremor, an involuntary shaking of the hands, the head or both. In many cases this is accompanied by a continuous rubbing together of the thumb and forefinger. Stooped posture, a mask-like face, trouble swallowing and difficulty performing simple tasks may all be seen at different stages of the disease. The tremors are most severe when the affected part of the body is not in use. There is no pain or other sensation other than a decreased ability to move. In severe cases, the person will be unable to walk smoothly due to an inability to swing the arms. Writing legibly and speaking clearly will also be affected. Depression often results.

Parkinson's disease affects more men than women at a ratio of three to two. It is estimated that one in every one hundred persons over age 60 will contract this condition. The specific cause of Parkinson's is not known. Predisposing factors include carbon monoxide poisoning, high body levels of noxious chemicals, brain infections (known as encephalitis) and certain drugs such as the ones used in treatment of schizophrenia. Medical treatment involves the use of various drugs such as Levodopa, Sinemet and Deprenyl. There is no medical cure for the condition.

In dealing naturally with Parkinson's, complementary health care practitioners aim to rule out toxic heavy metal excess body burden (e.g., lead, mercury, cadmium, etc.), food and chemical allergies and gastrointestinal parasitic/fungal infection. There is ample evidence for the negative neurological effects of mercury dental amalgams. Replacing your fillings may be beneficial. There is now a lab test (Elisa/Act blood test) for mercury hypersensitivity which is nearly 100 percent reliable. Hair mineral analysis as well as comprehensive digestive stool analysis are two other lab tests that may also be revealing.

Nutritional literature has reported that excess amounts of manganese may cause Parkinson-like symptoms. In people who self-prescribe megadoses of manganese, toxicity may result from the accumulation of it in the liver and central nervous system. Hair mineral analysis as well as blood testing can uncover cases of manganese excess in the body.

Cases that have been treated for long periods of time with the drug Levodopa may develop deficiencies in vitamin B6, folic acid and vitamin B12. Supplementation of these vitamins may be necessary to prevent worsening of the symptoms of the disease. Many people over the age of 60 have problems with absorption of vitamin B12. In these cases, taking the vitamin in either sublingual form or as an injection is preferable.

Other supplements that may be helpful in treatment include choline, inositol, lecithin, niacinamide, vitamin C, vitamin E, coenzyme Q10 and tyrosine. These nutrients are all involved in the body's synthesis of acetylcholine and dopamine. Herbal remedies that may be tried include ginseng and horsetail, both of which can be taken in capsules or made into a tea. A nutritional evaluation by a naturopath or nutritional doctor may help pinpoint these and other potential deficiencies or toxicities. Combined with conventional medical therapy, a good nutritional supplement program will help produce optimal results.

According to a 1989 Israeli study published in *ACTA Neurologica Scandinavia*, high levels of iron were found in the brains (substantia nigra) of Parkinson's disease patients. It is thought that excess iron leads to increased free radical pathology and accelerated cell death in Parkinson's disease. Both vitamin C and E as well as the amino acid derivative N-acetyl-cysteine are free radical scavengers and can remove excess iron from the body. So can properly conducted intravenous chelation therapy.

Restless Legs

Restless leg syndrome involves an irresistible urge to move the legs. It is thought that folic acid deficiency causes the problem. A 1976 study published in the Canadian Medical Association Journal showed that patients responded well to high doses of folic acid. The doses used were 35 to 60 mgs daily. Other studies indicate that vitamin E, iron and L-tryptophan supplementation is helpful.

Many sufferers have either a poor ability or no ability to absorb folic acid from the foods they eat. In a surprising number of cases even megadoses of folic acid pills remain unabsorbed. A series of folic acid injections would be helpful until the bowel regains the ability to absorb the vitamin more naturally. It's almost as if folic acid deficiency causes malabsorption of folic acid. Shots are required to break the vicious cycle.

In my practice I have had considerable success using megadose folic acid therapy for restless leg syndrome, cervical dysplasia (e.g., abnormal Pap tests), depression, anemia and anxiety. Treatment works best when those receiving folic acid also eliminate coffee, tea and caffeine-containing soft drinks from their diets. Iron status also must be normalized. Folic acid is found in large amounts in green leafy vegetables, root vegetables, wheat germ, whole grains, liver, organ meats and yeast. The birth control pill may increase the need for folic acid. The same is true for anticonvulsant medication like dilantin.

The best laboratory test for diagnosing a greater need for folic acid is called the Neutrophil Hypersegmentation Index (NSI). This is a blood test that reveals folic acid inadequacy before symptoms such as restless legs and cervical dysplasia develop. This test can be ordered by any doctor when he orders a CBC (complete blood count) as part of routine blood tests. You can be deficient in folic acid with a "normal" folic acid blood level so be careful about lab test interpretations that do not report the NSI. The best tests for determining iron status include serum iron and ferritin levels.

Tinnitus

Tinnitus, or ringing in the ears, is an extremely common complaint, particularly among the elderly. Rarely, it is accompanied by dizziness or vertigo (Meniere's disease). Tinnitus may occur as a symptom of nearly any ear disorder, including obstruction of the external auditory canal by wax and foreign bodies; infectious disease involving the outer, inner or middle ear; eustachian tube obstruction; allergies; otosclerosis (hardening of the ear drum); noise-induced hearing loss and trauma (e.g., as in the case of a skull fracture). Low frequency vibratory clicks, pops, roarings, etc., are usually due to contraction of muscles of the eustachian tube, middle ear, palate or pharynx and are not considered to be in the same category.

Tinnitus may also be associated with high blood pressure, hardening of the arteries, anemia, hypothyroidism, the candidiasis hypersensitivity syndrome, heavy metal toxicity (lead, mercury, aluminum and cadmium), carbon monoxide exposure, aspirin and certain drugs (diuretics, antibiotics, quinine, alcohol). Dental fillings that use silver, mercury, copper and other metals may be responsible for a long list of neurological problems that include ringing in the ears. So can root canal work of all types. Hair mineral analysis, blood and urine testing and even special tests on the immune system may be required to diagnose this problem.

Medical treatment is directed at the underlying cause, but when this fails to correct the ringing, a number of safe, natural alternatives can be tried. For example, studies show that dietary measures taken to reduce blood levels of cholesterol and saturated fat help the flow of oxygen and nutrients to the inner ear. One study on a group of 1,400 patients demonstrated benefits in most cases of dizziness and tinnitus when saturated animal fats were reduced in the diet. Other studies show symptom improvement when patients eliminate sugar from the diet. Research dating as far back as 1954 has shown an association between inner ear problems and hypoglycemia. Other researchers report that salicylate-free diets benefit some cases of tinnitus. As with most diet therapies, biochemical individuality will dictate effectiveness.

Allergies, particularly food allergies, can cause fluid retention in the labyrinth. Excessive salt in the diet can do the same. If the ringing has some association with dietary intake, a trial therapy with an elimination diet is worth doing. Alternatively, food allergies can be determined through the use of a number of different types of blood tests. A salt-free diet should also be tried for at least six weeks.

Over the years, doctors have noted that supplementation of the diet with high doses of niacin (vitamin B3), or niacin combined with inositol and pyridoxine (vitamin B6), eliminates the ringing in many cases where the cause is unknown. Inner ear problems may also be helped by supplementation of vitamins A, D, calcium, magnesium, potassium, iodine, zinc and omega-3-EPA oils (found in cod, halibut, trout, salmon, mackerel, shark and swordfish).

Ginkgo biloba and ginger have also been found to be highly effective. Ginger has long been a popular remedy for nausea, motion sickness and dizziness. It frequently helps tinnitus too. Ginkgo biloba extract improves blood supply to the brain and increases the rate at which information is transmitted at the nerve cell. It also has a significant free radical scavenging effect and may allow improved oxygenation of tissues and enhanced tissue repair. There have been no reports of toxicity occurring with either of these herbs. For specific, individualized doses, consult your health care practitioner.

Depression

There are a variety of natural approaches to psychiatric problems, including amino acid therapies, balancing vitamins and minerals and the use of herbal medicines. For example, a number of recent studies by Bell and others have reported that there is a definite benefit to be gained by giving vitamin B12 to patients suffering from depression, fatigue and mental illnesses of other kinds. Herbs that may work as effective antidepressants include oat, St. John's wort, panax ginseng and valerian.

The effective therapeutic dose of vitamin B12 is highly variable from patient to patient. A trial therapy of 3,000 mcgs taken daily under the tongue (sublingual) or as a nasal gel may be effective after two or three weeks. If not, daily intramuscular injections may be worth a try until symptoms resolve.

Vitamin B12 is not the only natural therapeutic agent for the treatment of depression. Dr. Melvyn Werbach, professor of psychiatry at UCLA, in his new book, *Nutritional Influences on Mental Illness*, discusses the many nutritional causes of depression. These include the frequent consumption of caffeine or sugar and deficiencies of essential fatty acids, biotin, folic acid, other B-complex vitamins, vitamin C, calcium, copper, iron, magnesium or potassium. Depression can also be caused by excesses of magnesium, copper or vanadium, imbalances in amino acids and food and chemical allergies.

Hormonal influences may also play a part in depression. The thyroid, adrenal gland and the balance of male and/or female hormones may have a direct impact on mental health. A classic example is the successful use of progesterone (natural or otherwise) in the treatment of depression caused by premenstrual syndrome (PMS).

Although we supposedly get all the amino acids we need from the typical North American diet, many individuals must supplement some of the amino acids in order to prevent depression. The psychiatric/medical/biochemical literature is now filled with research on the use of natural mood-altering supplements such as tryptophan, tyrosine, phenylalanine, glutamine, choline and many others.

There are many causes of amino acid imbalance in the body, including food allergy, food intolerance, hypochlorhydria (low stomach acid) and pancreatic digestive enzyme insufficiency. A serum amino acid analysis can be done on the essential amino acids (isoleucine, leucine, lysine, methionine, phenylalanine, threonine, tryptophan, valine and two conditionally essential amino acids, histidine and taurine). Labs that do this test report the results and supplementation requirements back to the physician that orders the test (see appendix). The patient can then be placed on a supplemental blend of the amino acids that will restore balance in the body.

Find a doctor or naturopath willing to test for biochemical individuality and prescribe natural therapies to turn depression around–without drugs.

Depression and Vitamin B12

A number of recent studies by Bell and others have reported a definite benefit to be gained by giving vitamin B12 to patients suffering from depression, fatigue and mental illnesses of other kinds.

The effective therapeutic dose of vitamin B12 is highly variable from patient to patient. A trial therapy of 3,000 mcgs taken daily under the tongue (sublingual) or as a nasal gel may be effective after two or three weeks. If not, daily intramuscular injections (3,000 mcgs daily) may be worth a try until symptoms resolve.

I must stress that vitamin B12 alone is not the only natural therapeutic agent for the treatment of depression. Dr. Melvyn Werbach, professor of psychiatry at UCLA, in his new book, *Nutritional Influences on Mental Illness,* discusses the many nutritional causes of depression. These include the frequent consumption of caffeine or sugar, and deficiencies of biotin, folic acid, other B-complex vitamins, vitamin C, calcium, copper, iron, magnesium or potassium. Depression can also be caused by excesses of magnesium or vanadium, by imbalances in amino acids and by food allergies. Other effective nutritional antidepressants include lithium, rubidium, phenylalanine, tyrosine, tryptophan, S-Adenosyl-L-methionine and hypericin (from St. John's wort).

Serotonin is a very important brain biochemical and must be present at optimal levels to prevent depression. One natural way of increasing serotonin in the brain is to take its amino acid precursor, tryptophan (on prescription). Tryptophan is an essential amino acid found in high amounts in fish, meat, dairy products, eggs, nuts and wheat germ. It is also found in lesser amounts in the herb camomile, long recognized for its soothing effects. People who have trouble digesting high protein foods may not be getting the tryptophan they need from their diets. As a result, brain serotonin levels may get low and lead to depression, obsessive compulsive disorders, mania, anxiety, insomnia, premenstrual syndrome, obesity and eating disorders like bulimia and anorexia.

If your doctor prescribes tryptophan, make sure it is balanced by other amino acids. It's best to get a plasma amino acid analysis done before taking high dose supplements of any amino acid. Tryptophan is made more effective by also supplementing with vitamins B3 (niacinamide), B6 and C. It's uptake in the brain is enhanced by taking it with a high carbohydrate meal (e.g., pasta, fruit, vegetables or starches). Foods which contain preformed serotonin also help brain uptake of tryptophan. These foods include bananas, walnuts and pineapples.

If digestion is poor, supplemental betaine and pepsin, glutamic acid, apple cider vinegar, Swedish bitters, pancreatin, vegetable enzymes, lactobacillus acidophilus or other digestive aids may need to be used. A naturopath or holistic doctor can order tests like a CDSA (comprehensive stool and digestive analysis) to assess for the different types of maldigestion. Specific therapy could then be implemented to optimize the digestive system.

Food allergies, candida infection, parasites and toxic heavy metals may all have deleterious effects on digestion and, hence, tryptophan absorption or utilization. A comprehensive biochemical/nutritional evaluation by a doctor familiar with the natural approach would certainly be a good idea.

Natural Therapies for Winter Depression
Seasonal affective disorder (SAD) or "winter depression" occurs in the fall and/or winter and clears spontaneously in the spring. The cause of this type of depression is still not well understood. One theory is that decreased exposure to sunlight increases the pineal gland's secretion of the hormone, melatonin. Increased levels of melatonin are associated with increased sleepiness. Symptoms occur from as early as October to as late as May.

Symptoms of SAD include sadness, depression, withdrawal, apathy, irritability, sleep disturbances (sleeping more and waking unrefreshed), decreased physical activity, weight gain, increased appetite, fatigue, craving for carbohydrates and decreased sexual drive.

Incandescent and fluorescent artificial lighting is deficient in the complete, balanced spectrum of sunlight needed by the body for the optimal absorption of nutrients. This type of "mal-illumination" is not only associated with depression but with chronic fatigue, a suppressed immune system and cancer. In most cases, light therapy by daily exposure to full spectrum lights (similar to real sunlight) successfully eliminates the symptoms of winter depression. Healing is further enhanced by complementary nutritional and botanical therapies.

Avoid red meat, caffeine products, alcohol, spicy foods, fried foods, fatty foods, salty foods, sweets and sugar. Eat foods that are high in B-complex vitamins and vitamin C such as citrus, brewer's yeast, spirulina, chlorella, blue-green algae, beets, carrots, artichokes, cucumbers, parsnips, parsley and watercress. Herbal teas made from licorice root, St John's wort and panax ginseng can help boost energy levels.

The amino acids tryptophan and tyrosine (available on prescription) can be used as natural antidepressants. Nervous system function is also optimized by B-complex vitamins (especially B6), vitamin C, vitamin E, calcium, magnesium and omega-6 fatty acids (e.g., evening primrose oil). Discuss these therapies with a doctor or natural health care practitioner.

A "Lump" in the Throat

Globus hystericus is a sensation of a mass or lump present in the throat at all times. There is usually no detectable organic cause. Conventional doctors tend to either dismiss the patient or prescribe tranquilizers like xanax. I do not agree with either approach. The muscles in the esophagus are not damaged; they are probably in spasm and can be helped by balancing biochemistry.

Magnesium deficiency may result in globus hystericus. The usual cause of magnesium deficiency is poor diet and stress. Depending on the severity of the deficiency, a lack of magnesium may result in muscle spasms, palpitations, high blood pressure, insomnia, irritability, anxiety, cramps, pain and even seizures. Blood tests for magnesium will not be helpful in revealing a magnesium deficiency unless the problem is severe.

Hair analysis may be more helpful, but it too is not completely reliable. Magnesium levels can be improved by eating large amounts of raw greens and avoiding sugar, coffee, tea, cola drinks, chocolate and pills that contain caffeine.

It is also beneficial to supplement the diet with liquid or encapsulated magnesium citrate, aspartate or gluconate. Watch out for diarrhea as a possible side effect. If there is no history of kidney problems, taking even 100 tablespoons of magnesium a day is safe. The body just gets rid of the excess through the kidneys and bowel. If you get diarrhea from magnesium supplementation, reduce the dose by half or more. Along with the magnesium, take a daily B-complex supplement that contains at least 100 mgs of vitamin B6. Give this combined therapy at least six weeks to work.

There are other natural supplements that help with irritability and spasm. These include calcium, potassium, zinc, brewer's yeast, lecithin, octacosanol and vitamin E. In people with low or absent stomach acid secretion, injections of B vitamins, especially vitamin B12, may dramatically improve nervous system function. Often, magnesium sulphate injections will stop spasm when oral supplementation fails.

Herbal or homeopathic remedies such as camomile, hops, lady's slipper, passion flower, skullcap, wood betony, St. John's wort and valerian may also be of help in some cases.

It may take several weeks to see changes for the better with nutritional, homeopathic or herbal supplement programs. If there is no progress after about three months, see a naturopath or nutrition-oriented doctor for assessment.

Lithium Problems

Lithium is a mineral that, like other minerals, is important for health. When used in very high doses to treat manic-depressive illness, there is a chance that the kidneys and the thyroid gland will be affected. It is not uncommon for lithium users to develop low thyroid function—hair loss, severe fatigue and flu-like illnesses may be the resulting symptoms. The solution then is to supplement thyroid gland function.

When taking one mineral in very high doses it is important to balance it with other minerals or deficiencies may develop. In particular, check for subnormal levels of zinc, copper and selenium on hair mineral analysis.

Ask your doctor to order thyroid function tests (T3, T4, TSH, anti-thyroid antibodies, anti-microsomal antibodies), kidney function tests, cholesterol, HDL-cholesterol, blood tests for iron and ferritin and a hair mineral analysis. This will give a good indication of what minerals are out of balance and if anything needs to be done about thyroid function. Get regular lithium blood levels done by your doctor.

Neck Muscle Spasms

Torticollis and tremor may be associated with excessive caffeine or sugar intake. Common sources of caffeine include coffee, tea, chocolate, carbonated soft drinks and over-the-counter medications for pain, flu, colds, headaches and weight loss. Sugar causes a variety of biochemical changes leading to muscle spasms and other nervous system abnormalities commonly referred to as reactive hypoglycemia.

Torticollis or tremor can also be caused by mercury excess in the body. Sources may include contaminated seafood and the erosion of the common silver (mercury) dental filling. Oral chelation with high doses of selenium, vitamin C, vitamin E, garlic and N-acetyl-cysteine can help rid the body of toxic heavy metals such as mercury, cadmium, lead, aluminum, arsenic and copper. Getting a hair mineral analysis is a good way of determining whether or not toxic heavy metals are present in the body above acceptable levels.

A more accurate test to see whether or not mercury hypersensitivity (not toxicity) is contributing to symptoms is the Elisa/Act test. This blood test can measure both cell mediated and humoral (antibody) reactions by the immune system to mercury or other toxic heavy metals. If the test is positive, consider replacing silver mercury fillings and use the oral chelation supplements mentioned above.

A trial therapy of high doses of vitamin B complex, especially vitamin B3 (niacinamide), may help with symptom relief. Other supplemental nutrients that may be of help include calcium, magnesium, potassium, zinc, brewer's yeast, lecithin, octacosanol and vitamin E. In people with low or absent stomach acid secretion, injections of B vitamins, especially vitamin B12, may dramatically improve nervous system function. Often, magnesium sulphate injections will stop spasm or tremor when oral supplementation fails.

Herbal or homeopathic remedies (in tea, capsule or tincture form) such as camomile, hops, lady's slipper, passion flower, skullcap, wood betony, St. John's wort and valerian may also be of help in some cases. It may take several months to see changes for the better with nutritional, homeopathic or herbal supplement programs. Work closely with a naturopath to get to the bottom of the problem.

Torticollis and Dystonia

Spasmodic torticollis is an involuntary turning of the head and it may be the first symptom of dystonia. In young adults, torticollis may last several years and then resolve spontaneously. Remission is less likely when torticollis occurs during middle age. The head movements are made worse with walking or during activities that require a fixed gaze, such as reading or watching television. With dystonia, the sternocleidomastoid muscle may hypertrophy (become enlarged). Other neck muscles are involved leading to muscle coordination abnormalities.

Conventional medical approaches to treatment aim at symptom control with drugs and are generally ineffective. Some of the drugs prescribed for dystonia are diazepam, carbamazepine, baclofen, clonazepam, propranolol, lithium, haloperidol, levodopa, bromocriptine, tricyclic antidepressants and anticholinergics. There is an experimental therapy that consists of local injections of botulinum toxin (a potent neurotoxin) into muscles that exhibit abnormal fiber discharge. Temporary relief has been reported in some cases, but nothing of a longstanding nature can be expected.

Torticollis and tremor may be associated with excessive caffeine or sugar intake. Common sources of caffeine include coffee, tea, chocolate, carbonated soft drinks and over-the-counter medications for pain, flu, colds, headaches and weight loss. Sugar causes a variety of biochemical changes leading to muscle spasms and other nervous system abnormalities commonly referred to as reactive hypoglycemia. Make sure the diet is free of both simple sugars and caffeine.

Torticollis or tremor can also be caused by mercury excess in the body. Oral chelation with high doses of selenium, vitamin C, vitamin E, garlic and N-acetylcysteine can help rid the body of toxic heavy metals such as mercury, cadmium, lead, aluminum, arsenic and copper. Getting a hair mineral analysis is a good way of determining whether or not toxic heavy metals are present in the body above acceptable levels. A more accurate test to see whether or not mercury hypersensitivity (not toxicity) is contributing to neurological symptoms is the Elisa/Act test.

A trial therapy of high doses of vitamin B complex, especially vitamin B3, may help. Other supplemental nutrients that may be of help include calcium, magnesium, potassium, zinc, brewer's yeast, octacosanol and vitamin E. In people with low or absent stomach acid secretion, injections of B vitamins, especially vitamin B12, may dramatically improve nervous system function. Often, magnesium sulphate injections will stop spasm or tremor when oral supplementation fails.

Herbal or homeopathic remedies such as camomile, hops, lady's slipper, passion flower, skullcap, wood betony, St John's wort and valerian may also be of help in some cases. They may work just as well as some of the drugs prescribed for dystonia, without the side effects.

Tics and Tourette's Syndrome

Tourette's syndrome is a neurological disease characterized by involuntary muscular movements, tics and uncontrollable, sometimes inappropriate, vocal sounds. In severe cases, there may be head shaking, shoulder jerking, arm flapping, foot stamping and the shouting of obscene words. It begins in childhood between the ages of 2 and 16, but those affected can expect to live a normal lifespan. Although the cause of Tourette's syndrome is unknown, research suggests that there may be a biochemical imbalance which affects neurotransmitter systems in the brain. Approximately 70 percent of all cases run in families.

An increased incidence of obsessive-compulsive behavior, attention deficit disorder (hyperactivity) and other abnormalities have been reported in Tourette's patients. Symptoms such as these have also long been associated with either food or environmental allergies. One paper in a leading allergy journal reported that many Tourette's syndrome patients have high blood levels of IgE, a sign of allergic disease. In other words, the symptoms of Tourette's syndrome may be those of undiagnosed allergies.

One Russian study published in 1984 found that concentrations of serum and 24-hour, urine-free amino acids were significantly abnormal in Tourette's syndrome patients. Amino acids are the basic building blocks of dietary proteins and act as neurotransmitters or precursors to neurotransmitters in the brain. It is highly probable that certain brain neurotransmitters are out of balance in people with Tourette's syndrome. Neurotransmitters are like hormones and are necessary in order for the brain cells to receive and send messages. It is interesting to note that hypoglycemia, allergies of all kinds and the candida syndrome are all benefited by specific amino acid supplement therapies. Tourette's syndrome may also prove to benefit if amino acid levels are balanced.

The best way of determining whether or not an individual is suffering from an imbalance in amino acids is to get a fasting plasma amino acid analysis done. Results of such a test can aid in designing a balanced amino acid formula that can be taken as a supplement to optimize neurotransmitter function. Several laboratories in the United States provide such a service. A listing is provided in the appendix.

Tics in general are helped by high doses of vitamin B complex, especially vitamin B3 (niacinamide). Other supplemental nutrients that can control tics include calcium, magnesium, potassium, zinc, brewer's yeast, lecithin (phosphatidyl choline), octacosanol and vitamin E. In people with low or absent stomach acid secretion, injections of B vitamins, especially vitamin

B12, may dramatically improve nervous system function. Often, magnesium sulphate injections will stop tics when oral supplementation fails. Herbal or homeopathic remedies such as camomile, hops, lady's slipper, passion flower, skullcap, wood betony, St. John's wort and valerian may also be of help in some cases.

Although none of these supplemental nutrients or herbs have a direct impact on the disease process in Tourette's syndrome, they are complementary to medical management. They are virtually free of side effects and may make living with this illness more bearable.

Standard drug therapies include haloperidol, clonidine and pimozide. Supportive psychotherapy for the condition is of limited use. Studies are currently underway on the drugs clomipramine and prolixin that treat the obsessive-compulsive symptoms of Tourette's syndrome. For more information on medical treatments, contact the following groups: National Organization for Rare Disorders (NORD), Tourette's Syndrome Association and National Institute of Neurological Disorders and Strokes (see appendix).

Huntington's Disease

Huntington's disease is an inherited degenerative neurological disease characterized by obstinacy, moodiness, apathy and choreiform movements. Huntington's has an insidious onset. Symptoms begin appearing between ages 30 and 50. Signs and symptoms do not occur until well into childbearing years. Choreiform movements are distinctive, irregular, spasmodic, involuntary movements of the limbs and facial muscles, usually beginning in the arms, neck and face, progressing from mild fidgeting to facial grimaces, hesitant speech, severe neck muscle spasms and irregular trunk movements. Gait is wide based and prancing and euphoria is common. Advanced Huntington's produces swallowing problems, dementia and an inability to walk. The condition is medically incurable, and treatment is directed at symptom control only, with various tranquilizing drugs and muscle relaxants.

Naturopathic and nutritional therapies are of some benefit in symptom control. A diet high in fiber and complex carbohydrates provides many nutrients that optimize nervous system health. Red meats, chicken, fish, dairy and other animal products are best avoided. Some important nutrients are calcium, magnesium, manganese, phosphorus, iodine, tryptophan and B vitamins. Therapeutic foods include brewer's yeast and rice bran; beneficial juices include celery, carrot, prune, black cherry, beet, cucumber, celery, parsley and spinach.

Helpful nutritional supplements to consider are B-complex vitamins, especially vitamin B3, choline, vitamin B6 and B12. The B vitamins seem to be most effective when injected intramuscularly on a fairly regular basis. These, and amino acids like tryptophan and GABA (gamma amino butyric acid), can help replace or reduce the dosages of prescription tranquilizers and muscle relaxants. Herbal remedies that may be beneficial are black cohash, passion flower, St. John's wort and mistletoe.

Aside from nutrition and herbal medicine, there are reports of symptom control of Huntington's using homeopathic remedies, electroacupuncture and various other types of "energy medicine." Since most of these are safe, there is no harm in a trial therapy with the guidance of a homeopathic doctor.

Stopping Tears

Excessive eye tears may be due to a variety of eye diseases. Sometimes, the tearing is due to allergies to dust or other airborne substances. If an eye specialist (ophthalmologist) can offer no solutions, it's worth while trying some safe and effective complementary medicines. If possible, purchase an air purifier/ionizer unit for the bedroom and other often-used rooms. Homeopathic eye drops are effective if the source of the problem is an airborne allergen or a chemical irritant.

Yarrow, in either a tea or tincture form, can be very helpful in treating chronically watering eyes. Vitamin C is also a good remedy for this problem. It's best to use buffered vitamin C crystals (calcium, sodium or potassium ascorbate). Take a high potency bioflavonoid supplement containing either quercetin, hesperidin, rutin or hesperidin. Additionally, the highly potent bioflavonoid pycnogenol could be supplemented.

If all this fails to produce good results within six weeks, try using eye drops made up from potassium ascorbate and bioflavonoids. These can be purchased from pharmacies, but may require a doctor's prescription.

Bad Temper

A bad temper may be related to poor blood sugar control. To control blood sugar levels well, eliminate all refined carbohydrates, sugars, coffee, tea and alcohol. A diet high in fiber and complex carbohydrates is usually ideal for the treatment of both hypoglycemia and adult-onset diabetes.

Most people who suffer from anxiety, irritability (bad tempers) and insomnia, and who also happen to suffer from blood sugar imbalances, benefit from high-dose niacinamide (not niacin), chromium and B-complex vitamin supplementation.

If this supplementation is ineffective after several weeks, I suggest biochemical testing be requested from a natural health care practitioner. This may include hair mineral analysis, amino acid analysis and food allergy testing. A personalized health program can then be prescribed to balance the system more exactly.

Charcot-Marie-Tooth Disease

Charcot-Marie-Tooth disease is an inherited motor and sensory neuropathy. It was formerly termed peroneal muscular atrophy. Type I disease is characterized by more severe segmental demyelination, and hence greater slowing of nerve conduction velocity, than is type II. Onset is usually in the teens, and there is slow, progressive weakness and wasting of the peroneal muscle groups with a lack of distal reflexes. Mild sensory impairment develops later, and eventually the process spreads to involve the upper extremities.

There are no reports of any types of treatments that may help prevent its progress. On the other hand, neuropathy and muscle wasting is often slowed by zinc, magnesium, ginkgo biloba extract, coenzyme Q10 and B vitamins, particularly B1, B2, B3, B5, B6, biotin, folic acid, choline, inositol and B12. These are some of the nutrients most important in nerve health and maintenance. Food sources include brewer's yeast, organ meats, whole grains, blue-green algae, sea vegetables, spirulina, berries, nuts and legumes. Evening primrose oil and other sources of essential fatty acids are also beneficial in the treatment of neuropathy.

In those over age 65, or with malabsorption problems, vitamin B12 and other nutrients may become deficient despite an excellent diet. As one ages, a number of things might develop, including a low or absent secretion of stomach hydrochloric acid, a deficiency of intrinsic factor (a substance secreted from the stomach which helps with vitamin B12 absorption), a bacterial flora overgrowth in the small intestine or a malabsorption due to excess antacids or previous stomach surgery. In these cases, oral supplementation with vitamins and minerals may not be enough. Supplementation with Swedish bitters, betaine or glutamic acid hydrochloride and pepsin may or may not be effective. Regular magnesium and B vitamin injections are required in most cases to control the problem.

Other treatment modalities to consider are acupuncture, electrical muscle stimulation, chiropractics and homeopathy.

Lou Gehrig's Disease

Amyotrophic lateral sclerosis (ALS) is a rare motor neuron disease characterized by progressive degeneration of corticospinal tracts and anterior horn cells of the central nervous system. The symptoms vary according to the part of the nervous system most affected. The disease generally occurs after age 40 and is more common in males. In most cases, muscular weakness and wasting (atrophy) begins in the hands and spreads to the forearm and legs. Throat muscles may be affected, making speech and feeding difficult. Prognosis is poor with death usually occurring within five years of diagnosis. There is no effective medical treatment except physiotherapy to help slow down muscle deterioration. All current drugs, injections, etc., are experimental and the risk (side effects) must be compared with the possible benefit in each case.

The cause of ALS is unknown. There are many theories, one being that a virus is responsible for the disease. Studies indicate that there are biochemical imbalances in ALS. These include both amino acid and mineral imbalances.

Several recently published articles conclude that ALS patients have a defective glutamic acid (glutamate) metabolism. One double-blind study showed that supplementation of the diet with branch chain amino acids for one year had a significant benefit in maintaining strength in extremity muscles and the ability to walk. Supplementation of the diet with branch chain amino acids (valine, leucine and isoleucine) is harmless and may help in the long-term prevention of muscle deterioration. A fasting plasma amino acid analysis would determine which amino acids are high or low in the system and would then guide amino acid therapy with respect to supplemental dosages.

Studies have also revealed that ALS patients may have abnormally high levels of manganese, mercury and aluminum in their systems and low levels of calcium and magnesium. A combination of blood, urine and hair mineral analysis can help determine the body's mineral balance. Diet change and mineral supplementation can then help restore balance.

Another theory about the cause of ALS is mercury toxicity (hypersensitivity) from dental fillings. There are some anecdotal reports on the benefit of replacing mercury dental fillings with non-metal fillings. No studies, however, support the testimonials. Mercury is a lethal substance that has been associated with hundreds of serious nervous and immune system problems.

Muscle Deterioration

Muscle loss or deterioration can be due to various nerve/muscle diseases. There may be a problem with the nerves supplying the area of the body that is affected. If a neurologist can make no specific diagnosis, consider a natural approach to healing the tissues.

Nutrients of special importance to muscles include all the amino acids (including the branched chain amino acids, lysine, carnitine, arginine and ornithine), calcium, phosphorus, manganese, sulphur, silicon, iodine, selenium, vitamin E, vitamin B12 and inositol. Studies also indicate that muscle health may be enhanced by supplementation with phosphatidyl choline, glutamic acid, glycine, lipase, pancreatin, wheat germ oil, coenzyme Q10, ginkgo biloba and bromelain. If B12 malabsorption is a problem, a series of vitamin B12 injections should help normalize muscle health.

A thorough nutritional evaluation should be done to determine body levels of at least the nutrients discussed above. The need for diet change and supplements can be determined by a combination of physical examination, diet history, blood tests, urine tests and hair mineral analysis.

Muscular Dystrophy

Muscular dystrophy is a group of diseases characterized by progressive muscle weakness and degeneration without nerve degeneration. Duchenne's muscular dystrophy is the most common type of these inherited disorders. Progressive muscle weakness initially leads to a waddling gait, toe walking, frequent falls and difficulty standing and climbing stairs. The shoulder muscles are affected later, and most patients are confined to a wheelchair by the age of 12.

Lab tests show very high blood levels of the muscle enzyme CK. The diagnosis can also be made by muscle biopsy, which will show muscle atrophy in cases of MS. Scoliosis and muscle contractures are common. Death usually results in the teens or twenties, most often from infections.

Studies done on those with muscular dystrophy indicate that it is helpful to balance many vitamins and trace minerals, especially selenium and vitamin E. Nutrient balancing helps prevent the rapid progression of muscle degeneration and reduces the severity of the symptoms of the disease.

Nutrients of special importance include calcium, phosphorus, manganese, sulphur, iodine, selenium, vitamin E, vitamin B12 and inositol. Studies also indicate that muscle health may be enhanced by supplementation with phosphatidyl choline, glutamic acid, glycine, lipase, pancreatin, wheat germ oil, coenzyme Q10 and bromelain.

Each case has to be dealt with on an individual basis. A thorough nutritional evaluation should be done to determine body levels of at least the nutrients discussed above. The need for diet change and supplements can be determined by a combination of physical examination, diet history, blood tests, urine tests and hair mineral analysis.

Multiple Sclerosis

Multiple Sclerosis (MS) is a disease that affects different parts of the nervous system through the destruction of the myelin sheaths-the structure that cover the nerves. The inflammatory response produces any number of symptoms, including blurred vision, staggering gait, numbness, dizziness, tremors, slurred speech, bowel and bladder problems, paralysis and sexual impotence in men. MS usually occurs in persons between the ages of twenty-five and forty. The disease may disappear for long periods of time, then return with acute symptom flare-ups. It progresses slowly and, in many cases, may last several decades. On the other hand, in a minority of cases, it can develop rapidly and progress unremittingly until death. There is no universally accepted treatment for MS. Hormone (ACTH) injections are often used in acute exacerbations, as are immunosuppressive drugs. These, of course, have severe side effects. When asked about the role of nutrition in MS, most conventional medical doctors still claim there is no benefit to any diet changes. I disagree.

Although the definitive cause of MS is unknown, a growing number of scientific studies suggest that nutrition may be a very important factor. Nutrition-oriented health care practitioners have noticed that early MS can be helped by optimizing nutritional status with respect to essential fatty acids, amino acids, minerals such as zinc, selenium and magnesium, and B vitamins, especially vitamin B12 and folic acid.

In my practice, I have noted tremendous subjective improvements in many MS patients after a series of vitamin B12 and folic acid injections. Not only did all these patients have greater energy after vitamin B12 and folic acid treatments, but, objectively, there were improvements in nerve conduction studies done by neurologists. Spontaneous remission? Not likely, because both vitamins have been demonstrated to improve nerve cell function. It is indeed possible that some cases of MS are really B vitamin deficiencies in disguise.

Most cases of MS (over 80 percent according to one 25-year study) improve on a low saturated fat diet (Swank diet for MS). Researchers have also reported that symptoms improve when food intolerances (allergies) are eliminated. In my experience, the most common hidden food allergies appear to be wheat, milk, eggs, yeast and corn. Testing and treatment of these allergies may unlock the door to recovery for many MS sufferers.

Supplements that are very effective in both prevention and treatment of MS include fish oil (omega-3-EPA) and evening primrose oil capsules. Dosages depend on the severity of the illness and the patient's tolerance for these supplements. Alternatives include flax seed oil, oil of borage and black currant oil. Vitamin E and other antioxidants (vitamin A, beta-carotene, B-complex vitamins, vitamin C, zinc, selenium, pycnogenol and others) are also beneficial.

Hypersensitivity to toxic heavy metals such as mercury can produce all the symptoms of MS; so can Lyme disease. Testing for these two possibilities is certainly worth while. Some dentists have advocated the replacement of mercury dental fillings with non-metal fillings as a therapy for MS. Although the testimonials that support the replacement of the common mercury filling in MS patients are legion, it is still a highly controversial topic. In my practice, I have had at least a dozen MS victims improve drastically after replacement of mercury dental fillings. Unfortunately, an equal number have had no change in their health status as a result of this sort of treatment. Hair mineral analysis and urine tests can screen for excess body burdens of mercury, as well as other toxic heavy metals that may interfere with the immune system. High levels can usually be offset by supplementation with vitamin C, selenium, garlic, cysteine, methionine and other sulfur-containing compounds. If you are one of those people with a mouthful of dental hardware, get yourself a copy of *Eliminating Poison in Your Mouth*, by Klaus Kaufmann—and find a dentist familiar with the mercury problem.

Some authors also believe that MS can be benefited by anti-candida treatment. This too is controversial. In situations where all else has failed and the patient is in the early stages of the disease, trial therapy with a yeast-free diet and natural antifungal remedies may be warranted.

Finally, European and South American doctors have reported successful results with the use of ozone therapy. So, as you can see, there are plenty of reasons to adopt a more positive, hopeful attitude when dealing with this serious disease.

Bell's Palsy

Bell's palsy is a condition in which there is sudden paralysis of the facial nerve on one side of the face. The cause is usually unknown, and the majority of cases recover completely within a few weeks to a few months without any specific medical treatment. In about 20 percent of the cases, the paralysis is so severe and prolonged that a course of prednisone (synthetic cortisone) is given.

To minimize swelling, fluid retention and inflammation, it is best to avoid salt and all animal products. Fish, seafood, poultry, milk, cheese, all dairy products, eggs, beef, lamb and pork are not only all high in sodium but also contain thousands of other pro-inflammatory fats and chemicals. Nutritional supplements may help speed recovery for Bell's palsy. These include B-complex vitamins (especially vitamins B1 and B3), vitamin C, chelated calcium, chelated magnesium, ginkgo biloba extract and coenzyme Q10. Vitamin B12 injections (oral supplementation is unlikely to be as effective as injections) and magnesium sulphate injections (in severe cases) may also be helpful.

Herbal remedies that may also be effective include oat, valerian and St. John's wort. This approach is best implemented by a medical doctor familiar with nutritional therapies. Side effects are minimal and treatment success is usually very rewarding. In my experience, the B12 shots alone work quickly (within two weeks) in nearly all cases.

Insomnia

A natural therapy exists for just about every symptom for which a drug is prescribed, and the natural therapy is often superior to the prescription drug. There are receptors in the brain for drugs like dalmane, a tranquilizer from the benzodiazepine family of drugs. Niacinamide (vitamin B3) in high doses can attach to the same receptors and thus help induce sleep.

Stress is a major factor in sleeping disorders; it may be desirable to change things in one's lifestyle and environment that could be contributing to insomnia. Ensure that there are no medical conditions associated with insomnia before taking any prescription drugs. One unsuspected cause of sleep disorders is hypothyroidism (low thyroid function). Counselling and stress reduction techniques such as meditation, aerobic exercise and relaxation may be helpful. There are also some nutritional factors to consider.

Insomnia and other nervous disorders are made worse by excessive caffeine or sugar intake. Make sure the diet is free of both simple sugars and caffeine. Insomnia can often be helped by a trial therapy with high doses of vitamin B complex, especially vitamin B3 (niacinamide), B6 and inositol. In practice, the combination of niacin and inositol (often used to help lower blood cholesterol levels) is an excellent sleep inducer. Other supplemental nutrients that can induce sleep include calcium, magnesium, potassium, zinc, brewer's yeast, lecithin, octacosanol and vitamin E. In people with low or absent stomach acid secretion, injections of B vitamins, especially vitamin B12, may dramatically improve nervous system function. Magnesium sulphate injections will help nerves relax when oral supplementation fails. Some studies indicate that insomnia may also be related to a deficiency in iron and copper. Blood and hair mineral analysis can be of help to reveal these and other nutritional deficiencies.

Herbal or homeopathic remedies such as camomile, hops, lady's slipper, passion flower, skullcap, wood betony, acid phosphoricum, St. John's wort and valerian may also be of help in some cases.

The amino acid tryptophan is very effective for insomnia (1,000 to 3,000 mgs before bedtime). Although it is a natural substance, it requires a doctor's prescription in Canada. Foods high in tryptophan include bananas, figs, dates and nut butters. To date, none of these foods require a doctor's prescription. Camomile herbal tea also contains tryptophan. Drinking lots of this tea may be very soothing for a hyperactive nervous system and can significantly help any sleep disorder. It may eventually require a prescription the way things are going in Canada. So, stock up and enjoy camomile while it's still on the market.

Another sleep remedy that has received a great deal of attention in the past few years is melatonin. This pineal gland hormone has proven benefits in seasonal affective disorder (SAD) and jet lag symptoms. Melatonin is available from some pharmacies or from the offices of most naturopaths or holistic doctors. Foods high in tyramine may prevent sleep by increasing the brain levels of adrenalin. These foods include cheese, alcoholic beverages, chocolate, sauerkraut, bacon, ham, sausages, eggplants, potatoes, tomatoes and tobacco. In rarer situations, insomnia can be caused by mercury excess in the body. Sources may include contaminated seafood and the erosion of silver (mercury) dental fillings. High doses of selenium, vitamin C, vitamin E, garlic and N-acetylcysteine can help rid the body of toxic heavy metals such as mercury, cadmium, lead, aluminum, arsenic and copper. Getting a mineral analysis (blood, urine and hair) is a good way of determining whether or not toxic heavy metals are present in the body above acceptable levels. See a naturopath or holistic doctor for an assessment before resorting to potentially harmful sleeping pill prescriptions.

Cataracts

Cataracts are the result of a process of clouding or opacification of the crystalline lens of the eye. They are the leading cause of impaired vision and blindness in North America, affecting approximately four million people. Over 40,000 cases of blindness are directly attributed to cataracts, and cataract surgery is the most frequent major surgery performed on Medicare patients. Cataracts may have some relationship to a variety of eye diseases, diabetes, ultraviolet light or radiation exposure, injury or surgery, viral infections, toxic heavy metal excess in the body (especially cadmium, bromine, cobalt, iridium and nickel), heredity, galactosemia (milk sugar toxemia) and advancing age.

Cataracts are caused by free radical damage to the sulphur-containing proteins in the lens. Free radicals are defined as any highly reactive molecule that can react with and destroy body tissues. The lens protects itself from free radical damage with antioxidants (free radical scavengers) like superoxide dismutase (SOD), catalase, glutathione, methionine, vitamin A, beta-carotene, vitamin B2 (riboflavin), vitamin E, vitamin C, bioflavonoids, zinc and selenium. Studies show that cataract formation may be retarded and vision abnormalities like floaters improved by increasing the intake of antioxidants.

This can be partially done with diet: avoid sugar, white flour products, milk, rancid or high fat foods and processed foods, all of which are sources of free radicals; eat more legumes, garlic and onions, the high sources of sulphur-containing amino acids; yellow vegetables (for carotenes) and fresh fruits and raw vegetables for their vitamin C. Other foods that are high in nutrients that help retard cataracts are spinach, cloves, water chestnuts, yams, lycium, black beans, and endive. Fresh juices that are recommended are combinations of carrot, spinach, beet, cucumber, endive and parsley. Cataract sufferers should avoid direct sunlight and bright lights and wear protective sunglasses when outdoors.

Vitamin C is a very important antioxidant for the eye. It is concentrated in amounts 30 to 50 times greater in the aqueous humor of the eye than in the blood. Studies show that vitamin C levels are greatly reduced or absent in the lens with a cataract and that supplementation (1,000 mgs or more daily) can halt cataract progression. Bioflavonoids, especially pycnogenol and quercetin, also provide strong antioxidant protection. In high doses, vitamin C and bioflavonoids help replace the use of antihistamines—drugs that may make cataract symptoms worse.

Glycine, glutamic acid and cysteine are the three amino acids that make up the antioxidant glutathione (also referred to as GSH), found in very high concentrations in a healthy lens. Low GSH levels are found in all cases of cataracts and can be increased by supplementing the amino acid precursors, glycine, glutamic acid and cysteine. An ancient Chinese herbal formula called Hachimijiogan helps raise the levels of GSH, thereby preventing cataracts. Hachimijiogan contains alismatis rhizome, rehmanniae root, cornus fruit, dioscoreae rhizome, hoelen, mountain bark, cinnamon bark and aconite root.

Supplementation of superoxide dismutase (SOD) does not raise the blood levels of this important antioxidant. One effective way to raise SOD blood levels is to supplement with zinc, copper and manganese, its co-factor minerals. The amino acid lysine, important in collagen formation, may be helpful in lens repair and in the inactivation of viruses thought to cause damage to the lens.

A natural health care practitioner can help with prescribing a personalized regime of vitamin, mineral and herb supplements designed for both cataract prevention and optimum eye health.

Chronic Pain Relief Naturally

A frequently unsuspected cause of chronic pain is nutrient deficiency. Deficiencies in vitamins A, B-complex vitamins, especially vitamin B12, vitamin C and magnesium can be easily reversed by oral supplementation or intramuscular injection.

Natural analgesics include DLPA (DL-phenylalanine), magnesium, niacin, niacinamide, L-tryptophan, vitamins B1, B6, vitamin B12 and vitamin C. Megadoses far above the RDA are usually required to produce an analgesic effect when any of these are taken orally. In resistant cases, intravenous or intramuscular injections are necessary to get a result. Herbs such as alfalfa, capsicum, cloves, camomile, comfrey, slippery elm, burdock, devil's claw, white willow, wintergreen, valerian, yarrow, echinacea and feverfew are also often effective in chronic pain control. Combination products containing some or all these herbs are available at most health food stores.

When pain becomes chronic and unresponsive to medical measures, one should consider the possibility of food or chemical allergy detection and treatment. Allergies can affect the nervous system in a direct way. Whenever one eats a food to which one is sensitive, the immune system makes antibodies against that food. Complexes of antibodies with the food substance in the blood are formed. These complexes set off a chain of chemical reactions that lead to inflammation or irritation of nerve tissue. Detection and elimination of the offending foods may be the only way to both prevent and alleviate the pain.

6

Women and Complementary Medicine

This chapter deals with some of the most important women's health issues. For those who want more information, I highly recommend Dr. Carolyn DeMarco's book, *Take Charge of Your Body: A Woman's Guide to Health*.

When I went through medical school in the 70s I was soundly indoctrinated with the following "facts" about women's health:

1. Hysterectomies are the preferred treatment for endometriosis and fibroids. Hysterectomies are sound preventive medicine. After all, beyond childbearing age, the uterus is an unnecessary organ. Removing the uterus may well be a good way to help prevent cancer of the uterus.

2. Episiotomy at chidlbirth is a routine procedure to ensure the safety of normal deliveries.

3. All women entering menopause must be put on synthetic female hormones to prevent osteoporosis and other effects of aging.

4. Nutrition has nothing to do with most gynecological problems.

5. The birth control pill is the safest and most effective form of birth control. Natural birth control methods are next to worthless.

6. Once a caesarean section, always a caesarean section.

7. PMS is not a real, clincial condition. Most women can be told, "It's all in your head." It should be treated with psychotherapy, salt restriction, diuretics, tranquilizers and antidepressants.

8. Due to the availability of the most modern equipment and highly skilled obstetricians, the use of midwives and home births are both dangerous and irresponsible. The pursuit of natural childbirth is a myth promoted by quacks. Midwifery is outdated and potentially as harmful as the use of chiropractic treatments for back pain.

9. All women should get ultrasounds when pregnant and mammograms once they reach the age of 40.

All these "facts" have been proven by sound scientific studies to be wrong. Despite this, the medical profession continues to batter women with dangerous drugs and unnecessary surgery while doing nothing whatsoever for the prevention of diseases such as breast cancer. There is a place for conventional gynecology, but only in conjunction with the naturopathic approach.

Perils of the Pill

Some doctors are of the belief that women need a prescription to furnish them with the hormones so inadequately supplied by nature. This is a viewpoint that has been challenged by many doctors, myself included. Over the past 15 years, I have often said that the single biggest cause of generated business at the doctor's office is the birth control pill. High dose, medium dose or low dose, the story is the same—lots of visits to doctors' offices to be examined, get Pap tests, treat all the resulting side effects and get prescription refills. I also have to admit to you that I am rather biased in favor of doing as little as possible to meddle with nature, especially in completely healthy young women.

Numerous studies have documented the fact that the pill creates vitamin and mineral deficiencies (folic acid, zinc, B6, other B vitamins) leading to depression, fatigue, abnormal food cravings, anorexia, migraine headaches, anemia, vision changes and dozens of other side effects.

Any woman who has ever read *The Yeast Syndrome*, by Trowbridge and Walker, or *The Yeast Connection* or *Chronic Fatigue Syndrome and the Yeast Connection*, both by Dr. William Crook, knows that taking the birth control pill causes an increase in the population of candida (yeast) in the bowel as well as in the vagina. Over the years, I have helped hundreds of women eliminate and prevent yeast vaginitis attacks by simply having them stop taking the pill. Recurrent vaginal, bladder and other types of infection are more common in birth control pill users. Food allergies and eye, nose, ear and sinus problems are also more common, possibly because of the increased yeast population.

Many women who are on the birth control pill for extended periods of time complain of increased weight gain, fluid retention, headaches and breast pain. Stopping the pill often reverses these problems. Numerous cases of intractable obesity and eating disorders may stem from the vitamin and mineral deficiencies generated by the pill.

Irrespective of diet, smoking or other drug intake, the birth control pill changes the concentrations of coagulation factors in the blood, adding to the risk of thromboembolism (blood clotting disorders), high blood pressure and stroke. This may be a rare event, but what woman wants to be a 27-year-old stroke victim thanks to the pill? The many lawsuits that have been started by victims of the pill support this fact.

The pill creates a higher incidence of PMS with symptoms such as chronic fatigue, fluid retention, loss of libido, depression, anxiety, craving for sweets, sleep disorders and personality changes.

The incidence of breast cancer in women is escalating. It is well known that many cases of breast cancer are estrogen sensitive, meaning that they grow in response to estrogens like those in the birth control pill. Cancer specialists, therefore, often take breast cancer patients off estrogens entirely. In fact, one of the recognized treatments for breast cancer is tamoxifen, a drug that suppresses the effects of estrogen in the body and prevents the spread of cancer.

Herbal Birth Control

At this time, I cannot recommend any natural product for worry-free, reliable contraception. However, the following herbs have known or suspected contraceptive properties:

American ginseng	Gromwell
Ashwaganda	Plantain
Blessed thistle	Rosemary oil
Chaparral	Shepherd's purse
Cinchona bark	Stevia
Cotton root	White pepper

Unfortunately, there are no studies or guidelines on reliability, contraceptive dosages, success percentages, failure rates, etc., for any of these herbs. Some, like gromwell have been documented to induce abortion.

Natural progesterone precursors like chaste berries, sarsaparilla and wild yam root are another natural birth control option. When any of these are taken, they increase the body's levels of natural progesterone. In a cream form, applied to the skin once or twice daily before ovulation, natural progesterone has contraceptive properties. It basically prevents sperm from entering the uterus. Once again, reliability and success and failure rates for such contraception have never been accurately documented. Unlike the other herbs mentioned earlier, natural progesterone cream is safe to use at any time during a woman's cycle, as well as during pregnancy and while breast feeding.

Water Retention

Edema, or water retention, is an abnormal accumulation of fluid in various organs, cavities or tissues of the body. Edema is not a disease in itself but a symptom of specific disorders.

The best treatment for edema is to identify the underlying cause. Edema in the legs and ankles occurs when the veins fail to maintain pace with the arteries. There are over 30 predisposing factors that can lead to edema. It is a common problem for people who stand in one position for too long, who wear restrictive garments, who have weak legs (especially calf muscles), who consume excess salt, or who are sensitive to warm weather. Certain high blood pressure medications (beta-adrenergic blockers) can cause edema. So can protein deficiency or imbalance, varicose veins, premenstrual syndrome, obesity, high blood pressure, the oral contraceptive pill, pregnancy, liver disease, thyroid disease, adrenal gland problems, various forms of heart disease, pancreatitis, kidney disorders—the list goes on. It is very important to exhaust all the medical causes for edema before doing anything else.

Once this has been done, one should look into the possibility of nutritional-biochemical imbalances. For example, some nutrition-oriented doctors have found that a significant number of people suffering from edema of unknown origin have hidden or delayed food allergies. Many women are put on diuretics to control their tendency for fluid retention. Weight fluctuations are very often associated with fluid retention problems and are usually indicators of unsuspected food allergies. Changing the diet to avoid or to rotate the allergic foods frequently causes the elimination of the fluid excess and may significantly help those with chronic weight problems. Wheat and other grains are the most common offenders, but any food can produce fluid retention in susceptible individuals.

The diet should also be analyzed for excessive sodium or salt intake. Inadequate water intake, believe it or not, may cause edema. Studies have also shown that suboptimal intakes of certain nutrients may also be involved. These include bioflavonoids (found in garlic, onions, chives, cherries, peppers and the white covering of citrus fruits,) and the vitamin B1, vitamin B5 (pantothenic acid), vitamin B6, gamma linoleic acid (from evening primrose or flax seed oil), iodine, magnesium (especially from deep green leafy vegetables such as parsley and spinach) and vitamin C. Eating more of the foods containing these nutrients will be of some help. Frequently, doctors prescribe these nutrients in supplemental form, occasionally in megadoses. Herbal diuretics such as uva ursi, juniper berries, shavegrass, cornsilk, queen-of-the-meadow, buchu, cranberries, watermelon seeds, horseradish, nettle, sassafras and parsley are safe, as long as the recommended doses are not exceeded.

The problem with diuretic drugs such as furosemide is that they may cause a loss of potassium, magnesium, zinc and other trace minerals from the body. People on such drugs should be monitored by their doctors for mineral imbalances.

In cases of poor muscle tone from many years of sedentary behavior, some practitioners recommend therapeutic massage or shiatsu treatment. Aerobic exercise or rebounding on a mini-trampoline on a regular basis may improve lymphatic circulation. In short, there is a lot that can be done before resorting to prescription drugs (diuretics).

I caution, however, that none of these natural remedies should be tried without the supervision of a qualified health care practitioner and certainly not before all treatable medical reasons for edema have been ruled out.

Endometriosis

Endometriosis is a disorder that results from the presence of actively growing and functioning endometrial tissue (the name for the cells that line the uterus) in sites outside the uterus. Endometrial tissue can be widespread, and the usual endometriosis sufferer has multiple sites, including the ovaries, the urinary bladder, the appendix, the small bowel, the large bowel, scars from previous abdominal incisions, the umbilicus and even the liver, gallbladder and kidneys may be involved.

Endometriosis is a disease that occurs during the reproductive life of women. It affects approximately 15 percent of all women, and many journals report that its incidence is increasing. The typical patient is in her late twenties or early thirties and is either single, has married late or has voluntarily delayed childbearing. Users of the birth control pill seem to have a slightly lower incidence of endometriosis while those using intrauterine devices (IUDs) have a significantly higher incidence. An estimated 40 percent of women who undergo hysterectomy have endometriosis.

Without intervention, endometriosis ceases almost entirely after menopause. Retrograde menstruation and implantation is still the most popular and widely accepted theory on the cause of the disorder. Although retrograde menstruation occurs in most women, the actual development of endometriosis is dependent on many other factors, including the health of the immune system which, in turn, is dependent on nutritional status.

An alternative theory about endometriosis has recently been advanced by Dr. David Redwine. He believes that endometriosis is caused by an embryonic defect in cell differentiation, as opposed to retrograde menstruation. Accepted theory states that lesions bleed monthly, whereas Dr. Redwine theorizes that they do not. Dr. Redwine has developed a new surgical treatment for endometriosis called "near-contact" laparoscopy. Based on his studies, he reports little recurrence of lesions following removal of both typical and atypical lesions. Dr. Redwine claims that endometriosis is a positionally static disease, while conventional gynecologists claim it is a progressive disease. Conventional thinking is that endometriosis primarily affects women over age 30, while Dr. Redwine believes it affects all females regardless of age. Accepted theories hold to the idea that endometriosis is associated with menstruation, is prevalent black lesions in the pelvis and that it causes infertility. Dr. Redwine believes that endometriosis is independent of menstruation, is associated with multicolored lesions and is not an actual cause of infertility. He maintains that removal of typical and atypical lesions by his special surgical techniques provides complete relief for 75 percent of cases.*

The most obvious symptom of endometriosis is painful menstrual periods. About 15 to 20 percent of sufferers report no pain or discomfort, but their endometriosis may be associated with infertility or a pelvic mass. Gynecologists have traditionally treated endometriosis with pituitary gonadotrophin hormone inhibitors such as danazol, or with surgery—as radical as complete hysterectomy and oophorectomy (removal of the ovaries). At present, the medical profession as a whole does not promote any treatments for endometriosis involving lifestyle change, diet or nutritional supplements. Research, however, has linked several nutritional imbalances and lifestyles to setting the stage for the development of endometriosis.

For example, epidemiological studies show that a low iodine intake may produce a state of increased pituitary gonadotrophin activity, which may lead to the development of endometriosis as well as endocrine disorders such as hypothyroidism (low thyroid function). It is also known that strenuous exercise decreases the risk for endometriosis. Although these associations exist, there have not as yet been any studies demonstrating that endometriosis can be ameliorated by either iodine supplementation or strenuous exercise. It is safe to say, however, that optimizing the iodine in one's diet is desirable. Good food sources of iodine include kelp, dulse, Swiss chard, turnip greens, watercress, pineapples, pears, artichokes, citrus fruits, egg yolks and seafoods. If the diet available is poor, supplementation of iodine with sea kelp or dulse tablets (no higher than 150 mcgs of iodine daily) is a good alternative. Overdoing iodine supplementation can be as disastrous as not getting enough. Signs of excessive iodine supplementation may include acne and inflammation of the thyroid gland (thyroiditis).

A 1985 study by Ylikorkala and Makila reported in the *American Journal of Obstetrics and Gynecology* showed that patients with pelvic endometriosis

---

* For more information on Dr. Redwine's studies, write to Nancy Petersen, St. Charles Medical Center, 2500 N.E. Neff Road, Bend, OR 97701 or call 503-382-4321.

may have elevated levels of chemicals that increase pain and inflammation. Other studies have reported moderate imbalances in prostaglandin levels in women who suffer from endometriosis. It is known that supplementation with either flax seed oil, borage oil, black currant seed oil, omega-3 EPA oils (e.g,. salmon oil) or evening primrose oil can inhibit the action of pro-inflammatory chemicals in the body and optimize prostaglandin hormone levels. A number of health care practitioners have been recommending flax seed oil, evening primrose oil and omega-3-EPA oil supplements as complementary treatments for sufferers of endometriosis. This would not interfere with any medical therapy. Since therapeutic intake levels of these supplements are usually safe, they're certainly worth a six-month trial therapy.

Essential fatty acid therapy should be complemented by vitamin E (400 IU to 1,000 IU), vitamin B complex, vitamin C, bioflavonoids, calcium and magnesium. These and other antioxidant vitamins and minerals may be important in the prevention of adhesion formation in endometriosis. Recent studies indicate that free radicals are involved in some aspects of the disease process. For those more interested in getting these essential oils from diet alone, two recent books, *The Omega-3 Phenomenon*, by Dr. Donald O. Rudin and Clara Felix, and *The Omega-3 Breakthrough*, by Julius Fast, are very thorough with respect to menus and recipes. They're definitely worth reading.

Herbal remedies that have been used successfully in the complementary medical treatment of endometriosis include dong quai, black cohosh, damiana, cramp bark, false unicorn, gentian, licorice, gotu kola, sarsaparilla, saw palmetto, sqaw vine, wild yam, raspberry leaves and Siberian ginseng. It is important to avoid caffeine, chocolate, salt, sugar, animal fats, fried foods and processed foods. These either rob the body of essential trace minerals, aggravate female problems or create imbalances in essential fatty acids.

Some authors believe that one of the major reasons we are seeing more endometriosis is because of the excess estrogen we are getting in beef, chicken, turkey and all dairy products. They also believe that women would be better able to handle excess toxins, such as the hormones in animal products, if the colon were kept healthy and regular. For more information on how to optimize elimination, see the section on constipation in this book.

Lastly, daily exercise can provide a marked improvement. This should include nothing more strenuous than walking or stretching because severe cases may be aggravated by anything more strenuous. It is well known that heavy exercise in women over long periods of time (e.g., as in marathon runners) may not only eliminate menstrual pain, but cause some women to stop having periods altogether, or until the heavy exercising is drastically reduced. Women suffering from endometriosis need to assess their physical fitness, as there is clearly some connection between this disease and exercise.

Treating endometriosis does not necessarily guarantee a cure for infertility. Fertility is a complex subject that is dealt with elsewhere in this book.

Menopause and the Wellness Viewpoint

Menopause is a natural event in every woman's life. It is not a "deficiency disease," a "deterioration," an "estrogen starvation" or any other of a long list of archaic, patriarchal medical labels. It is a process of change and transition as a woman's body sheds its child-bearing potential and adjusts to lower levels of hormones. Menopause starts around the late forties, when periods start to get more irregular, and finally stops altogether at an average age of 50 (earlier in black and non-European women). In the healthy female, once the ovaries stop producing the female hormones, the adrenal glands eventually produce enough hormones to maintain balance. During this transition period, hot flashes, vaginal dryness, depression, loss of libido and other menopausal problems prompt women to visit their doctors.

Doctors disagree about whether all menopausal women should be on hormones, or whether hormones should be reserved for women with severe hot flashes, vaginal dryness or those at high risk for bone loss and heart attacks. Some prescribe synthetic estrogen, with or without progesterone, to all their menopausal patients. Others, however, maintain that only in rare cases should women be prescribed synthetic hormones, and that symptoms can be controlled entirely by natural means. Doctors also disagree about the length of time hormones should be taken. The extremist pharmaceutical view holds that menopausal women should be on hormones until death.

Despite the grandiose claims of the drug lobby, there is little evidence to support the use of estrogen for the prevention of heart disease, osteoporosis or any other disease. Long-term studies on the effects of estrogen and progesterone on healthy postmenopausal women have never been done. An editorial in the *New England Journal of Medicine* (August 27, 1992) puts it this way: "Since the long-term safety of hormone replacement therapy has not yet been fully elucidated, there is need for other effective therapies for the prevention and treatment of osteoporosis."

Low estrogen is but one of 40 factors involved in the development of osteoporosis. Exercise and vegetarian (low protein) diets have been shown to be far more important for osteoporosis prevention. Other major risk factors for osteoporosis development are cigarette smoking, excessive alcohol and caffeine intake, having a fair complexion, having had the ovaries removed (or other causes of early menopause), a positive family history of osteoporosis, never having been pregnant, digestive disorders, overactive endocrine glands (especially hyperthyroidism) and drugs such as cortisone, diuretics, anti-seizure medications and anticoagulants (blood thinners).

Some of the many negative effects of estrogen replacement therapy during menopause include abnormal Pap tests, abnormal bleeding with resulting iron deficiency, candida (yeast) infections, circulation problems, high blood pressure, abnormal blood clotting (thrombosis), migraines, strokes, increased risk of coronary artery disease, weight gain and fluid retention. Some women who take prescription estrogens complain of acne, skin color changes, bloating, a loss of libido, depression and an increased sensitivity to light. Others complain of menstrual pattern changes, chest pain, difficulty breathing, eye pain, vision changes, a loss of coordination, increasing breast lumps and painful urination.

The use of estrogen hormone by itself is associated with a three to four times increased incidence of uterine cancer. To lower the potential cancer risk, doctors usually add a progesterone prescription for ten days out of every cycle. Unfortunately, this causes menopausal women to continue to bleed monthly for as long as they are on hormone replacement therapy. Other common side effects of progesterone therapy include migraines, bloating, breast tenderness and depression.

Hormone replacement therapy is linked to an increased risk of breast cancer. According to Dr. Sidney Wolfe in an article in the *Health Letter of the Public Citizen Health Research Group*, "If a woman used estrogen pills for 15 years, she had a 30 percent excess rate of breast cancer. If used for 25 years, a 'goal' toward which many doctors are pushing their patients, there would be a 50 percent increased risk of breast cancer...." Women have now been exposed to both long-term hormone treatment in the form of the birth control pill and long-term hormone treatment in the form of estrogen replacement. No one really knows what the combined effect might be on the intricate workings of the female reproductive system. There are several ongoing studies to evaluate the specific interaction, but the results won't be available for ten to twenty years. Many doctors feel that medicating a natural life process with potentially toxic drugs cannot be justified on the basis of some very questionable research. Certainly, there are no safety and efficacy studies that are conclusive enough to warrant the wide-scale drugging of a normal, healthy female population.

Menopausal symptoms can be controlled naturally and without any significant side effects. Osteoporosis and coronary artery disease can be prevented and even reversed by diet and lifestyle changes alone. The ideal diet for menopausal women is vegetarian. There are many reasons for this, the major one being that animal proteins, with their high phosphorus content, cause the body to lose large amounts of calcium and other minerals. For more information on vegetarian diets and a list of studies that support this type of diet in osteoporosis/heart disease prevention and treatment, see *Diet for a New America* and *May All Be Fed*, both by John Robbins.

Most menopausal symptoms, including hot flashes, can be treated successfully with supplemental vitamins, minerals and herbs. Some herbs contain estrogenic substances, but at levels of estrogen activity 400 times less than pharmaceutical compounds. These include dong quai, licorice, black cohosh, fennel and a long list of soya products. Other herbs that are helpful for menopausal symptoms include damiana, raspberry, sage, Siberian ginseng and gotu kola. Several food supplement companies make combinations of these herbal remedies (e.g., St. Francis Herb Farms, Nature's Sunshine, Enrich International). Natural vitamin E also contains traces of estrogens, making it an ideal menopausal supplement. The same can be said about brewer's yeast.

Dr. John Lee has found that the use of a natural progesterone cream applied to the skin will prevent bone loss even without the addition of estrogen. More and more health care practitioners are recommending creams containing natural progesterone, found in plants such as European mistletoe and Mexican wild yam, as the single most important substitute for the synthetic approach to menopausal symptoms. Studies done by gynecologists, internists and other types of doctors conclude that progesterone is far more important than estrogen in both the prevention and treatment of osteoporosis (see the book *Natural Progesterone* by Dr. John R. Lee).

Synthetic estrogens in pill or cream form may increase the risk for breast and uterine cancer and have virtually no impact on remineralizing an already osteoporotic skeleton. Yes, estrogens slow down osteoporosis. They do not, however, reverse it like natural progesterone. Progesterone is the precursor of many hormones, such as estrogen, cortisol, aldosterone and leutinizing hormone. It also promotes a more efficient use of thyroid hormone by the body. Aside from its role in reversing osteoporosis, progesterone cream protects against breast cancer, decreases fibrocystic breast disease and reduces the incidence of ovarian cysts. It prevents fluid retention, fat deposits, vaginal dryness and urinary bladder infections. Women who suffer from both stress and a loss of libido will benefit from the use of progesterone cream.

Oral progesterone is not as effective as the natural progesterone cream. The cream absorbs through the skin and goes directly to where it is needed by the body. The transdermal route ensures that the progesterone bypasses the liver for more efficient delivery to receptor sites. It can be applied once daily into soft tissue areas such as the chest, breasts, under arms, inner thighs or abdomen. The total monthly dosage is 1,000 mgs (equivalent to approximately 1/2 teaspoon daily). There are no side effects. Remember that progesterone is produced naturally by the body at levels as high as 400 mgs daily during pregnancy. Negative side effects are only associated with chemically altered forms of natural progesterone. The usual source of natural progesterone is an extract of Mexican wild yam.

Do not confuse natural progesterone cream with "progestins" or "progestagens," which are associated with many significant side effects. With natural progesterone cream, the body uses only what it needs and no excess is allowed to build up. Natural progesterone is initially absorbed into the body's fat tissues and takes about three or four months before blood levels increase significantly. The benefits of progesterone cream may, however, be seen much earlier. To help alleviate severe hot flashes, natural progesterone cream can be applied as often as every 15 minutes, until hot flashes disappear. In addition to natural progesterone cream, vaginal dryness and itching during menopause can be controlled by using vitamin E cream or calendula in flax seed cream.

Synthetic estrogen stimulates candida growth in the large bowel. So do anabolic steroids, cortisone-like drugs, sugar, white flour products and broad-spectrum antibiotics. For more information on candida, boosting immunity, fighting fatigue and other chronic health problems including chronic fatigue syndrome, see *Chronic Fatigue Syndrome and The Yeast Connection*, by Dr. William Crook.

For women who cannot go off synthetic estrogens for real or imagined reasons, vitamin E (400 IU to 1,200 IU daily) and evening primrose oil capsules (six to nine capsules a day) will help prevent some of the circulatory complications of synthetic estrogen therapy (e.g., abnormal blood clotting, etc.).

Bioflavonoids are plant substances that exist together with vitamin C in nature. They prevent estrogens from being broken down too rapidly in the body, thereby avoiding some of the unpleasant hot flash symptoms. Bioflavonoids are abundantly available in citrus fruits, garlic, onions, peppers, cherries, currants, buckwheat and many other foods. In supplemental form, look for bottles containing rutin, hesperidin, catechin, quercetin or pycnogenol on your health food store shelves.

Bee pollen (2 to 12 capsules daily) and boron (2 mgs 3 times daily) are other natural supplements that help women during menopause. Boron supplementation, for example, raises serum estrogen levels. One study demonstrated that boron supplementation produced estrogen blood levels identical to estrogen treated women whose diets were not supplemented with boron. Boron supplementation does not pose the same cancer-causing risks as synthetic estrogen replacement therapy (e.g., uterine or breast cancer). It is non-toxic. For a personalized program of diet and supplements, consult a natural health care practitioner.

Osteoporosis and Nutrition

Osteoporosis is a major health problem. Approximately one-third of all North American women suffer from this bone demineralization condition that may ultimately result in fractures. The most frequently affected sites are the hips, vertebrae and wrists. Bone mass begins to decline after age 35, reaching its peak around the time of menopause. Bone demineralization continues thereafter at a slower rate.

The medical approach to osteoporosis treatment and prevention centers around estrogen, Tums, prescriptions for calcium and pep talks about gobbling up more dairy products. Fluoride supplementation, although unproven and potentially toxic, is still popular in some medical circles as is megadosing with vitamin D. Despite conventional therapy and edicts by dietitians and dairy bureaus, fractures and bone loss still occur at an alarming rate.

Studies done by gynecologists, internists and other types of doctors conclude that progesterone is far more important than estrogen in both the prevention and treatment of osteoporosis. Dr. John Lee has found the use of a natural progesterone cream applied directly on the skin will prevent bone loss even without the addition of estrogen. Natural progesterone cream is derived from an extract of wild yam and has no toxic effects. Better still, you do not need a doctor's prescription as it is available at most health food stores just for the asking. (For more information on natural progesterone, see the section Menopause and the Wellness Viewpoint.)

Synthetic estrogens in pill or cream form may increase the risk for breast and uterine cancer and have virtually no impact on remineralizing an already osteoporotic skeleton. While estrogens slow down osteoporosis, they do not reverse it like natural progesterone.

Risk Factors For the Development of Osteoporosis Are:
- Cigarette smoking
- Excessive alcohol and caffeine intake
- High protein diet (encourages high mineral losses in the urine)
- Low calorie weight-loss diets
- High milk and dairy product consumption
- Drinking distilled water exclusively (my own observation)
- Having a fair complexion
- Physical inactivity
- Excessive physical exercise
- Weightlessness for extended periods of time (*avoid space shuttle trips!*)
- Having had the ovaries removed (*or other causes of early menopause*)
- A family history of osteoporosis
- Never having been pregnant
- Diuretics (water pills)
- Anti-seizure medications
- Anticoagulants (blood thinners)
- Antacid abuse, anti-ulcer drugs
- Digestive disorders leading to trace mineral malabsorption
- Overactive endocrine glands (especially hyperthyroidism)
- Long-term use of prescription steroids like prednisone
- Vitamin and mineral deficiencies

Vitamin D is required to absorb calcium from the small intestine. Deficiency can come about when there is reduced exposure to sunlight, decreased dietary intake or a malabsorption problem of one kind or another. Excess vitamin D can lead to the breakdown of bone, but is rarely seen even in elderly patients prescribed 50,000 IU per month. Taking one halibut liver oil capsule daily (400 IU of vitamin D) is sufficient for prevention in most people with good intestinal function. It certainly can do no harm.

Studies show that many other nutrients are involved in osteoporosis development. Bone is, after all, active, living tissue continuously forming and being broken down. It is not just an inanimate collection of calcium crystals. As with all our body tissues, bone is sensitive to diet and lifestyle habits. The typical western diet—high in refined carbohydrate, animal protein and fat, canned and processed foods—has been linked to a greater incidence of osteoporosis simply because such a diet is inadequate in a large number of nutrients. It is also excessively high in phosphorus, a mineral that in large amounts antagonizes calcium in the body. Interestingly enough, the foods most often recommended for healthy bones—milk and dairy products—are also excessively high in phosphorus and may actually promote osteoporosis. I strongly recommend avoidance of all animal proteins, including eggs and dairy products. Statistics world-wide support vegan diets as optimal for osteoporosis prevention and treatment. A good example of a vegan diet is the McDougall Plan.

The protein matrix upon which calcium crystallizes is called ostoecalcin. Studies show that vitamin K is required by the body to make osteocalcin. Several other vitamins are important for bone health. These include vitamin A, folic acid, vitamin B6, vitamin B12 and vitamin C. Because these vitamins are required in numerous biochemical reactions in bone (connective) tissue, a lack of them increases osteoporosis severity. The same can be said for minerals such as magnesium, manganese, boron, strontium, silicon, zinc and copper. Silicon, for example, is found in high concentrations in growing bone. It strengthens connective tissue and may be crucial in osteoporosis prevention.

Boron supplementation raises serum estrogen levels. One study demonstrated that boron supplementation produced estrogen blood levels identical to estrogen-treated women whose diets were not supplemented with boron. Boron supplementation does not pose the same cancer-causing risks as synthetic estrogen replacement therapy (e.g., uterine or breast cancer). It is non-toxic. Unfortunately, many people are deficient in this mineral simply because of poor soil quality. Consider panax ginseng as another source of naturally occurring estrogen (estriol). Not only does ginseng help control hot flashes, it may be a very valuable adjunct to the prevention and treatment of osteoporosis. Individual requirements for these nutrients will vary from woman to woman, depending on biochemical make-up, activity and stress levels. Focusing only on calcium, milk, vitamin D and estrogen therapy is not enough.

To find out whether you have a problem with osteoporosis, ask your family doctor to order bone density studies on you. This is a non-invasive test (covered by Medicare in most provinces) similar to an x-ray but far more specific in that it will indicate whether or not osteoporosis is an issue in your health. Without such a test you really have no way of knowing where you stand and how far you have to go with diet and lifestyle changes. Also, consider getting blood, urine and hair mineral analyses done to determine your body's current mineral levels.

Male/Female Hormone Imbalances

The appearance of oily skin and acne in women past the teenage years is a major concern since it is often treated by dermatologists with potent broad-spectrum antibiotics and other drugs. The underlying problem in these situations is often a hormonal imbalance. Another possibility is mal-digestion—an incomplete breakdown of several foods with resulting bowel toxemia. Chronic candida overgrowth in the large bowel may also be involved. A variety of lab tests can help confirm these possibilities.

Male hormones may be a little too active and, hence, hair loss may occur. There are some natural ways of rebalancing your hormones. One of these is through the use of natural progesterone, an extract of Mexican wild yam. The best way of using this product is as a cream which allows the progesterone to absorb into the bloodstream through the skin. Progesterone then converts into many other hormones in the body, including estrogens. The net effect is a rebalancing of male and female hormones. Natural progesterone is also important to optimize thyroid hormone function.

Saw palmetto is very effective in the management of more stubborn cases of oily skin and acne because of its ability to reduce the levels of dihydrotestosterone, the male hormone responsible for stimulating acne development. Other natural hormone balancers are dong quai, black cohosh, damiana, bee pollen, natural vitamin E and the mineral boron. For bowel detoxification, consider a combination of burdock, slippery elm, Turkish rhubarb and sheep sorrel. Echinacea, aloe vera juice (whole leaf, cold processed), berberine and lactobacillus acidophilus all have natural antibiotic effects and can help clear up oily skin and acne.

A very effective topical option is tea tree oil, derived from the Australian native tree *Melaleucea alternifolia*. It has a variety of antimicrobial activities and has been used successfully in the treatment of many different skin conditions, especially those associated with fungal or candida infections.

Theories about the direct effects of food on the development of comedones (blackheads) and acne have not been proven. However, many doctors involved in nutritional medicine report that food allergy or hypersensitivity is involved. Studies do support some basic dietary guidelines for prevention. All refined carbohydrates and processed foods should be eliminated.

These include chocolates, sweetened cereals, candy bars, cakes, cookies and other junk foods. High fat foods, particularly those containing trans-fatty acids like margarine, shortening and other hydrogenated vegetable oils, should be limited. Fried foods of most kinds fall into this category.

Foods high in iodine (white flour products, heavily salted foods) can cause acne in some people and should be eliminated for those that are iodine-sensitive. Limit cow's milk consumption due to its high hormone content. Food allergy testing should be considered if there is any question about specific offending foods. See a naturopath or holistic medical doctor for a professional opinion.

Hair Loss in Women

Hair loss in women is a fairly common problem related to aging. Sometimes, a low thyroid condition causes excessive hair loss and is reversible with thyroid hormone replacement therapy. It can also be the result of a greater need for estrogen and progesterone. These female hormones are available naturally from a variety of sources, dietary and herbal.

Eating more foods with a high content of safe estrogens might be helpful. These include soy products (soy milk, tofu, etc.), wheat germ, bee pollen, brewer's yeast, alfalfa and yams. Natural progesterone cream (from an extract of Mexican wild yam) and natural estrogen cream (from soy beans) could both be rubbed into the skin and the scalp to help increase blood levels of both hormones. A two-ounce jar of either cream will last about one month, and a trial therapy could be done for at least six months.

Some herbs contain estrogenic substances. These include dong quai, licorice, black cohash, damiana, raspberry, sage, Siberian ginseng and gotu kola. Several food supplement companies make combinations of these herbal remedies. Natural vitamin E also contains traces of estrogen. Bioflavonoids are plant substances that exist together with vitamin C in nature. They prevent estrogens from being broken down too rapidly in the body. Bioflavonoids are abundantly available in citrus fruits, garlic, onions, peppers, cherries, currants, buckwheat and many other foods. In supplemental form, look for bottles containing rutin, hesperidin, catechin, quercetin or pycnogenol.

Many essential nutrients are involved in healthy hair growth. These include vitamin A, biotin, inositol, vitamin B12, PABA, other B-complex vitamins, unsaturated essential fatty acids (from evening primrose, flax seed, rice bran, borage, black currant or fish), vitamin E, coenzyme Q10, DMG (dimethylglycine), silica, zinc, copper, iron, iodine, cysteine and methionine. A naturopath or a medical doctor familiar with nutritional evaluations can provide an individualized diet and supplement program.

Calcium Confusion

The body has a built-in homeostatic mechanism to continuously keep blood levels of calcium within a normal range. In other words, blood levels will be normal in the face of very low or very high calcium intakes. If intake is low, calcium comes out of bone to normalize the blood levels. This all takes place with the help of several organs and glands, including the kidneys and parathyroids. To properly test for calcium adequacy a combination of dietary intake determinations, 24-hour urine test for calcium, blood ionized calcium level and hair mineral analysis should be done. If these indicate an imbalance, parathyroid function and other tests should be done. If calcium tablets provide relief of aching muscles and joints, chances are high that there is a greater need for calcium at that particular time. Since calcium is so often in a state of flux, needs for it will be different depending on the circumstances.

Many factors lead to chronic calcium deficiency. These include inadequate intake, hormonal imbalances (e.g., as occurs in pregnancy), thyroid disease, parathyroid disease, kidney disease, gastrointestinal malabsorption, food allergies (milk being a very common one), excessive protein (phosphorus) intake, inactivity (sedentary behavior), excessive fat intake, vitamin D deficiency, drugs such as diuretics, cigarette smoking, excessive alcohol intake, excess sugar intake and stress.

A diet high in oxalic acid (soybeans, kale, spinach, rhubarb, beet greens, chard and cocoa) may interfere with calcium absorption. Excess zinc, magnesium, fiber and iron can also interfere with calcium absorption. High phosphorus sources in the diet (red meats, soft drinks, refined grains like white bread) are common calcium inhibitors.

Dairy products are a calcium source, but by no means the only ones. Contrary to popular belief, women do not need milk or dairy products to be well nourished with respect to calcium. Other excellent sources include salmon, sardines, seafood, asparagus, broccoli, cabbage, collards, dulse, almonds, figs, filberts, mustard greens, parsley and other green leafy vegetables. If you consume a large variety of these calcium sources, there is no need to use dairy products. Consult a naturopath or nutritional doctor to develop a health program based on objective tests.

Osteoporosis and Silica

According to Passwater and Cranton, silica is concentrated in the body in sites of active calcification in the bones. In their book, Trace Elements, Hair Analysis and Nutrition, they state that "calcium and silicon are probably concurrently necessary for bone formation." Silica is, in fact, necessary for calcium absorption. This would obviously be important for bone healing after a fracture.

Patients over 70 years of age usually have a hard time with protein digestion and trace mineral absorption because of low secretion of stomach hydrochloric acid. In a 70-year-old osteoporotic lady, this is most likely the case. This can be confirmed by a comprehensive stool and digestive analysis and hair mineral analysis. If stomach acid deficiency is the problem, appropriate digestive aids (e.g., stomach bitters, apple cider vinegar, citric acid, betaine and pepsin HCL, etc.) can be prescribed based on the degree of hypoacidity.

Candida

The long-term use of the birth control pill, estrogens, steroids and antibiotics such as tetracycline can lead to the development of the yeast syndrome (candidiasis). A candida overgrowth in the digestive system can lead to odd or irregular food intolerances, intractable pain and numerous other health problems, including eczema, recurrent vaginitis and other pelvic problems. Biochemical testing would have to be done in order to confirm this diagnosis.

See a naturopath or medical doctor familiar with the yeast syndrome to get a thorough assessment and individualized treatment plan. Do not start on any treatment until this is done. The subject of candida has been beaten to death in at least two dozen popular books. For more information on this twentieth century epidemic, consult the following books:

The Missing Diagnosis (Orian Truss)
Candida (Luc de Schepper)
Candida: A Twentieth Century Disease (S. S. Lorenzani)
Candida Albicans (L. Chaitow)
The Yeast Syndrome (J. P. Trowbridge and M. Walker)
The Yeast Connection (W. G. Crook)
Chronic Fatigue Syndrome and the Yeast Connection (W. G. Crook)

Endless Candida

Whether the remedies are natural or not, months of barely successful candida treatments are usually a sign that something else needs to be addressed. Remember, candida is a secondary, opportunistic infection caused primarily by a weakened immune system. There may be concurrent parasitic infections, bacterial infections and a long list of other health problems that need treatment. These include vitamin and mineral deficiencies, protein and amino acid imbalances, toxic heavy metal accumulations (e.g., mercury, lead, cadmium, etc.), immunodeficiencies, food and chemical allergies, hypothyroidism, adrenal insufficiency and other hormonal imbalances like progesterone deficiency.

One does not pass on candida infections to healthy people. All healthy people carry candida on their skin and in their gastrointestinal tracts. It is only when the immune system is compromised that the so-called candida syndrome develops.

Many cases of subclinical hypothyroidism are behind endless candida diagnoses and treatments. Synthetic thyroid prescriptions are not necessarily the right way to treat such cases. Although conventional lab tests for thyroid problems may be entirely normal, these cases respond well to natural desiccated thyroid hormone prescriptions. See *Hypothyroidism: The Unsuspected Illness*, Dr. Broda Barnes' book on the use of natural thyroid hormone.

Still others do better with time-released liothyronine (T3) prescriptions. For more information on T3, consult *Wilson's Syndrome: The Miracle of Feeling Well*, by Dr. Denis Wilson. Wilson's syndrome treatment can sometimes get complicated. Supervision by a medical doctor on a regular basis is required, mainly to decide on dosages and to monitor for side effects.

My advice to people on seemingly endless candida treatments is to encourage your doctor or naturopath to do some detective work on your behalf. Tests to consider include more extensive vitamin, mineral and amino acid analysis, Elisa/Act blood tests for food, chemical and toxic heavy metal hypersensitivities, comprehensive stool and digestive analysis (CSDA) for digestive function, flora balance and parasite detection. Look into the possibility of treating Wilson's syndrome and other hormone imbalances.

The RU-486 Madness

Thirty years after the introduction of the birth control pill we are seeing long-term side effects like cancer, heart disease, high blood pressure and strokes. Although feminists may be quite excited about "absolute reproductive freedom," there is really no such guarantee with RU-486, the latest in a long line of potentially hazardous chemicals. RU-486 is better known as "the abortion pill." This drug seriously disrupts normal human physiology and biochemistry. To believe it will have no harmful long-term effects on health is wishful thinking.

Some of the short-term documented side effects of RU-486 include heavy blood loss, anemia requiring transfusions, abdominal pain, nausea, vomiting and death. Scientists speculate that it may have serious long-term health effects on the immune system, the endocrine system and fertility. Despite the negative publicity generated by RU-486 around the world, the National Cancer Institute of Canada will study its use in the treatment of breast cancer at a dozen hospitals across Canada.

There are a number of reports suggesting that RU-486 is endorsed as safe and effective by the American Medical Association. This is the same association that lost a major lawsuit because it advised member physicians not to associate with chiropractors. Remember that approximately half of the physicians in the United States are not members of the AMA. Like most physicians, I would certainly think twice about anything endorsed by the AMA.

Supporters of RU-486 also claim that it is endorsed by the "prestigious" *New England Journal of Medicine.* As with virtually all medical journals, most of it's revenues come from advertising by drug companies.

Promoting the myth that RU-486 is a safe drug is a way of getting around the issue of abortion clinics. The use of drug company-sponsored "studies" to promote RU-486 as a money saver for the health care system is nothing more than an endorsement of experimentation with the lives and fertility potential of women. The drug remains illegal in Canada and the United States.

Responsible birth control can be effectively practiced without the use of drugs or surgery. The answer is to fund health education and preventive techniques, not experimentation with dangerous products like RU-486.

Abortion and Breast Cancer

Studies by Pike and Henderson at the University of Southern California reported that a woman who aborts her first pregnancy increases her risk of getting breast cancer by 140 percent! These are shocking statistics and, no doubt, bad news for abortion lobbyists who have managed to hide them successfully from the public. This kind of information should be part of any family planning counselling. Unfortunately, like the RU-486 (abortion pill) issue, the truth about the disastrous side effects are never mentioned by its proponents. The public has the right to know that abortion by knife or drug has serious long-term health consequences.

While we're on the subject, the public has the right to know that the routine prescription of estrogens to menopausal women also increases the risk of breast cancer. Guess what many women with breast cancer are prescribed? They're prescribed a drug called tamoxifen, which blocks the cancer-stimulating effects of estrogen. With this knowledge you have got to be asking why doctors are prescribing estrogen to women who are most at risk for developing breast cancer.

Women have now been exposed to both long-term hormone treatment in the form of the birth control pill and long-term hormone treatment in the form of estrogen replacement. If we now compound this with abortion, the standard North American diet and the increased use of carcinogens in our food supply, it's no wonder we have a breast cancer epidemic. Women have been brainwashed into believing the bunk that without prescription estrogens their bones will collapse and they'll die of an early coronary. Hogwash! None of this is proven. Women deserve better than to be bullied into birth control pills, abortions, RU-486, routine mammograms and estrogen prescriptions for the menopause. There are safe, natural alternatives to all of these.

Natural Infertility Treatments

Over three million visits each year to North American physicians are for infertility. The demand for treatment is increasing and the cost, both financial and emotional, can severely strain relationships. Infertility is defined as the absence of conception after one year of regular intercourse without the use of any contraceptive. About 15 percent of all couples experience conception problems and the percentage is growing. Men are responsible for the problem at least 40 percent of the time.

In women, some of the causes of infertility are failure to ovulate, tubal disease, endometriosis, cervical disease, pituitary gland failure, ovarian failure, long-term effects of the birth control pill, other hormonal imbalances (e.g., hypothyroidism), endometrial failure, sperm antibodies, hostile cervical mucus, recurrent miscarriages, chronic illness or infection (e.g., chlamydia), and nutritional deficiencies.

Most gynecological infections with resulting infertility stem from microbes that have crept into the vagina and/or uterus from the large bowel. Stool cultures for these potential problems may help make the diagnosis, and treatment could then be aimed at balancing the large bowel flora with supplements like lactobacillus acidophilus.

In men, infertility can be caused by an inadequate sperm production or poor sperm motility. This may be due to environmental toxins, radiation, drugs, heavy metal exposure, cigarette smoking and street drug use.

Studies show that sperm counts have declined steadily over the past 50 years. During this period of time, our civilization has experienced the introduction of over 70,000 chemicals in our food, water and air. Radiation, stress, poor diet and lifestyle habits all contribute to low sperm counts or poor sperm motility.

Other causes in men include varicocele, undescended testis/testes, infectious disease and endocrine (glandular) diseases affecting the hypothalamus, pituitary and the testes. Nutrient deficiencies also have a role to play. An obstruction of the seminal tract will decrease or stop the passage of sperm from the testes to the urethra for ejaculation. This may be due to congenital abnormalities, urethral stricture and infection of the epidydimis, testes, seminal vesicles, urethra, prostate or vas. All such correctable medical conditions should be ruled out.

One rational measure that may be of significant help to infertile couples is the avoidance of recreational drugs. Substance or drug abuse may affect neuroendocrine and gonadal function, leading to infertility and sexual dysfunction. Recent studies indicate that women who smoke marijuana have a slightly elevated risk for infertility, secondary to abnormalities in ovulation. Cocaine use is associated with a greater risk of infertility due to the abnormalities the drug causes to the fallopian tubes. Amphetamine abuse is thought to have the same effect on fertility as cocaine. Marijuana, cocaine and heavy cigarette smoking all decrease sexual capabilities by damaging the tiny blood vessels that supply blood to the penis. Coffee and other caffeinated products (soft drinks, chocolate, analgesics, etc.) decrease sperm production. Elimination of caffeine raises sperm count.

The two most frequently prescribed drugs for the treatment of ulcers, cimetidine and ranitidine, have both been reported to decrease sperm count and produce impotence as one of their side effects. The average sperm count is between 120 to 350 million per cubic centimeter. A low sperm count is one below 40 million per cubic centimeter.

A healthier diet and supplemental vitamins, minerals and amino acids may also be of significant help to infertile couples. Malnutrition or a suboptimal nutritional state can result in the failure of ovulation and menstruation. Anorexia nervosa is not the only cause of malnutrition in North American females. It is estimated that up to 50 percent of all women who complain of a loss of periods suffer from the effects of dieting.

Studies indicate that simple lifestyle changes, such as stress reduction, avoidance of excessively vigorous exercise and maintaining one's recommended body weight, may help restore fertility in some women. For example, heavy, prolonged exercise (e.g., marathon running) can lead to a cessation of periods. Menstruation may resume once the exercise program is reduced.

Recurrent miscarriages have been reported to be caused by deficiencies in essential fatty acids, zinc, manganese and vitamin E. Iodine deficiency may be an unsuspected cause of infertility. Along with infertility, iodine deficiency may cause spontaneous abortion, stillbirths and perinatal mortality. Iodine may be important for egg maturation and its release for fertilization and implantation. Toxin overload from the diet may also be responsible for some miscarriages. Heavy metal toxicity may affect ovulation. Hair mineral analysis can reveal possible heavy metal poisoning with lead, mercury, cadmium, arsenic, aluminum or copper.

It is well worth while following a sensible diet. This means getting plenty of fresh fruits, vegetables, whole grains and legumes. It also means avoiding refined carbohydrates, coffee, tea, alcohol and foods with artificial additives. Excessive amounts of vitamin A have been linked to congenital malformations. How much is too much depends on the given individual. Women trying to get pregnant should avoid supplementation with vitamin A unless they have a documented deficiency of this vitamin. Since cigarette smoking destroys many vitamins and minerals, it is important that any infertile couple do their best to quit this negative health habit.

Food deprivation in men leads to a loss of sex drive and structural changes to reproductive tissue leading to infertility. Obesity, on the other hand, can be associated with a low sperm count and impotence. Folds of fat may raise the temperature of the testicles, lower testosterone levels and elevate female hormone levels. Optimal weight and healthy diet should not be overlooked in the male partner of an infertile couple.

Juices that would be helpful in cases of infertility in women include carrot, beet, spinach, celery and parsley. In men, fertility can be enhanced by eating more oatmeal, dates, kelp, dulse and other seaweeds, black beans, kidney beans, yams, lycium fruit, peanuts, walnuts, wheat germ and brewer's yeast. Juices that would be beneficial include celery, oatstraw, carrot and spinach.

Reports from around the world support the use of supplemental nutrients to enhance fertility in both men and women. In women, the most important supplement appears to be vitamin B6 (pryridoxine). Recommended dosages vary, but according to one study by Dr. G.E. Abraham, optimal B6 supplementation is between 100 and 800 mgs daily. Vitamin B6 at such dosages causes a significant increase in progesterone levels. This may, in part, also help explain its effectiveness in the treatment of premenstrual syndrome (PMS).

In men, the most important supplemental nutrients to enhance fertility are vitamin C, zinc and L-arginine. Vitamin C helps prevent sperm from clumping or sticking together, thus improving the chances for fertility. Safe and effective dosages are between 2,000 and 6,000 mgs daily. Zinc supplementation has been shown to increase both sperm count and sperm motility. Effective dosages are between 100 and 200 mgs daily. Low sperm counts and poor motility are also helped by supplemented L-arginine (4,000 mgs daily). Arginine is found in high amounts in the head of the sperm. Other nutrients that have been shown to improve sperm counts include essential fatty acids, chromium, selenium, copper, vitamin E, coenzyme Q10 (200 mgs daily) and B-complex vitamins. Side effects of any of these supplements are negligible in comparison to fertility enhancing drugs and hormones. Since sperm formation takes almost three months, it will take at least this amount of time before seeing the benefits of a nutrient supplementation program. Nutritional assessment and treatment of imbalances by a qualified health care practitioner would be ideal.

There is a long list of herbs known to enhance fertility in women. They include angelica, borage, raspberry, wild clover, nettle, chaste tree, Siberian ginseng, licorice, serenoa repens, sarsaparilla, damiana, squaw vine, wild yam, panax ginseng, ho shou wu, dandelion, black cohash, alfalfa, motherwort, cramp bark and milk thistle. For men, recommended herbs are oat, false unicorn root, black cohash, pumpkin, panax ginseng, damiana and saw palmetto. Many herbal companies market formulations containing three or more of these herbs in tincture or capsule form. Check with a local health food store or herbalist.

Painful Periods

Menstrual cramps (dysmenorrhea) can be primary (functional) or secondary (acquired) to various pelvic conditions. Primary dysmenorrhea occurs in ovulatory cycles without any obvious pathology in the genital tract. In many cases of primary dysmenorrhea, women may be constipated as a direct result of poor diet, candida overgrowth or inadequate water intake. If the stools do not evacuate frequently enough, estrogens can be reabsorbed from the bowels, leading to higher estrogen levels. Menstrual cramps can become severe when there is a hormonal imbalance (i.e., the amount of estrogen relative to progesterone is too high in the body). Successful treatment of candida will often improve almost any kind of chronic gynecological condition.

Secondary dysmenorrhea occurs as a complication of other abnormal pelvic conditions, such as endometriosis, uterine fibroids, PID (pelvic inflammatory disease) and fibrous adhesions. The majority of dysmenorrhea patients also have PMS (premenstrual syndrome) and the two syndromes are often treated simultaneously. Before you attempt any conventional or natural treatments, make sure you have seen a family doctor or gynecologist to determine the cause of the dysmenorrhea. Treatment can then be aimed at the specific source of the problem.

If the cause of the symptoms of primary dysmenorrhea has been termed "functional" or "of unknown etiology" there are several treatment alternatives. Conventional treatment consists of aspirin, non-steroidal anti-inflammatory drugs, codeine, other narcotics, tranquilizers, the birth control pill and, in rare cases, surgery (hysterectomy, presacral neurectomy). For many sufferers, this mindless approach seems to be readily accepted. For those with an interest in more natural remedies, there are a good number of more gentle alternatives to be found in the fields of nutrition, botanical medicine, homeopathy and chiropractic.

Nutritional management gets the best results when the person follows a high-fiber vegan diet. Eat as many greens as possible in order to increase dietary magnesium, a mineral that is very helpful in relieving spasm of any kind. Eating more seeds and nuts, flax seed oil and black currant oil will increase the dietary intake of the omega-3 and the omega-6 fatty acids which are known for their anti-inflammatory effects. Blackberries, beets, blueberries, parsley and raspberries are also beneficial because of their content of vitamin C and bioflavonoids, nutrients known to control bleeding. Therapeutic juices include carrot, spinach, beet and cucumber. Avoid coffee, caffeine-containing analgesics and known food intolerances. Supplements that have been found to help painful periods include:

Bioflavonoids (hesperidin, catechin, rutin, quercetin)

Bromelain (Crush the contents of a tablet or capsule into calendula or flax cream and insert in vagina to relax os.)

Calcium

Evening primrose oil

Magnesium (When pain is acute, magnesium sulphate can be self-injected or injected by a doctor or nurse who is not afraid of using vitamins or minerals.)

Natural progesterone cream (Can be applied to the skin anywhere on the the body. It has a very high success rate even in stubborn cases, and there are no side effects because the natural progesterone bypasses the liver.)

Niacinamide

Pycnogenol (proanthrocyanidins)

Vitamin B complex

Vitamin B6

Vitamin C

Vitamin E

Anti-spasmodic herbal remedies can be added if pains are not alleviated. Some of these are angelica, ginger, black cohash, wild yam, lobelia and valerian. Homeopathic remedies include belladonna, colocynth, magnesia phosphoricum and pulsatilla, but these and others are best determined for you by a homeopathic doctor. Some women benefit from aerobic exercise, some from doing qi gong, some from hydrotherapy or chiropractic treatments, diathermy, biofeedback, TENS and other physical therapies. Talk it over with a holistic doctor, naturopath or soon-to-be-enlightened family doctor.

PMS Relief

Premenstrual syndrome (PMS) is a term used to describe a condition occurring in many pre-menopausal women up to two weeks before menstruation (during the luteal phase of the menstrual cycle). It is one of the most common health problems affecting North American women, with as high as 90 percent incidence in women between the ages of 30 and 40. It is frequently a problem for women who have suffered from postpartum depression (depression after delivery of a baby) and in those who have had tubal ligations for birth control.

The symptoms of PMS are cyclical and vary from month to month in type and severity. There are several different types of PMS, depending on the predominant symptoms seen in a given individual and each is treated somewhat differently.

In PMS-A (anxiety), the most common complaints are anxiety, irritability and mood swings. This form of PMS responds best to vitamin B6 (100 to 300 mgs) and magnesium (300 to 400 mgs) along with an improved diet. By this I mean eating more fresh fruits, vegetables, legumes and seafood and less processed, sweetened and salted foods, including red meats. Red meats and dairy products may contain estrogen which aggravates PMS. From a biochemistry standpoint, it is thought that deficiency of vitamin B6 (pyridoxine) together with high estrogen levels causes a deficiency of serotonin in the brain.

Since serotonin is a soothing, mood-elevating substance, a deficiency leads to anxiety and depression. Women who take the birth control pill, which destroys vitamin B6 reserves, are prone to low serotonin levels and, hence, the psychological consequences. Many doctors and PMS clinics prescribe progesterone, a female hormone that antagonizes high estrogen levels. Unfortunately, this therapy is not without its side effects. Many women can benefit from a natural progesterone cream derived from Mexican wild yam. This non-ingested progesterone absorbs through the skin and can control all the symptoms of PMS without side effects. The usual effective dosage is 1/2 teaspoon applied to the skin daily for two weeks prior to menstruation.

PMS-H (heavy) is characterized by water retention, swelling of the hands and feet, abdominal bloating and premenstrual weight gain. Avoidance of excess sugar, salt and fat is important, along with stress reduction (meditation, visualization, etc.) and regular exercise. PMS-H also responds well to vitamin B6, progesterone cream and magnesium.

In PMS-C (craving), the major symptoms are cravings for various foods, especially sweets. There may also be heart palpitations, fatigue, dizziness and fainting. This form of PMS responds to a healthier diet as well as vitamin B6, progesterone cream, zinc, vitamin C and gamma-linolenic acid (GLA), which comes from the oil of evening primrose. It's a good idea to eat five or six smaller meals throughout the day, instead of three large ones, in order to stabilize blood sugar levels.

PMS-P (pain) refers to the type where the primary problem is breast tenderness and abdominal discomfort. Sufferers are benefited by vitamin E supplementation (150 to 600 IU). This is because vitamin E increases the body's synthesis of prostaglandin E-1, which antagonizes the hormone prolactin. An excess of prolactin has been reported in some studies to be associated with PMS. Research indicates that vitamin E is effective in controlling breast tenderness and other PMS symptoms, including mood swings, anxiety, confusion and headaches. Vitamin E, however, does not handle water retention, weight gain and abdominal bloating in PMS. Caffeine in coffee and tea aggravate breast tenderness during PMS and should be replaced by herbal teas or juices.

Finally, in PMS-D (depression), the major concern is depression which can, at times, be so severe that suicide is contemplated. Other symptoms of PMS-D are forgetfulness, crying, confusion and insomnia. In this type, gamma-linolenic acid (GLA) supplementation is beneficial as well as calcium and magnesium. As far as diet is concerned, it is important to avoid tyramine-containing foods such as cheese and red wine. Increased tryptophan intake (from higher protein in the diet, or a supplement) is helpful because tryptophan is converted into serotonin in the brain. As mentioned earlier, serotonin is a natural mood elevator.

These are arbitrary classifications of PMS and most cases have combinations of symptoms. Double-blind studies show that premenstrual syndrome responds favorably to candida therapy. Women who do not respond to nutritional management alone should try an anti-candida program which may include the use of psyllium seed powder, digestive enzymes, hydrochloric acid, olive oil, garlic, lactobacillus acidophilus, taheebo (pau d'arco) tea, caprylic acid, fish oil concentrates or other natural remedies. In rare cases, mercury and other heavy metal toxicities should be suspected as possible contributing factors. Food allergy testing and elimination as well as thyroid function assessment may be crucial.

Many cases of subclinical hypothyroidism are behind chronic, intractable PMS. Although conventional lab tests for thyroid problems may be entirely normal, these cases respond well to natural desiccated thyroid hormone prescriptions. Still others do better with time-released liothyronine (T3) prescriptions.* (See section on Hypothyroidism.)

Natural metabolic boosters like kelp, tyrosine and ma huang may or may not be helpful, depending on individual biochemistry. Get an amino acid analysis done through a doctor. This will help decide whether or not tyrosine and other amino acids would be beneficial.

Recently, Dr. Attila Toth, of the Cornell Medical Center in New York, found many cases of severe PMS related to bacterial infections. Women in his clinic were prescribed an antibiotic (Doxycycline) for one cycle and were found to have a dramatic improvement in symptoms. It is speculated that bacterial infection (chlamydia) might cause inflammation of the ovaries and endometrium, leading to hormonal imbalances that result in symptoms of PMS.

In my experience, over 80 percent of cases of PMS respond well to diet, supplements and lifestyle changes. Individualized homeopathic remedies may also be very effective in a large number of cases. Doctors dealing with these cases have their hands full, but with persistence all cases respond to therapy. If possible, get an evaluation done by a naturopath or nutrition-oriented medical doctor before experimenting with various treatments.

Mammography

The subject of mammography seems about as emotionally charged as the subject of whether or not babies should drink cow's milk. The female breast is an emotional item irrespective of the context.

A Canadian study concluded that mammography as a screening device does nothing to lower the death rate from breast cancer. It is reasonable, therefore, that many physicians, myself included, find the idea of screening for breast cancer by mammography to be a highly questionable practice.

* If you or your doctor are having difficulties with the treatment protocol, try calling the Wilson's Syndrome Foundation (1-800-621-7006).

All this is not to say that mammography is worthless. When either the doctor or the patient discovers a breast lump and there is concern about whether it is a benign or malignant lump, mammography can be a very helpful diagnostic test. Few will argue about the use of mammography for diagnostic purposes. But the value of its use as a preventive health screening tool remains to be proven.

Some radiologists in the United States have been researching the use of MRI (magnetic resonance imaging) as a safer and more effective alternative to mammography. However, the widespread use of MRI for breast cancer screening is still many years away.

Currently, the best way to screen for breast disease is with periodic breast self-examination and examination by a physician. The best prevention against breast cancer is a healthy diet and lifestyle.

Breast Enlargement

Assuming that there are no breast tumors, large breasts may be the result of hereditary factors, excessive female hormones or fibrocystic breast disease. There's little that can be done about heredity, but it may be helpful to cut down on the intake of foods containing high amounts of female hormone, especially beef, pork, eggs, chicken and all dairy products. An overall fat reduction in the diet (to 10 to 15 percent of caloric intake) is recommended. Avoid alcohol, sugar and white flour products.

Eliminating caffeine from the diet (coffee, tea, colas, chocolate, analgesics) helps prevent breast cysts. Supplementation with iodine (from kelp or dulse), selenium, silicon, vitamin B6, vitamin E (800 IU or more daily), evening primrose oil and pineal gland extract (melatonin) may help shrink some of the swelling from breast cysts. Aerobic exercise and weight training will boost circulation and enhance chest wall muscle tone. One is never too old to get started. The overall effect after several months would be a slimmer breast appearance.

Fibroids

Fibroids are benign tumors of the myometrium of the uterus and are the result of estrogen stimulation. They may also be termed fibromyomas or leiomyomas. Fibroids occur in 25 percent of women over age 35 and are often asymptomatic. For most cases nothing needs to be done; the fibroids shrink, along with the entire uterus once menopause is reached. They may, however, bleed excessively, leading to iron deficiency anemia, and cause pelvic pain, cramps or bloating. Bleeding can be prevented by more careful attention to diet and lifestyle as well as supplementation with iron and vitamin K. (Excessive bleeding from fibroids may also be related to subclinical hypothyroidism. See the section on hypothyroidism in this book.) Pregnancy and estrogen therapy increases their growth. Most conventional doctors treat fibroids with a hysterectomy, provided that pregnancy is not desirable. This treatment, however, is not cast in stone.

The best therapeutic diet to follow is a high-fiber vegan diet consisting only of fruits, vegetables, whole grains and legumes. Particularly therapeutic foods are beets, carrots, artichokes, deep yellow and dark green vegetables (these are particularly high in vitamin K), sweet potatoes, yams, squash, peaches, apricots, citrus fruits, parsnips, dandelion greens and watercress. Carrot, spinach, beet, cucumber and lemon juices are most effective. Foods high in omega-3 and omega-6 essential fatty acids have an anti-inflammatory effect and help prevent pain and cramping. These include flax seed oil, borage oil, rice bran oil, evening primrose oil and black currant seed oil.

Avoid foods known to stimulate tumor or cyst growth like meat, alcohol, hot sauces, spicy foods, fried foods, fatty foods, salty foods, synthetic sugar and white flour products. Cigarette smoking, food additives and food coloring should also be strictly avoided. Soy products, if eaten in excess, may also be a problem due to their content of estrogen-like substances (phytoestrogens). For more information on vegan diets see *Diet For A New America*, by John Robbins, and *Vegan Delights*, by Jeanne Marie Martin.

The following supplemental vitamins, minerals and herbs are recommended:

Vitamin A

Vitamin B complex

Bioflavonoids (hesperidin, rutin, catechin, quercetin, pycnogenol, which help prevent bleeding by stabilizing capillary walls)

Vitamin E (d-alpha-tocopherol acetate)

Vitamin K (prevents bleeding)

Zinc

Copper

Calcium

Magnesium

Potassium

Selenium

Silicon

Flax seed oil

Evening primrose oil

Slippery elm, sheep sorrel, burdock and Turkish rhubarb

Chaparral

Parsley

Red clover

Liquid chlorophyll

Goldenseal

Echinacea

Milk thistle, artichoke and tumeric (to cleanse the liver)

Kelp (iodine content helps with pain and swelling)

Progesterone cream (to prevent bleeding)

Dosages for nutritional supplements should be individualized, pre-scribed and supervised by a natural health care practitioner.

Ovarian Cysts

An ovarian cyst is a closed sac or pouch with a definite wall that pro-trudes from the ovary and contains fluid or solid material. Ovarian cysts are often asymptomatic. There may eventually be abdominal pressure, discomfort, pain with palpation and a sense of heaviness. Conventional medical treatment is surgery and is only needed if the cyst becomes symptomatic. If the cyst is malignant, surgery is usually done immediately.

The course of polycystic ovary syndrome is usually benign, the only problem often being infertility. Fertility is drug-induced (e.g., Clomiphene). Suppressing the pituitary gland release of LH with low dose birth control pills is another medical treatment.

Complementary nutritional therapy may help prevent enlargement of the ovarian cyst, but regular medical follow up should not be ignored. The best eating principle is a high-fiber vegan diet consisting only of fruits, vegetables, whole grains and legumes. Foods particularly therapeutic for ovarian cysts are beets, carrots, artichokes, deep yellow and dark green vegetables, sweet potatoes, yams, squash, peaches, apricots, citrus fruits, parsnips, dandelion greens and watercress. Carrot, spinach, beet, cucum-ber and lemon juices are most effective. Foods high in omega-3 and omega-6 essential fatty acids have an anti-inflammatory effect. These include flax seed oil, borage oil, rice bran oil, evening primrose oil and black currant seed oil.

Avoid foods known to stimulate tumor or cyst growth, like meat, alco-hol, hot sauces, spicy foods, fried foods, fatty foods, salty foods, synthetic sugar and white flour products. Cigarette smoking, food additives and food coloring should also be strictly avoided. Soy products, if eaten in excess, may also be a problem due to their content of estrogen-like sub-stances (phytoestrogens). For more information on vegan diets see *Diet For A New America*, by John Robbins, and *Vegan Delights*, by Jeanne Marie Martin.

Dosages for nutritional supplements should be individualized, pre-scribed and supervised by a natural health care practitioner.

The following supplemental vitamins, minerals and herbs are recommended:

Calcium

Chaparral

Copper

Echinacea

Evening primrose oil

Flax seed oil

Goldenseal

Kelp (iodine content helps with any cystic condition)

Liquid chlorophyll

Magnesium

Milk thistle

Parsley

Potassium

Red clover

Selenium

Silicon

Slippery elm, sheep sorrel, burdock and Turkish rhubarb combination

Vitamin A

Vitamin B-complex

Vitamin C

Vitamin E (d-alpha-tocopherol acetate)

Wild yam (helps control spasm and ovarian pain and can be used periodically when needed)

Zinc

Recurrent Bladder Infections and Incontinence

Recurrent bladder infections and incontinence are common complications of hysterectomy or pelvic surgery of other kinds. It's important to drink large amounts of spring or mineral water (at least eight glasses daily). Avoid sugar, white flour products, coffee, tea and alcohol, all of which encourage the growth of bacteria.

Cranberry juice (fresh, unsweetened, not the commercial type available at supermarkets, which is laced with sugar) has a good, natural antibiotic effect. Juicing fresh, raw cranberries mixed with other fruit juices or carrot juice is not only effective but quite tasty. Adding one or two tablespoons of pure ascorbic acid crystals (vitamin C in a powdered form) to each eight ounces of cranberry juice (about three or four times times daily or as tolerated without getting very loose bowel movements) will enhance the antimicrobial effect.

Other supplemental nutrients that may be important to prevent infection are vitamin A, beta-carotene, zinc, selenium and bioflavonoids like rutin, hesperidin, pycnogenol and quercetin. Herbal remedies that can be used and alternated on a four-day basis include garlic, echinacea, goldenseal, St. John's wort, lomatium, pau d'arco, chaparral, propolis, capsicum, burdock, red clover and astragalus. These are available in tincture or capsule form, either alone or in combination.

A good lactobacillus acidophilus and bifidus culture (friendly bacteria) taken on a regular basis may also be important for prevention. Bee pollen and ma huang (ephedra) can help in stopping or normalizing urinary flow. They both have a beneficial effect on the nerves associated with bladder continence.

Interstitial Cystitis

Interstitial cystitis is a chronic condition caused by inflammation of the space between the urinary bladder lining and the bladder muscle. There are a variety of causes, but in cases of interstitial cystitis, bacteria are generally not found in the bladder so antibiotics are ineffective. This is in contrast to the more common bladder infections caused by bacteria originating in the large bowel. It is important to get a urine culture done to determine if bacteria are present before starting antibiotic prescriptions. Bacteria may presensitize the bladder so that various promoters (certain drugs, foods, hormones and viruses) start the chronic disease process. Interstitial cystitis is a progressive disease that can range in severity from microscopic ulcers to a completely scarred bladder. It is an environmentally induced illness that frequently responds to diet and lifestyle changes.

Patients with interstitial cystitis can usually control symptoms of frequency, burning, painful intercourse and pelvic irritation by avoiding high acid forming foods and those that contain high amounts of tyrosine, tyramine and aspartate. Eat more of the alkaline forming foods. If symptoms improve, challenge occasionally with low acid forming foods. For a guideline, see the food lists at the end of this section.

Foods high in tyrosine, tyramine, tryptophan and aspartate include beer, brewer's yeast, canned cheeses, chicken livers, chocolate, corned beef, mayonnaise, aspartame, pickled herring, saccharine, sour cream, soy sauce, wines and vitamins or minerals buffered with aspartate. It is also possible that hidden allergies to wheat, milk and other commonly eaten foods may cause recurrent bladder irritation.

Stress in general worsens symptoms of interstitial cystitis. Meditation, relaxation and various forms of psychotherapy may be very helpful. Drugs that may be promoters of the disease include over-the-counter cold medicines and some long-lasting cough drops. Amphetamine-like diet pills may also be involved.

Cranberry juice and vitamin C supplementation may be very helpful in the treatment of acute bacterial bladder infections, but make interstitial cystitis symptoms worse. Instead, take one to two tablespoons of sodium bicarbonate powder in water every four hours as needed for pain relief. Sodium bicarbonate alkalinizes the urine and prevents acids from interacting with sore and damaged tissues. Also, take about 500 mg of calcium carbonate every six hours. This also helps in alkalinizing the urine. Drink lots of clear fluids, especially water, since diluting the urine prevents harmful elements from interacting with damaged tissue. Also, experiment with ice packs or heating pads to see which helps best.

Supplemental vitamins and minerals that may be very helpful in the treatment of interstitial cystitis include vitamin A, beta-carotene, vitamin B6, calcium ascorbate (a buffered form of vitamin C), vitamin D, vitamin E , calcium, magnesium, selenium, cysteine, cystine, glutathione, methionine, PABA (para-aminobenzoic acid), taurine and dimethylglycine (DMG) and essential fatty acids like evening primrose oil, flax seed oil and borage oil. Although this may seem like an awesome list of vitamin and mineral supplements, many companies have most of these available in three or four combination products, available at most health food stores.

Try the dietary restrictions and the vitamin and mineral supplements for at least one month to see if symptoms come under better control. Consult a nutrition-oriented health care practitioner for appropriate supplementation dosages, supervision and follow up.

Highest Acid Forming Foods/Chemicals:

Antibiotics	Fried foods of any kind	Processed cheese
Barley	Hazelnut	Pudding/jams/jellies
Beef	Ice cream	Soybeans
Brazil nut	Lobster	Sugar/cocoa
Carob	Malt	Vinegar
Cottonseed meal	Pheasant	Walnut

High Acid Forming Foods/Chemicals:

Aspartame	Crustacea	Pistachio seed
Barley groats	Green pea	Pomegranate
Casein (milk protein)	Lard	Pork
Carrots	Legumes	Psychotropic drugs
Cheeses	Maize	Rye
Chestnut oil	Nutmeg	Saccharin
Chick peas	Oat bran	Snow pea
Chicken	Palm kernal oil	Soy milk
Corn	Peanut	Veal
Cranberry	Pecan	Yeast/hops/beer/wine

Low Acid Forming Foods/Chemicals:

Adzuki beans
Aged cheese
Alcohol
Almond oil
Antihistamines
Balsamic vinegar
Benzoate
Black tea
Buckwheat
Cashew oil
Chard
Cow milk

Farina/semolina
Goat milk
Goose
Lamb
Lima beans
Navy/red beans
Pinto beans
Plum
Prune
Safflower oil
Shell fish
Seitan

Sesame oil
Spelt/teff
Tapioca
Tofu
Tomato
Turkey
Vanilla
Wheat
White beans
White rice

Lowest Acid Forming Foods/Chemicals:

Amaranth
Brown rice
Canola oil
Cherimoya
Chutney
Coffee
Cream
Curry
Dates
Eggs
Fava beans
Figs

Fish
Gelatin
Goat cheese
Grape seed oil
Guava
Honey/maple syrup
Kasha
Kidney beans
Millet
MSG
Persimmon juice
Pickled fruit

Pine nut
Pineapple
Pumpkin seed oil
Rhubarb
Rice vinegar
Sheep cheese
Spinach
String/wax beans
Triticale
Venison
Wild duck
Yogurt

Lowest Alkaline Forming Foods/Chemicals:

Algae
Apricot
Avocado oil
Banana
Beet
Blueberry
Brussel sprout
Chive/cilantro
Coconut oil
Currant
Ghee (clarified butter)

Ginger tea
Grain coffee
Grape
Human milk
Jicama
Lettuces
Linseed oil
Most seeds
Oats
Okra
Olive oil

Quinoa
Raisin
Squashes
Strawberry
Sucanat
Sulfite
Turnip greens
Umeboshi vinegar
Wild rice

Low Alkaline Forming Foods/Chemicals:

Apple	Ginseng	Sake
Almond	Green tea	Sesame seed oil
Apple cider	Mu tea	Sprouts
Bell pepper	Mushroom	
Blackberry	Papaya	
Cauliflower	Peach	
Cherry	Pear/avocado	
Cod liver oil	Pineapple juice	
Collard greens	Potato	
Eggplant	Pumpkin	
Evening primrose oil	Rice syrup	
Fungi	Rutabaga	

High Alkaline Forming Foods/Chemicals:

Broccoli	Honeydew	Parsley
Canteloupe	Kale	Parsnip
Chestnut	Kohlrabi	Pepper
Cinnamon	Loganberry	Poppy seed
Citrus	Mango	Sea salt
Endive	Mineral water	Soy sauce
Garlic	Molasses	Spices
Ginger root	Mustard green	Taro
Grain beverage	Olive	

Highest Alkaline Forming Foods/Chemicals:

Baking soda	Nori/kombu	Table salt
Burdock	Onion	Tangerine
Daikon	Other sea vegetables	Umeboshi plums
Hydrogenated oil	Persimmom	Wakame
Lentils	Raspberry	Watermelon
Nectarine	Sweet potato/yam	Yam

Silicone Implants

Silicone breast implants were first used by Japanese women after World War II. In North America, they were first used for augmentation mammoplasty (breast enlargement) in 1962. Over two million women have since had breast implantation with silicone. Recent research concludes that silicone causes a connective tissue disease referred to as systemic sclerosis. Women who suffer from systemic sclerosis complain of chronic fatigue, muscle and joint inflammation and chronic pain. This iatrogenic (doctor-caused) disease is the direct result of an immune system reaction to a foreign, toxic substance. In some cases, signs and symptoms can be partially or completely reversed by surgical removal of the silicone implants. In many cases, however, symptoms persist due to widespread dispersal of leaked silicone throughout the body.

There is no specific, recognized treatment for the long-term effects of silicone implants, but one can dramatically improve the function of the immune system through good nutrition, antioxidant supplementation and supportive herbal or homeopathic remedies. The immune system requires healthy levels of zinc, calcium, magnesium, potassium, selenium, germanium, silicon (different from silicone), iron, beta-carotene, vitamin C, vitamin E, vitamin A, B-complex vitamins (especially vitamins B5, B6 and B12) and all the essential amino acids. Testing for vitamin, mineral and amino acid levels may open the door to a speedier recovery.

Studies have also shown that refined carbohydrates (glucose, fructose and sucrose), have a depressant effect on the immune system as early as an hour after eating them. Removing sugar and white flour products from the diet is often helpful.

A hypoallergenic rotation diet with 70 percent of calories coming from complex carbohydrates (whole grains, fruits, vegetables and legumes) is best. Avoid caffeine, alcohol and processed foods. If possible, get food allergy, candida and chemical allergy testing done by the Elisa/Act blood test. (See list of natural immune system boosters on following page.)

Natural Immune System Boosters:

Adrenal extract
Astragalus
Baptisia
Blue-green algae, barley green, spirulina, green kamut and other whole green
Burdock, slippery elm, sheep sorrel, Turkish rhubarb combination
Carnitine
Chaparral
Coenzyme Q10
DHEA
DMG (dimethylglycine)
Echinacea
Garlic
Ginkgo biloba
Goldenseal
Green foods
Kelp, dulse and other seaweeds
Kola nut
Lactobacillus acidophilus and bifidus
Licorice
Liothyronine
Lomatium
Ma huang
Methionine
N-acetyl-cysteine
Natural progesterone
Pau d'arco (taheebo)
Phenylalanine
Pokeweed
Propolis, bee pollen, royal jelly
Pycnogenol
Red clover
Shiitake mushroom
Siberian ginseng
St. John's wort
Thymus gland extract
Tyrosine
Whole leaf aloe vera juice
Yarrow
Yerba maté

Consult a naturopath or medical doctor familiar with nutrition for a personalized program of diet and natural supplements.

7
Skin, Hair
and Nails

The health of the skin, hair and nails is a reflection of internal processes. For example, eczema can be caused by an unsuspected allergy to eggs, wheat or dairy products. Psoriasis could be the result of an essential fatty acid deficiency. Hair loss could be due to, among many other things, either too much vitamin A or not enough. Brittle or soft nails could be due to a greater need for silicon or iron. The list goes on.

It often seems more than ridiculous to me and my patients that a visit to the dermatologist for eczema, psoriasis, seborrhea, hives and a host of other rashes ends with a prescription for a cortisone cream. Not only does this fail to address the source of the problem (allergy, infection, toxicity, deficiency, etc.), but it leads to a permanent dependence on a drug with significant side effects. There is a more rational and effective way to deal with skin, hair and nail problems. It involves looking at the health of the whole individual, not just the skin, scalp or nails. This chapter deals with this holistic approach.

Optimizing Skin Health

The health of your skin, the body's largest organ, may be dependent on stress, emotional factors, heredity, proper nutrition, the immune system (e.g., food and chemical allergies) and the digestive system, especially with respect to assimilation of nutrients and elimination of waste materials. Like the kidneys and the bowels, the skin excretes toxins present in the body.

To optimize skin health, the diet should be as natural as possible. Avoid chemicals, processed foods, high-fat junk foods, caffeine, alcohol and sugar in any form other than fresh fruit. Animal products, including all dairy products and eggs, contain fats that can often aggravate skin problems. They may also be loaded with drugs like antibiotics, steroid hormones, nitrates and other toxins. Organic fruits, vegetables, whole grains, seeds, nuts and legumes are best, provided one knows there are no allergies to these.

Healthy skin requires adequate amounts of water, many vitamins, minerals and other food factors. One of the most important of these, especially for dry, flaky skin, is the essential fatty acid found in seeds (sesame, pumpkin), nuts (pine, walnut) and oils (flax, canola, olive).

Beta-carotene, vitamins A, C and E, zinc, selenium and other antioxidants can prevent skin damage caused by sun exposure. Antioxidant supplements may provide a great deal of protection against both sunburn and skin cancer. They may also be important in the healing process of any skin disorder or trauma. Aloe vera creams, gels and juices are effective for both prevention and treatment of sun-damaged skin. It is also important to avoid exposure to the sun (especially between 11 a.m. and 4 p.m.) and to use sun block creams.

The amino acids, B-complex vitamins (especially biotin), vitamin D, bioflavonoids, silicon and many other trace minerals are also important for the health of the skin. Some people develop deficiencies in these and other nutrients because of a number of digestive problems. The most common of these are low stomach acid, low pancreatic enzyme levels, candida over-growth and bacterial flora imbalance in the large bowel. If possible, see a natural health care practitioner for testing and treatment with natural remedies.

Acne

Theories about the direct effect of food on the development of comedones (blackheads) and acne have not been proven. However, many doctors involved in nutritional medicine report that food allergy or hypersensitivity is involved. Studies do support some basic dietary guidelines for prevention. All refined carbohydrates and processed foods should be eliminated. These include chocolates, sweetened cereals, candy bars, cakes, cookies and other junk foods. High-fat foods, particularly those containing trans-fatty acids like margarine, shortening and other hydrogenated vegetable oils, should be limited. Fried foods of most kinds fit into this category. Foods high in iodine (white flour products, heavily salted foods) should be eliminated for those that are iodine-sensitive. Limit cow's milk consumption due to its high hormone content.

Many published studies support the use of supplemental nutrients and herbal remedies. These include vitamin A, vitamin E, vitamin C, chromium, selenium, zinc picolinate, brewer's yeast, lactobacillus acidophilus and vitamin B6. The herb echinacea has a long history of use in inhibiting inflammation, promoting wound healing, stimulating the immune system and killing bacteria. Goldenseal has detoxifying and antimicrobial properties. It also stimulates the immune system. Drinking aloe vera juice on a regular basis may also work wonders in given individuals. Effective dosages depend on the severity of the problem and the tolerance of the individual to higher than RDA doses of the individual nutrients. Serenoa repens, an extract of saw palmetto, is very effective in the management of more stubborn cases because of its ability to reduce the levels of dihydrotestosterone, the hormone responsible for stimulating acne development.

In some particularly stubborn cases, a bowel cleansing (detoxification) program may be necessary, with supplementation of friendly lactobacillus bacteria. In cases where hormonal imbalances may be at the root of the problem, supplementation with essential fatty acids (e.g., omega-3-EPA and evening primrose oil), vitamin E and vitamin B6 in large doses are beneficial. It is essential to have a naturopath or doctor familiar with nutritional medicine suggest the safe and effective doses and monitor progress.

The use of topical vitamin A, aloe vera and calendula creams may be of great immediate cosmetic relief in most cases. Another very effective topical option is tea tree oil, derived from a native Australian tree *Melaleucea alternifolia*. It has a variety of antimicrobial properties and has been used successfully in the treatment of many different skin conditions, especially those associated with fungal or candida infections.

Finally, alpha hydroxy acids, the most effective of which is glycolic acid, are acknowledged by dermatologists and plastic surgeons as the best products to use to both cleanse and exfoliate the skin. These naturally occurring, non-toxic substances are derived from sour milk, grapes, citrus fruits, apples and sugar cane. When used in conjunction with EGF (epidermal growth factor), a protein the skin uses to protect against injury from burns and cuts, glycolic acid is efficacious and free of side effects. Most of these supplemental nutrients and creams are readily available from health food stores, pharmacies and other distributors.

Acne Rosacea

Acne rosacea occurs in adults as a pimple-like eruption on the forehead, cheeks, nose, and chin in association with facial flushing and small blood vessel abnormalities. There may be pustules, seborrhea and an enlargement of the soft tissues of the nose (rhinophyma). It occurs three times more often in women than men, but the most severe forms are seen in men. The basic cause is unknown, but there is a high correlation with low or absent hydrochloric acid secretion by the stomach and hidden food allergies or intolerances.

If tests for low stomach acidity (e.g., gastric analysis or comprehensive stool and digestive analysis) confirm the problem, then supplementation with stomach acidifiers may be of help for this skin condition. These acidifiers include glutamic acid hydrochloride, betaine hydrochloride, Swedish bitters, apple cider vinegar, B-complex vitamins, especially vitamin B2 (riboflavin) and vitamin B6 (pyridoxine). In severe cases, a bowel detoxification program may be necessary (juice fasting with or without colonic irrigation, psyllium seeds, bentonite, aloe vera, acidophilus and other bowel cleansers). Most naturopaths are experts in bowel detoxification programs and may help start the sufferer on the road to recovery.

Food allergy testing, elimination and control are also vital in returning the skin to its natural state. Most sufferers report reactions with coffee, alcohol, hot beverages, spicy foods, iodine and nuts, but any food may aggravate the skin condition depending on the biochemical uniqueness of the individual. Other factors that may trigger attacks in susceptible individuals include stress, excessive heat or cold, sunlight and certain prescription medications that dilate the blood vessels in the face. For more information on food allergies, testing methods and treatments, see the section Food Allergies and Allergy Testing.

Another nutritional problem that has been found in some cases of acne rosacea is low or insufficient pancreatic lipase. If serum lipase levels are low, or a CSDA test reveals a fat malabsorption problem, supplementation with pancreatic digestive enzymes (pancreatin) may be beneficial. Many trace minerals (especially zinc), essential fatty acids and the fat-soluble vitamins depend on adequate amounts of pancreatic digestive enzymes for absorption. In other words, if there is a deficiency of pancreatic enzymes, vitamins A, D, E, K, essential fatty acids and zinc may be very poorly absorbed despite megadose supplementation. Although it may be a truism that you are what you eat, in the case of acne rosacea it may be more accurate to say you are what you absorb.

Chemically-altered vitamin A (available by prescription) has been shown to be highly effective for rosacea. Unfortunately, it can cause side effects (liver toxicity, fetal malformations) and is not recommended. A three- to six-month trial therapy with high doses of natural antioxidants is more desirable. These should include natural vitamin A, beta-carotene, vitamin C, vitamin E, vegetal silica or silica gel, chelated zinc, selenium and B-complex vitamins, especially vitamin B2 (riboflavin).

Careful monitoring of liver and kidney function tests would help avoid any potential side effects from megavitamin doses. I should note here that several medical journals have reported cases of acne rosacea that were triggered by high dose supplementation with vitamin B6 and B12. This, however, is extremely rare. Supervision of megavitamin therapy by a qualified health care practitioner is highly recommended.

Many people plagued by various forms of acne have been raving about the benefits of lactobacillus acidophilus supplements. Several excellent brands can be found at your local health food store in capsule or powdered form. These should not be confused with either yogurt or acidophilus milk, neither of which contain adequate amounts of viable organisms to have a therapeutic effect in even mild cases of acne.

Herbal remedies that may be helpful for their natural antibiotic effects include echinacea, goldenseal, calendula, capsicum, chaparral and aloe vera. Calendula and aloe vera may be effective taken both orally (capsule or tincture form) and topically (a cream or gel). Some dermatologists and natural health care practitioners are claiming resolution of rosacea with the use of a skin care treatment that uses alpha hydroxy acids, the most effective of which is glycolic acid. These naturally occurring, non-toxic substances are derived from sour milk, grapes, citrus fruits, apples and sugar cane. When used in conjunction with EGF (epidermal growth factor), a protein our skin normally uses to protect against injury from burns and cuts, glycolic acid is efficacious and free of side effects. Visit your naturopath or nutrition-oriented medical doctor to help clear up this very distressing skin condition the natural way.

Vitiligo

Vitiligo is a skin condition characterized by areas of depigmentation (white spots) associated with a loss of pre-existing melanin (pigment) and melanocytes (pigment forming cells). It may be associated with an endocrine (adrenal or thyroid) imbalance, but the nutritional literature suggests that the cause is a lack or insufficiency of hydrochloric acid production by the stomach. Certain infections (leprosy, syphilis and pinta) may also damage melanocytes and produce hypopigmented lesions. Vitiligo usually appears in otherwise healthy persons, but several systemic, autoimmune disorders occur more often in patients with vitiligo than in the general population. These disorders include thyroid disease (e.g., hyperthyroidism, Grave's disease and thyroiditis), Addison's disease/adrenal insufficiency, pernicious anemia, alopecia areata (patchy baldness) and diabetes.

Achlorhydria (no acid) or hypochlohydria (low acid) leads to dozens of nutrient deficiencies. This is because most high protein foods need acid for digestion. If acid is low or absent, amino acids, vitamins and minerals are poorly absorbed. The best recognized nutrient deficiency caused by low or deficient stomach acid is vitamin B12 deficiency. This deficiency leads to pernicious anemia and can usually only be rectified by regular vitamin B12 injections.

Low stomach acid may be the result of heredity, extended use of drugs such as antacids, anti-ulcer medications (cimetidine, ranitidine and others), infection in the gut or food allergies (especially to milk and dairy products). Doctors specializing in nutritional medicine can do several tests to determine the etiology (e.g., comprehensive digestive and stool analysis).

If the cause of low stomach acid is heredity, a variety of things can be tried. These include supplements of glutamic acid hydrochloride, betaine hydrochloride, pepsin, apple cider vinegar, lemon juice, stomach bitters, pantothenic acid (vitamin B5), vitamin C, PABA and pyridoxine hydrochloride (vitamin B6). These supplements are usually safe, but may, on occasion, lead to too much acidity and the development of gastritis or ulcers. All are best taken directly before each meal or in the middle of each meal.

Many studies support the use of natural anti-inflammatory supplements for the autoimmune diseases. Example include cold-pressed flax seed oil, gamma linolenic acid (GLA found in evening primrose oil, black current seed oil and oil of borage) and omega-3-EPA (found in trout, cod, halibut, mackerel, salmon, shark, herring and other seafoods). Increasing these in the diet (or taking them in encapsulated supplement form) while decreasing the intake of saturated animal fats can have a remarkably good anti-inflammatory effect.

Vitamins such as A, B-complex, C and E as well as beta-carotene and bioflavonoids can be supplemented in higher than RDA doses because of their antioxidant properties that help prevent certain aspects of autoimmune disease. The recommended intake doses for all these nutrients would have to be determined for the individual by a qualified health care practitioner based on appropriate biochemical tests. Tests that would be of particular value include blood, urine and hair mineral analysis.

There are many way to stimulate the body's natural production of cortisone. This is not a replacement for prednisone or other therapeutic steroids, but can help the body minimize its dependence on this synthetic steroids. This is done by nutritional support of the adrenal glands with the following natural supplements:

Pantothenic acid (vitamin B5) . . . . *500 to 3,000 mgs daily*
Vitamin C . . . .*6,000 mgs or more daily (depending on bowel tolerance)*
Magnesium citrate . . . .*400 mgs daily*
Potassium citrate . . . .*400 mgs daily*
Zinc citrate . . . .*90 mgs daily*
Raw adrenal concentrate . . . .*100 to 300 mgs daily*
Bioflavonoids . . . .*1,000 mgs daily*
Licorice root capsules or tincture . . . .*100 to 300 mgs daily*

Siberian ginseng and DHEA (an extract of wild yam) and evening primrose oil (or borage and black currant) also provide adrenal support. DHEA (dehydroepiandrosterone) is the most abundant androgen (male hormone) produced by the adrenal cortex. DHEA has weak androgenic activity and can be found in almost any organ, including the testes, the ovaries, the lungs and the brain. Testosterone is synthesized from DHEA. In animal studies it has been shown to reduce body weight without food reduction (anti-obesity effect). DHEA also has an anti-tumor property, is anti-diabetic, cholesterol lowering, anti-atherogenic, anti-autoimmune and immune stimulating. Animal studies also suggest that it prevents aging. Work out an individualized dosage schedule and supplement regime with a naturopath or health care practitioner.

There are a growing number of studies that demonstrate the relationship between food allergies (hypersensitivity) and autoimmune diseases. People who react adversely to all foods (i.e., pan-allergic) may have an intestinal tract parasitic or fungal (candida) infection that needs to be investigated and treated before starting on a food allergy elimination program. Although one cannot say that parasites or candida cause autoimmune diseases, many nutrition-oriented physicians have reported successes when either the candida or parasitic infection was cleared first. Look into some of these possibilities with a natural health care practitioner.

Transplantation (autologous mini-grafting) involves transferring normally pigmented skin by means of small punch grafts to non-pigmented areas. Repigmentation results from the spread of melanin to non-pigmented areas and melanocyte recolonization. This is a very specialized procedure.

Total Hair Loss

The cause of alopecia universalis (total body hair loss) and alopecia areata (patchy baldness) is unknown. The good news is that many cases recover spontaneously (without any treatment), though it can take several months or years. There is little proven nutritional treatment, but doctors in Poland have been successful with long-term, high-dose zinc supplementation.

In some cases, oral zinc supplements in tablet or capsule form fail to produce changes in the scalp condition. This may be because of selective malabsorption of zinc from the gastrointestinal tract. White spots on the nails or horizontal ridges ("washboard nails") may be signs of zinc deficiency. One way of determining zinc status in the body is to get a hair mineral analysis done. If hair analysis indicates a low level of zinc in the face of a normal to high intake of zinc in the diet, it may indicate a problem with zinc absorption. Those without body hair obviously cannot get hair analysis done. Finger and toenail samples will yield the same kind of information.

In cases where zinc gluconate or amino acid-chelated zinc tablets have failed to improve hair growth, a liquid zinc supplement such as zinc sulphate heptahydrate solution or zinc picolinate is recommended. Effective dosages are between 150 to 200 mgs per day. The only possible drawback to this might be a zinc-induced copper depletion. To prevent this, take a copper supplement, roughly in a ratio of 6 to 1 (zinc to copper). It is also advisable to reduce fiber intake from grain and legume sources and increase the intake of high protein foods, especially eggs and seafood (oysters, clams, mussels, cod, halibut, mackerel, salmon, shark, sardine, sole or trout). Liver is also a good source of zinc, as are all other organ meats. Excessive dietary fiber and hidden food allergies may inhibit zinc absorption. Avoid sugar, white flour products and other junk foods.

Also, pancreatic digestive enzyme supplements may be very important in some cases. These enzymes break down dietary protein, carbohydrate and fat such that more zinc and other minerals and vitamins are absorbed. Pancreatic enzymes (pancreatin) are available at most health food stores. The dosage is two tablets or capsules after each meal (three times daily), which should be sufficient to enhance zinc absorption from the gastrointestinal tract.

A recent clinical trial using supplements of shark oil concentrate (400 mg capsules of Squalene) showed a success rate of more than 70 percent in alopecia areata. The dosage used was one capsule three times daily after meals. No side effects were reported. The reason this supplement works is probably because the biochemical structure of Squalene resembles that of the steroid hormone scalp injections given by dermatologists.

It is thought that alopecia universalis is an autoimmune disease. This means that it may result from an abnormal immune system reaction of the body to its own tissues. Another way of looking at it is that the immune system has become hyper-reactive. The immune system may be reacting to many different foods and chemicals on a delayed basis without producing classic allergic reactions like hives or wheezing. Instead, the allergies may be manifesting themselves as hair loss, rheumatoid arthritis, lupus, scleroderma and a host of other autoimmune diseases. Knowing what foods or chemicals to avoid may help reduce some of the constant stress on the immune system.

Aside from the nutritional factors already mentioned, many essential nutrients are involved in healthy hair growth. These include biotin, vitamin B12, PABA (para amino benzoic acid), other B-complex vitamins, unsaturated fatty acids (evening primrose oil, flax seed oil, etc.), vitamin C, vitamin E, coenzyme Q10, dimethylglycine (DMG), silica, copper, iron, cysteine and methionine. See a naturopath or a medical doctor familiar with nutritional evaluations to get an individualized diet and supplement program.

Lichen Planus

Lichen planus is a recurrent lumpy rash that may involve the inside of the mouth in about half the cases. The cause of lichen planus is unknown, but stress and food allergies are thought to be a factor. Flare-ups and remissions are common and may occur for many years. Some drugs (quinacrine) and potentially toxic metals (arsenic, bismuth, gold, mercury, etc.) may cause very similar eruptions. Some of these toxic metals may be found in the common silver dental filling (amalgam). Hair mineral analysis and urine tests can screen for excess body burdens of toxic heavy metals that may have a damaging effect on the immune system and skin.

In the case of mercury, the Elisa/Act blood test can determine whether or not a person is hypersensitive to mercury. High levels can usually be offset by removal of the source and supplementation with vitamin C, selenium, garlic, cysteine, methionine and N-acetyl-cysteine. In some cases, replacement of dental amalgams with non-metal fillings is essential. High-dose vitamin A supplementation has been reported to be effective in the treatment of lichen planus. Due to potential side effects of vitamin A in megadoses, treatment should be supervised by a medical doctor who can monitor for toxicity by ordering regular liver function tests.

Most skin problems are helped by psychotherapy and stress reduction. There is also growing evidence that avoidance of hidden food allergies and improvement of bowel function and waste elimination is helpful. Also of benefit in most skin conditions is the supplementation of the diet with essential fatty acids (e.g., evening primrose oil, flax seed oil, black current seed oil, etc.), vitamin A, B-complex vitamins, vitamin E, zinc, calendula and aloe vera.

Aloe vera can be very effective when taken internally as a juice. Make sure to purchase aloe vera juice that is whole leaf and cold processed. This type is at least eight times more potent than aloe vera juices of other types. Aloe vera gel and natural progesterone cream used topically may be very effective for both the skin condition and the overall health of the immune system. Treatment is different in each case and depends mainly on biochemical individuality. See a naturopath or a medical doctor familiar with the natural approach for a personalized program.

Healing Sun-Damaged Skin

Actinic keratosis is an age-related skin condition that is the result of many years of overexposure to the sun. There is no association with thyroid disease. Fair-skinned blondes and redheads are particularly susceptible. Victims may not be getting enough antioxidants from their diet or from supplements to protect them from the damaging rays of the sun. Toxins accumulate under the skin over the years as a result of radiation damage. Periodic juice fasting can be done to rid the body of these toxins. The skin problem frequently improves or disappears as a result. For more information, see *The Joy of Juice Fasting* by Klaus Kaufmann.

Aside from using a powerful sun block, oral supplementation with antioxidant vitamins and minerals may help prevent the problem from worsening. These include aloe vera juice, calendula tincture, vitamin A, beta-carotene, vitamin B complex, vitamin C, bioflavonoids (e.g., pycnogenol), vitamin E, selenium, silica, zinc and glutathione. If the skin is on the dry side, add supplements of flax seed oil (or evening primrose oil) and biotin. Drink aloe vera juice daily. Optimal dosages of all these supplements depend on the health of the liver and kidneys and are best determined by a natural health care practitioner.

Taking high-dose oral antioxidants will improve the severity of the rashes over a period of three to six months. Somewhat faster results can be observed if vitamins A and E and aloe vera creams or lotions are applied directly to the skin daily.

Skin Cancer Prevention

It is important to keep in mind the fact that the skin is the largest organ in the body and that its health is a reflection of the health of the body in general. Measures aimed at optimizing total health will also enhance the skin's ability to resist cancer and other diseases.

There is growing scientific evidence that supplementation with certain vitamins and minerals helps prevent skin cancer by neutralizing the effect of free radicals initiated by sun or radiation exposure. Beta-carotene, vitamins A, C, E, zinc, selenium and other antioxidants can be very effective preventive agents. It is also important to avoid exposure to the sun (especially between 11 a.m. and 4 p.m.) and to use PABA-containing sun blocking creams. Antioxidant supplementation also provides a great deal of protection against both sunburns and skin cancer. They are also important in the healing process of any skin disorder or trauma.

Aloe vera creams, gels and juices are effective for both prevention and treatment of sun-damaged skin. Zinc oxide ointment is yet another natural topical remedy that can be applied to unprotected skin to prevent burns and cancer.

The amino acids, the B-complex vitamins (especially biotin), vitamin D, bioflavonoids like pycnogenol and quercetin, essential fatty acids, silicon, copper and many other trace minerals are also important for the health of the skin. Some people develop deficiencies in these and other nutrients because of a number of digestive problems. The most common of these are low stomach acid, low pancreatic enzyme levels, candida overgrowth and bacterial flora imbalance in the large bowel. If possible, see a natural health care practitioner for testing of biochemical individuality and treatment with natural remedies.

Purpura

Purpura is a condition characterized by bruising over any part of the body. There are many types of purpura, but all involve a defect in the capillaries, the platelets or other blood clotting factors. In Schonlein-Henoch purpura the bruising may be accompanied by joint and intestinal symptoms such as abdominal pain.

Elimination of allergic foods from the diet prevents the inflammatory response that manifests as flare-ups of the disease. Two nutritional interventions of proven benefit are food allergy treatment and supplementation with bioflavonoids. Bioflavonoids such as rutin, hesperidin, catechin, quercetin, eriodictyol and pycnogenol help strengthen the walls of capillaries thereby preventing bruising. They stabilize the mast cell membranes and thus block the series of reactions that are associated with almost any allergy.

Bioflavonoids are found in many foods, including citrus fruits (the white material just beneath the peel), onions, garlic, peppers, buckwheat and black currants. In supplemental form, they have been successfully used for many years as a treatment for pain, bumps, bruises and more severe athletic injuries. Bioflavonoids work together with vitamin C to protect blood vessels. They are also useful in the treatment of asthma and other allergic conditions.

Side effects of bioflavonoid supplementation even in megadoses are unlikely, but, due to the serious nature of Schonlein-Henoch purpura, it is important that even this natural therapy be supervised by a doctor. In other words, do not attempt this without medical supervision.

Bags Under the Eyes

Most doctors say that bags under the eyes are a hereditary condition that can only be corrected with plastic surgery. I do not, however, believe that this is the case for the majority who suffer from the condition. In children, the cause of dark circles or bags under the eyes is almost always food allergies. In adults, the story may be a little more complicated. Technically, the problem is termed edema (otherwise known as fluid retention), an abnormal accumulation of fluid in various organs, cavities or tissues of the body. Edema is not a disease in itself but a symptom of specific disorders. See the section Water Retention for detailed information on edema.

Cellulite Remedies

Cellulite is made up of fat and fluid. It accumulates as a result of hereditary factors, fat intake, a low level of physical activity, hormonal factors (thyroid, adrenal, ovaries, pituitary, etc.), sluggish brown-fat metabolism, drug use, nutrient imbalances, large and small bowel health, food allergies and other factors. Ideally, see a health care practitioner to isolate what areas need investigation and balancing. In severe cases, bowel detoxification programs may be necessary.

Although there are all kinds of anecdotal reports of tremendous results with various lotions, potions and natural supplements, there is very little objective evidence to support the claims. It is beneficial to follow a low fat, high complex carbohydrate diet (e.g., Pritikin, HCF diet). Such a diet is high in grains like brown rice, barley, whole wheat, whole rye, whole oats, corn and legumes (starchy beans). Seeds and nuts are allowed on a limited basis. Avoid beef and pork.

Go as far vegetarian as possible, using fish as a protein source instead of beef, pork and poultry. Avoid chips, fried foods and highly sweetened or salted junk foods. If you must drink milk, keep to skim. Cheeses should be limited to skim types as well. See the recipe section in this book for more details on menus and healthy recipes.

Exercise is very important. To see an effect on fat deposits, walk briskly or use a rebounder for about half an hour per day. This helps mobilize fats and stimulates the lymphatic channels to rid the body of stored fluid and waste. In some cases it takes months to move the fat out, so patience and a firm resolve are important. Massage therapy is also essential and will yield cosmetic changes for the better if done long enough (several dozen sessions are often needed).

Supplements which help limit fat absorption by the body include various types of high fiber products. The best of these are psyllium seed husks and powder, glucomannan, guar gum, aloe vera and dried fruits like prunes. Certain free-form combinations of amino acids have been shown to effectively burn off fat when taken in large doses. These include arginine, lysine, ornithine, carnitine, phenylalanine and tyrosine. Many different companies make combinations of these for body builders who want to build muscle. Since these amino acids release growth hormone, their net effect is to burn off fat and build greater muscle mass. Other supplements that could be helpful for cellulite reduction include blue-green algae, chlorella, barley green, green magma, spirulina, kelp, dulse, evening primrose oil, flax seed oil, vitamin C, vitamin E, B-complex vitamins, (especially vitamin B 6) zinc, chromium and manganese. Since everyone's needs for these nutrients is highly individual, discuss dosages with a health care practitioner before supplementing.

Women that follow a low fat diet, get regular exercise and massage therapy combined with an individualized supplement program are likely to improve their general health significantly within three to six months. Cellulite will be improved and, in some cases, eliminated. Results depend on too many factors to be able to make predictions on treatment success rates. The truth remains that for large numbers of women nothing but the surgeon's knife will rid the problem for certain.

Light-Sensitive Eyes

Avoid watching television for extended periods of time. Most eye specialists recommend frequent breaks away from the tube. Look away from the TV screen as often as possible. The same can be said for sitting in front of a computer terminal for long stretches of time. Also, the further away from the screen, the better. The eyes and body absorb less radiation that way.

Many prescribed and over-the-counter drugs can cause a hypersensitivity to light because of the damage they cause to the optic nerve, retina or other parts of the eye. These include allopurinol, antibiotics (streptomycin, sulfa drugs, tetracycline), anticoagulants, antihistamines, aspirin, indomethacin, steroids (including the birth control pill), diuretics, digitalis, diazepam, haloperidol, other psychiatric drugs and quinine. If you take any of these, consult your doctor for safer alternatives.

Light-sensitive eyes may be an indication of allergies. The condition may also be related to a greater need for nutrients, such as protein, vitamins A, B-complex, C, E, zinc and selenium. Maintaining healthy eyes depends on all these nutrients, many of which are not always readily available in the standard North American diet.

In my practice, I have found that most light-sensitive patients benefit from a supplement of vitamin A alone (50,000 to 100,000 IU daily). If this or any other nutrient is taken as a supplement, make sure to get regular follow-up supervision by a doctor. Although it is unlikely that vitamin A will become toxic at this level, rare cases of vitamin A overdose have been reported in some scientific journals.

Herbs that may be helpful in soothing light-sensitive eyes include camomile, eyebright and fennel. These can be made into herbal teas or can be used as hot compresses. Homeopathic eye drops are an ideal product to use for a long list of benign eye conditions, including light sensitivity. It is also highly advisable to avoid caffeine products, sugar, tobacco smoke, marijuana, alcohol and the chemicals found in processed or prepared foods. If you are not getting adequate sleep, this too may have something to do with your problem.

If all these recommendations fail to resolve the problem, consider getting tested for food and environmental allergies (dust, molds, grasses, etc.).

Dry Eyes

Dry eyes, in their most severe forms, can be associated with rheumatoid arthritis or rarer forms of arthritis. Deficiencies in vitamin A, vitamin B 2 and essential fatty acids can lead to eye dryness. When unassociated with any medical diagnosis or nutritional deficiency, dry eyes can be helped by oral supplementation of vitamin C, vitamin B6 and chelated zinc for at least two months. Evening primrose oil, flax seed oil, vitamin A and vitamin E are helpful as well. Also, it is important to drink at least eight glasses of water each day to guarantee good hydration.

Some cases of eye dryness are due to food allergies, most commonly to wheat and other gluten-containing grains (rye, oats, barley). Other allergies, especially to house dust and pets, can cause eye irritation and dryness. A good air purifier and ionizer can help reduce symptoms dramatically. I often recommend vitamin C and bioflavonoid eye drops, as well as combination homeopathic eye drops for allergies or irritated eyes. Also effective are high doses of Ester-C powder with bioflavonoids in fruit or vegetable juice, and bioflavonoids like pycnogenol and quercetin in high doses. For more information on allergies and testing procedures, see the section Food Allergies and Allergy Testing.

Geographic Tongue

Geographic tongue results from the rapid shedding and growing of the papillae on the tongue. The cause is unknown and medical treatment is usually not required because the problem is self-limiting. Sometimes, it is the result of vitamin B complex deficiency. In such cases, brewer's yeast or a good B-complex supplement clears up the problem. If this therapy is not effective after several weeks, have a doctor or naturopath check for the presence of a candida (yeast) infection or other infections in the mouth.

Diet changes can also make a big difference. Eliminate sugar, fried foods, salt, strong spices, animal fats, alcohol, black tea, coffee, chocolate, cola, other carbonated soft drinks and peppers of all kinds. These foods may irritate the tongue and further aggravate the burning.

Many of the natural remedies that help heal ulcers and gastritis may be helpful for a burning, geographic tongue. The amino acid L-glutamine is important in the healing of hyperacidity. Vitamin A, vitamin B6, buffered vitamin C, beta-carotene, vitamin E, chelated zinc, evening primrose oil and flax seed oil have all been shown to promote faster healing. Herbal remedies that have traditionally enjoyed success in healing excess acid include aloe vera, slippery elm, comfrey, camomile, goldenseal, peppermint and licorice. Echinacea (a herbal antibiotic) in high doses may have a good natural anaesthetic effect, irrespective of the cause. These remedies are all safe in the recommended dosages and are well worth trying before resorting to prescription drugs.

Peyronie's Disease

Peyronie's disease is the name given to a condition whereby the fibrous tissue of the penis becomes thickened and contracted (flexed). Studies indicate that the B-complex vitamin PABA (para-aminobenzoic acid) helps to decrease the fibrotic contracturing lesions.

The cause of Peyronie's is unknown, but some have speculated it could be the result of hardening of the arteries and poor oxygen supply to the genitals. Vitamin E and aloe vera juice supplementation seem to help, as does any therapy that increases oxygen and improves circulation in the body. Topical application of aloe vera gel often helps soften any scar tissue.

The best diet to follow would be vegan (no dairy or eggs). Other supplements that may be helpful include niacin, ginkgo biloba, coenzyme Q10, pycnogenol, evening primrose oil, quercetin, hesperidin, catechin, vitamin C, beta-carotene, zinc, selenium, silicon and glutathione. See a natural health care practitioner for a personalized program.

Nail Problems

Fingernail problems are common and may be the result of various diseases like psoriasis or nutritional deficiencies. In children, the problem usually responds fairly quickly to nutritional therapy. In adults, treatments may take a year or longer to work successfully.

A number of tests can help determine the cause of the problem when medical diagnoses have been ruled out. For example, fingernail clippings can be analyzed by laboratory techniques very much the same way that hair samples are analyzed. Analysis often reveals deficiencies in zinc, copper, boron, silicon, manganese, calcium, magnesium, selenium or a combination of several of these minerals. Mineral supplementation can then be started to correct the imbalances. For more information on fingernail mineral analysis, contact Anamol Laboratories (see appendix).

If fingernail analysis or other tests indicate a fungal infection, treatment with natural antifungals may help eliminate the nail problem. This includes supplementation with friendly bacteria (lactobacillus acidophilus), psyllium seed powder, caprylic acid, castor bean oil and the herb pau d'arco. Tea tree oil can be applied directly to the nails to kill off the fungi. The diet would also have to be changed to prevent growth of fungi (see the section Healing Foods for Healing Diets).

Blood tests can be done to determine whether or not there are deficiencies in vitamin A, vitamin B12, folic acid, protein or iron. Deficiencies in any of these nutrients may lead to dry, brittle or bumpy nails. Horizontal ridges and white spots are usually associated with zinc and protein deficiencies. Splitting nails with vertical ridges may be directly related to a low secretion of stomach hydrochloric acid. Low stomach acid is often the cause of poor mineral absorption. A CSDA test (comprehensive stool and digestive analysis) can help uncover this potential problem.

Since iron, copper, zinc, silicon, boron, protein, vitamin B12 and many other nutrients are dependent on adequate amounts of acid for absorption, they may all be deficient in someone with low stomach acidity. Treatment would then be to supplement a good acid source alongside meals. Examples of this are Swedish bitters, apple cider vinegar, betaine or glutamic acid hydrochloride, vitamin C and vitamin B6. Many nail problems also respond very well to herbs such as horsetail and black walnut. Other supplements that have been reported to be helpful are kelp and herbal calcium.

If the nail problems are caused by psoriasis, consider supplementation with essential fatty acids. Researchers have reported that psoriasis may be related to changes in the metabolism of dietary oils. Long-term dietary changes with respect to fat intake may produce improvement. Animal fat, especially from red meat and dairy products, must be reduced or eliminated. Fresh fruits and vegetables should be increased. Get your fats from fish, sesame seeds, flax seed or soybeans. Supplementation with zinc, evening primrose oil, flax seed oil, fish oils and emulsified vitamin A and vitamin E along with vitamin B6 and pancreatic digestive enzymes usually improves or eliminates psoriasis over a period of six months. See a naturopath or nutritional doctor for assessment of biochemical imbalance and supervision of natural therapy.

Psoriasis

Psoriasis is a common skin condition that results in red, scaly plaques on the arms, legs and trunk. It also affects the scalp, but rarely the face. The most common sites include the points of the elbows and knees. The toes and fingernails become dull and develop ridges and pits. It is most commonly seen in people between the ages of fifteen and twenty-five. The cause is unknown, and sufferers respond to a variety of medical treatments, including coal tar, steroid creams and ultraviolet light. Stress, anxiety, surgery, cuts, other illnesses, infections, drugs such as lithium, chloroquine and beta-blockers may all trigger attacks. Some studies have demonstrated that psoriasis benefits from fasting and from gluten-free, elimination and complete vegetarian diets. Food allergy detection and control may be very important in some cases. The condition lessens in severity in the summer. It may go into remission from time to time, but the possibility always exists that it will return.

Researchers have reported that most psoriasis sufferers have abnormal serum levels of free fatty acids. Long-term dietary changes with respect to fat intake may produce improvement. Animal fat, especially from red meat and dairy products, must be reduced or eliminated. Fresh fruits and vegetables should be increased. Get your fats from fish, sesame seeds, flax seeds or soybeans. Supplementation of the diet with flax seed oil is recommended.

Fish oils (omega-3-EPA oils) are especially helpful. Greenland Eskimos, who consume a large amount of these oils, have a very low incidence of psoriasis despite limited exposure to the sun. Many recent double-blind studies have shown that supplementation of the diet with 10 to 12 grams of EPA oils results in significant improvement in psoriasis. This is roughly equivalent to a daily intake of 150 grams of mackerel or herring. Cod liver oil or salmon oil capsules may be more palatable for those with less than a love for fish. The essential oils in these fish (and in flax seed and soybeans) interfere with the body's production of inflammatory chemicals that cause psoriasis lesions to swell and turn red. Red meats and dairy products do the opposite, and are best eliminated from the diet. It may take three to six months to see the full benefit of supplementation with essential fatty acids. The diet changes are not expensive and may actually reduce your total grocery bill.

Other supplements that have been reported to be helpful include vitamin A, folic acid, vitamin B12, selenium, zinc, evening primrose oil, digestive enzymes and vitamin E. Supervision by a naturopath or medical doctor familiar with potential side effects from high doses is advisable.

Herbal remedies that may be of help to psoriasis sufferers include silymarin, dandelion, goldenseal, sarsaparilla, yellow dock, lavender and chaparral. Topical application of poultices made from these herbs may be helpful. The medical literature also reports that some cases of psoriasis benefit from candida treatment. Finally, psychiatrists at McGill University have recently reported that stress reduction techniques such as meditation produce significant improvements in psoriasis symptoms.

Thin Skin

Thin skin may be the result of years of cortisone-type cream use. Many other drugs and chemicals can cause this problem as well. It may also be related to stress, food allergies, nutritional deficiencies and digestive function abnormalities (low stomach acid, low pancreatic enzyme levels, etc.).

To help improve the general health of the skin, diet should be as natural as possible. Avoid chemicals, animal products, processed foods, coffee, tea, alcohol and sugar in any form other than fresh fruit. Animal products, including all dairy products and eggs, contain fats that can often be the cause of skin problems. They may also be loaded with drugs such as antibiotics, synthetic hormones, nitrites and other skin toxins. Organic fruits, vegetables, whole grains, seeds, nuts and legumes are best.

Nutrient supplements that may be very helpful for both treatment and prevention of thin skin include essential fatty acids (e.g., evening primrose oil, flax seed oil, black current seed oil, oil of borage, etc.), vitamin A, B-complex vitamins (including biotin), vitamin C, bioflavonoids (pycnogenol, hesperidin, catechin, quercetin), vitamin E, zinc, calendula and aloe vera. Treatment depends mainly on biochemical individuality. Topically, calendula cream helps heal cuts and sores and prevent infections. So does topical vitamin E and aloe vera. See a naturopath or a medical doctor familiar with the natural approach for a personalized program.

Eczema

Eczema is usually treated by dermatologists with countless prescriptions for various cortisone-based creams. Dermatologists rarely prescribe remedies directed at the systemic source of a rash, preferring to suppress skin problems with assorted steroid lotions and creams. For many patients, this is acceptable practice. There are, however, natural alternatives.

Eczema is often the result of stress or emotional reactions. According to Dr. Louise Hay, skin problems represent anxiety, fear, being threatened; it's old, buried emotions. There is a strong psychosomatic component to eczema. Dr. Steven Locke compared the psychosomatic histories of 90 patients with disorders of the eczema family to 50 controls. He discovered that specific situations precipitated the onset or relapse of eczema. These included threats to life and existence, threats of loss of outside sources of support or disturbance to inner, established patterns, such as blows to self-esteem or conflicts over sex and aggressiveness. It would seem likely therefore that psychotherapy, meditation, visualization or relaxation techniques would be helpful in the treatment of eczema.

Aside from stress and emotional factors, nutritional deficiencies, food allergies and digestive function abnormalities (low stomach acid, low pancreatic enzyme levels, etc.) may be related to eczema. If possible, see a natural health care practitioner for biochemical individuality testing.

Diet should be as natural as possible. Avoid chemicals, animal products, processed foods, coffee, tea, alcohol and sugar in any form other than fresh fruit. Animal products, including all dairy products and eggs, contain fats that can often be the cause of skin problems. They may also be loaded with drugs such as antibiotics, synthetic hormones, nitrates, nitrites and other skin toxins. Organic fruits, vegetables, whole grains, seeds, nuts and legumes are best.

Nutrient supplements that may be very helpful for both treatment and prevention include essential fatty acids (e.g., evening primrose oil, flax seed oil, black current seed oil, oil of borage, etc.), vitamin A, B-complex vitamins (including biotin), vitamin C, bioflavonoids (pycnogenol, hesperidin, catechin, quercetin), vitamin E, zinc, calendula and aloe vera. Treatment depends mainly on biochemical individuality.

How to Stop Fingernail Biting

Fingernail biting may be a nervous habit related to stress. It may also be driven by biochemical imbalances. These imbalances may be the result of blood sugar problems (hypoglycemia) or nutritional deficiencies. In my experience, it is helpful to follow a diet high in fiber and complex carbohydrates. Avoid sugar, white flour products, processed foods, red meats and caffeine products (coffee, tea, soft drinks, chocolate). It's best to have at least three meals and two snacks daily of wholesome, chemical-free foods. For more information on this type of diet and sample menus, see the section by Jeanne Marie Martin in this book.

The most common nutrient deficiencies that I see in my practice that are associated with fingernail biting are zinc, iron, magnesium and B-complex vitamins. White spots and horizontal ridges on the fingernails may be a sign of zinc deficiency. Vertical ridges, on the other hand, are commonly observed with iron deficiency. Trial therapy with a supplement containing these nutrients is well worth doing. The biting habit may be under control with this approach within six weeks. If possible, work with a health care practitioner familiar with natural therapies.

Boils

Boils (carbuncles) are more likely to occur in people who eat a lot of refined carbohydrates (foods high in simple sugars and white flour products) and/or animal products. Other possible contributing factors include diabetes, immune system problems and dermatitis. In the case of recurrent boils, a hypersensitivity (allergy) to certain foods, especially dairy products, wheat, corn, alcohol, spicy foods, fried foods and high fat foods, should be suspected. Boils originate from infected hair follicles (folliculitis).

Try a vegetarian diet high in whole grains, fruits, vegetables and beans (legumes). If already on a vegetarian diet, try a fruit and vegetable diet or a short juice fast. Eliminate anything that contains sugar and white flour products. In severe, resistant cases, a bowel detoxification program using psyllium seed powder, aloe vera juice, pectin and other soluble fibers is necessary to remove the source of the toxins that initiate the series of reactions leading to boils.

Supplements that may be very helpful in high doses include vitamin A, B-complex, vitamin C, vitamin E, zinc, selenium, silicon, garlic and lactobacillus acidophilus. Effective herbal remedies include berberis, calendula, echinacea, goldenseal, St. John's wort, phytolacca and thuja. Calendula and silica gel can be applied directly to the affected areas for some relief. Consult a naturopath or doctor familiar with natural therapeutics for a personalized treatment program and advice on prevention.

Seborrhea

Seborrhea is a fairly common condition known to most as dandruff in adults and cradle cap in infants. It is a disorder of the oil-secreting sebaceous glands found in the scalp, face, chest and other parts of the body. Greasy patches that scale, crust, fissure and flake are characteristic of this annoying skin condition. Seborrhea may be a part of what has been referred to as the "acne-seborrheic complex" frequently seen in brunettes with a positive familial history. Seborrhea usually appears along the hairline, eyebrows, eyelids, behind the ears, the bridge of the nose and the sternum (breast bone). It is worse in the winter and aggravated by stress, fatigue and certain trigger foods.

Unsuspected food allergies may be at the bottom of seborrhea. Common culprits include dairy, wheat, caffeine, alcohol, yeast, fried foods, beef and pork. Detection of the food allergies, elimination of the offending foods and a rotation diet will clear up a large number of cases. Some cases will clear with the use of antifungal or anticandida remedies. Natural antifungal remedies include berberine, caprylic acid, olive oil, garlic, primrose oil, flax seed oil, psyllium seed husks or powder, castor bean oil, omega-3 fish oils and acidophilus.

Some cases of seborrhea are caused by a deficiency in vitamin A. Supplementing the diet with cod liver or halibut liver oil will help provide both vitamin A and D. Other nutrients known to be of help to seborrhea are B-complex vitamins (especially biotin, folic acid and vitamin B12) vitamin E, selenium, silicon, iodine and zinc. In older adults, vitamin B12 injections may be necessary because of low stomach acidity or deficiency of intrinsic factor. Effective herbal remedies are aloe vera juice or gel, pau d'arco, echinacea, goldenseal, red clover, chaparral, dandelion, kelp and silymarin. Selenium, tea tree oil, or biotin-containing shampoos can help control dandruff and speed healing. For a personalized diet and supplement program, see a natural health care practitioner.

Itchy Skin Solutions

Two Chinese herbs that can help with an itchy skin are wormwood and phellostatin. These herbs have been used successfully in the treatment of candida infections as well. Itchy skin is also helped by increasing water intake to at least eight glasses a day.

Nutrient supplements that may be very helpful for both treatment and prevention include essential fatty acids (e.g., evening primrose oil, flax seed oil, black current seed oil, oil of borage, etc.), vitamin A, B-complex vitamins (including biotin), vitamin C, bioflavonoids (pycnogenol, hesperidin, catechin, quercetin), vitamin E, zinc, calendula and aloe vera.

Treatment depends mainly on biochemical individuality and some trial and error. Topically, calendula and tea tree oil help heal cuts and sores and prevents infections. So does topical vitamin E and aloe vera. See a naturopath or a medical doctor familiar with the natural approach for a personalized program of natural supplements and herbal remedies.

Skin Rashes and the Gut Connection

Rashes are most often related to a greater need for biotin, zinc, silicon, selenium, vitamin A, vitamin E and essential fatty acids. They may also be the result of certain imbalances in the gut. Bowel permeability abnormalities (leaky gut syndrome) and/or dysbiosis (bowel flora imbalance) can cause skin problems of almost any kind due to the absorption of various toxins.

A fruit and vegetable diet (three weeks), or a short juice fast (three to five days) followed by only fruits and vegetables (three weeks) may be helpful. Also of benefit are the following supplements (take for about six weeks):

Biotin	Selenium
Chelated zinc	Silica gel
Flax seed oil	Vitamin A
	Vitamin E

If the supplement program helps, experiment with the doses to see how much of each nutrient is needed to prevent a recurrence. If the problem does not clear, I would suggest having a CDSA (comprehensive digestive and stool analysis) done. A naturopath or nutrition-oriented medical doctor can order the test to help diagnose infection (candida, parasites, flora imbalances), digestive enzyme problems or other functional problems. It may also be worthwhile to be tested for food allergies.

Scleroderma

Scleroderma is a chronic connective tissue disease of unknown cause. There are inflammatory, vascular and fibrotic changes in the skin and internal organs. The most commonly affected organs are the GI tract, esophagus, thyroid, kidney, heart, lungs and joints. Scleroderma is also called progressive systemic sclerosis (PSS).

The characteristic skin thickening and restriction (morphea) is the result of an overproduction of collagen. The disease is highly individual in terms of severity and progression. Some patients experience only skin problems for decades before visceral or organ involvement begins. Others develop generalized skin thickening and often lethal internal organ disease over a period of two years. The full manifestation of the disease is called the CREST syndrome: Calcinosis, Raynaud's phenomenon, Esophageal dysfunction, Sclerodactylia and Telangiectasia. Scleroderma is seen in women four times as often as in men and appears between the ages of 20 and 40.

Over the years, I have treated a number of patients with various connective tissue diseases using a strictly natural approach. The medical treatment may be continued while general health improves with the use of natural remedies.

Many studies support the use of natural anti-inflammatory supplements for connective diseases such as scleroderma and polymyosits. Examples include cold-pressed flax seed oil, gamma linolenic acid (GLA found in evening primrose oil, black current seed oil and oil of borage) and omega-3-EPA (found in trout, cod, halibut, mackerel, salmon, shark, herring and other seafoods). Increasing these in the diet, or taking them in encapsulated supplement form, while decreasing the intake of saturated animal fats can have a remarkably good anti-inflammatory effect. The diet needs to be as close to completely vegetarian as possible. Read *Diet For A New America* by John Robbins to get an idea about all the reasons for adopting new eating habits. Also, see the section Healing Foods for Healing Diets in this book.

Optimizing the body's trace mineral balance may be crucial. It is therefore necessary to avoid foods known to interfere with mineral absorption such as bran, coffee and tea. Minerals that may be involved include iron, zinc, copper, manganese, calcium, magnesium, boron, silicon and selenium. Excess lead and iron in the body can indeed cause a great deal of damage. If tests (blood, urine and hair) indicate that this is a problem, oral or intravenous chelation therapy may be necessary.

Vitamins such as A, B-complex, C and E, as well beta-carotene and bioflavonoids, can be supplemented in higher than RDA doses because of their antioxidant properties that help prevent certain aspects of inflammation. In my practice I have found that high doses of vitamin E in particular have a remarkable effect in calming a hyperactive immune system. The recommended intake doses for all these nutrients would have to be determined for the individual by a qualified health care practitioner based on appropriate biochemical tests. The medical literature documents the benefits of at least two natural food supplements in scleroderma: para-aminobenzoic acid (PABA) and vitamin E. DMSO(dimethyl sulfoxide) is a natural remedy that helps soften the skin in scleroderma.

Many sufferers have reported benefits from the use of certain herbs. Alfalfa, for example, has been extensively studied. It contains many important substances including saponins, sterols, flavonoids, coumarins, alkaloids, vitamins, amino acids, minerals, trace elements and other nutrients. Numerous clinical and anecdotal reports support its use as a natural anti-inflammatory substance. Other herbs that have been reported to have beneficial effects for their anti-inflammatory effects include devil's claw, comfrey, sassafras, licorice and ginseng. Like vitamin and mineral supplements, herbs are not without their side effects and are best administered and supervised by an experienced health care practitioner.

There are many ways to stimulate the body's natural production of cortisone. (This is not a replacement for prednisone, but can help the body minimize its dependence on synthetic cortisones.) This is done through nutritional support of the adrenal glands with the following natural supplements:

Bioflavoniods	Potassium citrate
Licorice root capsules or tincture	Raw adrenal concentrate
Magnesium citrate	Vitamin C
Pantothenic acid (vitamin B5)	Zinc citrate

Siberian ginseng and DHEA (an extract of wild yam), astragalus and evening primrose oil also provide adrenal support. Work out an individualized dosage schedule and supplement regime with your naturopath or health care practitioner.

There are a growing number of studies that demonstrate the relationship between food allergies (hypersensitivity) and connective tissue diseases.The Elisa/Act or RAST blood tests can pick up hidden allergies to any number of foods. Unfortunately, these tests cannot be done unless the patient has been off prednisone or other cortisone-like drugs for at least four days. Discuss the pros and cons of doing this with a doctor or naturopath.

For people who react adversely to all foods (i.e., pan-allergic), the possibility of an intestinal tract parasitic or fungal (candida) infection should be investigated and treated before starting on a food allergy elimination program. Although one cannot say that parasites or candida cause connective diseases, many nutrition-oriented physicians have reported successes when either the candida or parasitic infection was cleared first. This is particularly true in those cases where there is a history of long-term antibiotic use. Look into some of these possibilities with your health care practitioner.

Excessive Body Hair

Excessive body and facial hair is a common problem in women. Various clinics specializing in hair removal by electrolysis—and other less dignified means—have sprung up to take advantage of this epidemic of hair growth. Hormonal or glandular problems may be at the root of the problem, and conventional testing by a specialist (endocrinologist) is recommended. There are also a variety of harmless alternatives that may be of some help.

Excessive androgens in women can be antagonized by measures favoring increased estrogenic activity. Many commonly eaten, wholesome foods are high in estrogen-like sterols. If there is no specific diagnosed medical condition (e.g., fibroids, ovarian cysts, fibrocystic breast disease), eat more of the foods high in estrogen: cherries, apples, olives, plums, garlic, peanuts, soy products, coconuts, yeast products, carrots, alfalfa, anise, brown rice, licorice root, parsley, red raspberry, sage, oregano, eggplant, tomatoes, potatoes, peppers, barley, bulgur, oats, wheat and wheat germ.

Most importantly, lower the intake of saturated fat and cholesterol by eliminating red meats from the diet. Keep high-fat dairy products, especially cheeses, to a minimum. Avoid coffee, regular tea, alcohol, sugar and white flour products. The more vegetarian, the better. Essential fatty acids of the omega-3, 6 and 9 families should be supplemented in the form of flax seed, olive, evening primrose, black currant, rice bran or borage oils.

Some herbs contain estrogenic substances but at levels of estrogen activity 400 times less than pharmaceutical compounds. These include dong quai, licorice, black cohosh and fennel. Other herbs that lead to higher estrogen levels include damiana, raspberry, sage, ginseng and gotu kola. Natural vitamin E (derived from wheat germ or soy) also contains traces of estrogens. (Synthetic vitamin E does not have the same beneficial effect as the natural form.) The same can be said for brewer's yeast. Vitamin E and evening primrose oil will help prevent some of the circulatory complications of estrogen therapy (e.g., abnormal blood clotting, etc.). So will B-complex vitamins (especially B6), zinc and selenium.

Bioflavonoids are plant substances that exist together with vitamin C and protect estrogens. They prevent estrogens from being broken down too rapidly in the body, thereby increasing overall estrogen activity. They are abundantly available in citrus fruits, garlic, onions, peppers, cherries, currants and many other foods. In supplemental form, look for bottles containing rutin, hesperidin, catechin, quercetin or pycnogenol on your health food store shelves. Homeopathic remedies made from ovarian extracts may also be very effective in reversing androgen effects in women. A natural health care practitioner can help with specific doses and individualized natural therapy.

Keloids

A keloid is an abnormal overgrowth of fibrous tissue (a scar) where skin has been somehow damaged following trauma. The tendency to forming keloids may be hereditary. They are seen more frequently in black people. In some African tribes, keloids are deliberately formed by repeated self-inflicted wounds as part of tribal ritual. The conventional treatment of keloids is to surgically remove these scars and prevent new ones from recurring through the use of radiation, laser surgery and injections of corticosteroids. Unfortunately, even these very modern treatments are far from perfect and may take as long as two years to work.

From a complementary medicine point of view, foods rich in vitamin A, the B-complex vitamins, vitamin C, vitamin E and trace minerals, especially iodine should be consumed. A partial list includes whole grain breads, cereals and pastas, wheat germ, avocados, sea vegetables, apples, cucumbers, millet, rice bran and sprouts of all kinds. The most important fresh juices to use as often as possible are carrot, celery, lemon, cucumber, endive and pineapple.

The following supplements may also be effective:

Aloe vera juice	Iodine
Barley green	Pycnogenol (proanthocyanidins)
Bee pollen	Vitamin C
Blue-green algae	Vitamin E
Bromelain (pineapple enzyme)	Zinc
Calendula tincture	

Use daily topical applications (at different times) of calendula cream, aloe vera gel and vitamin E (break an 800 IU capsule of clear base vitamin E and apply directly to the keloid). Supervision of these remedies by a natural health care practitioner is ideal. As with any skin disorder, the best approach to the problem of keloids is a combination of the conventional and nutritional (complementary medicine) therapies.

Eyelid Injury

Chemical injury to the eyelids must often be corrected by surgery. On the other hand, taking high doses of antioxidant supplements may help with healing, whether or not surgery is ever done.

Vitamins and minerals that may be particularly helpful are beta-carotene, B-complex vitamins, vitamin C, quercetin, pycnogenol, N-acetyl-cysteine, ginkgo biloba extract, coenzyme Q10, vitamin E, zinc, selenium, silica gel and glutathione. Essential fatty acid supplementation (e.g., flax seed oil, evening primrose oil, borage oil, fish oils) may also be vital for skin repair.

Natural creams made with zinc oxide, aloe vera gel, calendula, flax seed oil, Na-PCA, vitamin A and E or EGF (epidermal growth factor) may be of help to the skin surrounding the eyes.

Skin Tags

A skin tag is a small pedunculated protrusion of skin. Technically, it is a benign tumor known as a fibroma. It is not associated with any form of cancer and its specific cause is nebulous. Skin tags seem to occur with greater frequency as one ages and to people suffering from hypoglycemia (low blood sugar). It is important to remember that the skin is one of the body's excretory organs. The bowel, kidneys, lungs and liver are the body's other organs of elimination. When the skin gets clogged from dead cells, soap accumulations and other debris, it is prevented from discharging toxins from the body. Waste material can get trapped, eventually leading to a variety of skin problems including skin tags.

To help the skin breathe properly, many health experts suggest regular skin brushing—about five minutes daily before bathing or showering, using a skin brush made from natural bristles. Regular washing will not remove the layers of dead skin, uric acid crystals, catarrh and other acid wastes that come up through the pores of the skin. Skin brushing not only helps eliminate toxins but also cleanses the lymphatic system, stimulates the bloodstream and improves circulation in general. All body areas can be brushed including the breasts, thereby helping to prevent abnormal lumps.

The basic principles for the prevention and treatment of any benign tumor would apply to skin tags. Most nutritional authorities advise eliminating all animal protein, dairy products (except yogurt and yogurt products), salt, sugar, white flour products, processed and packaged foods. The reasoning behind this is that these foods are difficult to digest, contain no enzymes and form toxins (oxidants or free radicals) in the large bowel and blood. Raw fruits and vegetables should make up about half of dietary intake. The remainder may include seeds, nuts, whole grain and cultured dairy products such as yogurt, buttermilk and kefir. One thing to seriously consider as a good way to detoxify is juice fasting. For details, see the *The Joy of Juice Fasting*, by Klaus Kaufmann.

There is good evidence to suggest that supplementation with antioxidants will help prevent tumors from occurring. These include vitamin A, beta-carotene, most of the B-complex vitamins, vitamin E, vitamin C, all the bioflavonoids (rutin, hesperidin, catechin, quercetin, pycnogenol), selenium, silicon, zinc, cysteine, glutathione, coenzyme Q10 and germanium. A health care practitioner familiar with their use can suggest appropriate doses.

Scientific and anecdotal studies have shown that many different herbs and food supplements are useful in both the prevention and complementary medical treatment of skin tags and other benign tumors. These include deodorized garlic, pancreatin, raw thymus extract, lactobacillus acidophilus and herbs such as barberry, dandelion, pau d'arco, chaparral, echinacea, horsetail, comfrey, ragwort, wood sage and the mixture of burdock, slippery elm, Turkish rhubarb and sheep sorrel. Drinking aloe vera juice on a regular basis is also beneficial. Topical use of silica gel after skin brushing may be particularly effective.

In her book *Health Through God's Pharmacy*, Maria Treben describes the use of poultices made with horsetail, Swedish bitters and calendula in the treatment of tumors. A naturopath or medical doctor familiar with herbal remedies can be of help in prescribing an individualized treatment plan.

Facial Veins and Capillaries

Low stomach acidity (hypochlorhydria) may be associated with unsightly veins and capillaries on the face. The exact mechanism of this is unclear. Milk, dairy products and antacid supplements containing calcium and magnesium may make low stomach acidity problems worse. Treatment is highly variable and is based on biochemical individuality.

Low stomach acidity can be caused by a deficiency in B vitamins, vitamin C and amino acids; by the use of drugs like the birth control pill, antacids and alcohol; by cigarette smoking and by eating foods to which your body is allergic. In some cases, heredity seems to be involved. A greater need for vitamin C and bioflavonoids like rutin, hesperidin, catechin, pycnogenol and quercetin may also be involved in many cases.

Betaine, pepsin, glutamic acid, bromelain, papain, apple cider vinegar, Swedish bitters, lemon juice and ascorbic acid would all be helpful in improving stomach acidity. There is no toxicity and no dependence developed, even if taken for long periods of time. The stomach will learn to secrete higher amounts of acid on its own, thanks to supplementation. The length of time for this to occur varies from a few months to several years.

Constipation, bloating and gas are the most common symptoms of low stomach acidity. However, using symptoms to assess stomach acidity levels is not very reliable. In taking any acid-promoting supplement, the danger of causing gastritis or ulcers is always of some concern. Symptoms like burning, diarrhea and abdominal pain after taking an acid supplement are warnings that you may be taking too much. Make sure to take the supplement with food and, if any side effects develop, reduce dosage, drink lots of extra water and see a natural health care practitioner at the earliest opportunity.

Varicose Veins

Varicose veins are dilated, tortuous superficial veins caused by poorly functioning valves. They may be hereditary, but are also associated with anything that increases pressure in the abdomen and pelvic veins, such as obesity, pregnancy, a sedentary lifestyle or a job requiring long periods of standing. Varicose veins are worse when standing and during menses. Elevating the legs frequently improves symptoms. Regular, brisk walking or the use of a rebounder (mini-trampoline) will help improve both lymphatic and venous flow.

As far as nutritional therapy is concerned, the most important thing to do is to increase fiber intake and speed bowel elimination. By doing so, pressure in the lower abdominal or pelvic areas is relieved. Both varicose veins and hemorrhoids are helped by a diet high in fiber and complex carbohydrates and low in sugar and fat. Short juice fasts using carrots, celery, spinach, parsley, beets and cucumbers, or fruits and vegetables only (vegetarian cleansing) may be beneficial. Paavo Airola recommends eating foods high in rutin, silicon, vitamin C and bioflavonoids, like buckwheat and all berries. Foods high in water-soluble fiber like psyllium seed, flax seed, apple pectin, guar gum and oat bran are also very effective. Other therapeutic foods for varicose veins are barley bran, eggplant and cabbage. It's best to avoid red meat, milk, dairy products, fried foods, caffeine, sugar, fatty foods and refined foods.

Supplemental vitamin B complex, vitamin C and bioflavonoids (especially rutin, hesperidin, catechin, pycnogenol, pronogenol, quercetin) may not necessarily reverse varicose veins, but might help with pain and prevent a worsening of the condition. Several herbs may be used both topically and taken internally to improve vascular integrity and prevent inflammation. The most important of these are calendula, camomile, ginkgo biloba and witch hazel.

Stretch Marks

Stretch marks on the body are associated with zinc deficiency. Zinc deficiency signs and symptoms are similar to the general signs of malnutrition and include growth retardation, infertility, delayed sexual maturation, low sperm count, hair loss, skin conditions of various types, diarrhea, weakened immune response, behavior and sleep disturbances, vitamin A nonresponsive night blindness, impaired taste or smell perception, impaired wound healing and white spots or horizontal ridges on the fingernails. A long list of skin diseases, including eczema, psoriasis and stretch marks can be helped by zinc therapy.

Stretch marks can both be prevented and treated by oral supplements of vitamin B complex (especially pantothenic acid), vitamin C and vitamin E. Puncture capsules of natural vitamin E (400 to 800 IU capsules) and apply directly onto the stretch marks at least once daily in addition to any vitamin E consumed orally. Aloe vera juice (whole leaf, cold processed), silica gel and calendula can be used not only topically but also internally for their healing properties throughout the body. It may take several months to see results.

Natural Remedies for Blisters

Sports like tennis, squash, golf, baseball and weight lifting are plagued by hand and foot blisters. Many safe and effective natural remedies are available for both treatment and prevention. Before using any topical solutions, bathe (but do not rub) the affected area in warm water.

Eat more vitamin C-rich foods (citrus, berries, cherries, peppers, onions, potatoes, greens and sprouts). Aloe vera juice in combination with cranberry or other fruit beverages high in vitamin C is helpful. Essential fatty acids found in seeds (flax), nuts (avocados), olives, fish and legumes are important for practically all skin conditions.

The following have either soothing, natural antibiotic, protectant, antioxidant or skin softening effects:

Aloe vera gel	Crushed chili peppers mixed in sesame oil
Arnica montana lotion or cream	St. John's wort lotion or cream
Calendula lotion or cream	Tea tree oil

Beneficial natural supplements include:

Aloe vera juice or capsules	Selenium
B-complex vitamins	Silicon
Beta-carotene	Vitamin A
Bromelain	Vitamin C
Coenzyme Q10	Vitamin E
Evening primrose oil	Zinc
Pycnogenol	

All these remedies are readily available from health food stores. For more information on any of these treatments, see a naturopath or holistic medical doctor.

8

Muscles, Joints and Ligaments

C onventional medical doctors have little, if anything, to offer people who are suffering from chronic muscle, ligament and joint problems. Musculoskeletal problems are handled far better by the chiropractic profession, massage therapists, naturopaths and acupuncture practitioners. Additionally, there are many safe and effective natural remedies that act as analgesics, muscle relaxants and anti-inflammatory agents. Prescription drugs for musculoskeletal disorders often have significant side effects like stomach ulcers and hemorrhage. In addition, they do nothing to either change the course of the disease or to get to the root of the problem. This chapter describes a natural approach to some of the most common musculoskeletal problems encountered in daily life.

Natural Relief for Sore Muscles

Stiff or sore muscles after exercise are a common complaint. People who sit most of the day and do not exercise regularly are more susceptible. Also at risk are those who consume too few magnesium-rich foods like green vegetables. Additionally, if one follows a high acid-forming (high phosphate) diet, which reduces calcium availability to the body, muscle soreness is a likely outcome. Some medications, especially diuretics, increase the loss of minerals, thereby making muscle soreness worse. A high alkaline-forming diet (high in fresh fruits and vegetables) helps prevent the loss of calcium, magnesium, potassium and other vital muscle nutrients.

Avoid Acid Forming Foods:

All animal foods, especially red meats and liver

Colas, soft drinks

Caffeinated beverages

Refined sugars

Excess grains

Highly processed foods high in phosphates

Increase Alkaline Forming Foods:

Alfalfa

Beets

Brewer's yeast

Carrots

Cornmeal

Fruits (especially apricots)

Honey

Leafy green vegetables (spinach, kale, lettuce, broccoli, celery, cucumber, sprouts)

Millet

Sesame seeds, pumpkin seeds

Yogurt, kefir

Consider Natural Food Supplements:

Calcium	Niacinamide (B3) and thiamine (B1)
Chlorophyll	Potassium
Cramp bark herb tea	Silicon
Lobelia herb tea	Vitamin C
Magnesium	Vitamin B complex, with extra niacin
Multi-mineral formula	Vitamin E

Topical Applications

A mixture of evening primrose oil, olive oil, sesame seed oil, or of flax seed oil, ginger juice, vitamin A and zinc oxide applied topically several times daily will help ease muscle discomfort. Hot packs, hot baths and local Epsom salts packs are also effective in many cases. Homeopathic combination creams (e.g., Traumeel, Myoderm, Zeel) applied before and after exercise can be surprisingly effective.

Regular stretching (yoga-type) prior to exercise, and warm baths before bedtime can prevent muscle soreness, stiffness and even cramps. Also, consider periodic visits for massage therapy, shiatsu or chiropractic treatments.

Arthritis and Nutrition

Arthritis is a disease of the joints characterized by pain, swelling, redness, heat, and, at times, structural changes. The two most common forms, osteoarthritis and rheumatoid arthritis, are more common in women than men.

Osteoarthritis involves the gradual deterioration of cartilage, usually in larger, weight-bearing joints like the hips, knees, and spine. This wear and tear is thought by doctors to be a normal and inevitable process in people age 55 and older. By the eighth decade, approximately 90 percent of all people have some degree of osteoarthritis.

Rheumatoid arthritis is a chronic joint disease affecting one or more joints, usually those of the hands and feet, particularly the knuckle and toe joints. The synovium and other parts of the joint may gradually become inflamed and swollen with tissue destruction and deformities occurring in the most severe cases. Rheumatoid arthritis, unlike osteoarthritis, is a condition that waxes and wanes, occurring as a single attack or as several episodes, leaving the victim increasingly disabled. The disease may also be associated with damage to the lungs, heart, nerves and eyes. Although this form of arthritis primarily affects those between the ages of 40 and 60, it can also affect children and teenagers (juvenile rheumatoid arthritis). The cause of the disease is unknown, but is considered to be an autoimmune process (components of the immune system attacking the joints).

Conventional medicine treats arthritis with anti-inflammatory drugs (most commonly aspirin) and physiotherapy. In severe cases of rheumatoid arthritis, more potent anti-inflammatory drugs are used: nonsteroidal anti-inflammatory drugs such as Indomethacin, cortisone-like drugs, anti-malarials, gold salts, penicillamine and even experimental cytotoxic drugs.

Although this approach may produce pain relief, it does little, if anything, to alter the arthritic process itself. Surgical removal of badly inflamed joint synovium (synovectomy), arthroplasty (joint realignment and reconstruction), tendon repair, arthrodesis (joint fusion) and even artificial joint replacement may be required .

Non-steroidal anti-inflammatory drugs (NSAIDS) are the most common therapy for arthritis. They are big business for the pharmaceutical companies. Unfortunately, they cause bleeding from the gastrointestinal tract in close to 25,000 people a year. What's more, there is now evidence that these drugs accelerate the destructive nature of the disease. Are there safer and more effective alternatives?

Nutritional approaches to arthritis seem to have the most supporting scientific research and documentation behind them. For example, weight reduction, particularly in those suffering from osteoarthritis of the hips, knees and ankles, may be very important. Losing weight will alleviate some of the stress on the joints. The main types of foods that should be reduced as much as possible are refined carbohydrates (sugar and white flour products) and animal fats (especially those found in red meats).

There are certain types of fats, however, which may, in higher than average intake amounts, act in the same way as standard anti-inflammatory drugs. Examples of this include cold-pressed flax seed oil, gamma linolenic acid (GLA found in evening primrose oil) and EPA (found in cod, halibut, mackerel, salmon, shark, herring and other seafoods). Increasing these in the diet (or taking them in encapsulated supplement form) while decreasing the intake of saturated animal fats can have a remarkably good anti-inflammatory effect.

The amino acid DL-phenylalanine has been shown to help release the body's own natural opiates (endorphins) and can provide substantial pain relief naturally. This product is only available in health food stores in the United States.

In osteoarthritis, optimizing the body's trace mineral balance may be crucial. It is therefore necessary to avoid foods known to interfere with mineral absorption, such as bran, coffee and tea. Minerals that may be involved in osteoarthritis include iron, zinc, copper, manganese, calcium, magnesium, silicon, boron and selenium. Vitamins such as A, B-complex, C and E, as well as beta-carotene and bioflavonoids, can be supplemented in higher than RDA doses because of their antioxidant properties. The recommended intake doses for all these nutrients would have to be determined for the individual by a qualified health care practitioner based on appropriate biochemical tests.

Many arthritis sufferers have reported benefits from the use of certain herbs. Alfalfa, for example, contains many important substances (saponins, sterols, flavonoids, coumarins, alkaloids, vitamins, amino acids, minerals, trace elements) that numerous clinical and anecdotal reports have shown to be helpful in arthritis treatment. Other herbs that have been reported to have beneficial effects for arthritis include devil's claw, yucca, white oak, comfrey and sassafras.

There are a growing number of studies that demonstrate the relationship between food allergies (hypersensitivity) and arthritis. The purported benefits of juice or water fasting for all types of arthritis may simply be because the fast eliminates the food or foods to which the person is allergic. For years, testimonial reports have suggested that some individuals are adversely affected by plants from the *Solanacea* group (the nightshades). These include tomatoes, potatoes, eggplants, peppers, paprika and tobacco. It certainly can do no harm for an arthritis sufferer to exclude these foods from the diet for at least two months to see whether or not avoidance has any impact on the disease process. For those who find the rigors of fasting and food elimination diets too inconvenient or risky, the RAST or Elisa/Act blood tests can pick up allergies to the nightshades and other hidden food hypersensitivities.

In some people that react adversely to all foods (i.e., pan-allergic), the possibility of an intestinal tract parasitic or fungal (candida) infection needs to be investigated and treated before starting on a food allergy elimination program. Although one cannot say that parasites or candida cause arthritis, many nutrition-oriented physicians and clinical ecologists have reported successes in the treatment of arthritis when either the candida or parasitic infection was cleared first.

Wearing copper bracelets may be beneficial to many arthritis sufferers. Double-blind studies have proven that copper from the bracelet can penetrate the skin and produce an anti-inflammatory effect. Assorted reports

294

have claimed beneficial effects with supplemental niacinamide (vitamin B3), the New Zealand green-lipped mussel (because of its mucopolysaccharide content), shark cartilage and DMSO.

Recently, double-blind, placebo-controlled trials conducted in Europe have shown that the harmless amino-sugar glucosamine is superior to the commonly prescribed arthritis drugs. Glucosamine is normally found in high concentrations in the joint spaces. It stimulates connective tissue production and repair of the arthritic joint. The safe and effective dosage of glucosamine sulfate for most arthritis victims is 2,000 to 3,000 mgs daily. No side effects have been reported.

There are no quick and lasting remedies that work in all cases. One of the most important things that must be stressed in any holistic program for arthritis is that treatment is long term. Sufferers should be prepared to actively involve themselves in all aspects of therapy and not just passively wait for something to happen. Any holistic approach requires a far greater degree of self responsibility than just taking aspirins. A holistic health care practitioner's guidance is usually essential.

Polymyalgia Rheumatica and Natural Anti-Inflammatories

Polymyalgia rheumatica is one of many different connective tissue diseases. It is in the same family of diseases as rheumatoid arthritis, lupus and temporal arthritis. It is rare and characterized by aching and stiffness, involving mainly the trunk and larger joints (especially the shoulders). In the early stages it resembles a bad case of the flu. Blood tests are usually normal, with the exception of a very high sed rate (a non-specific blood test that is an indicator of inflammation occurring somewhere in the body).

Conventional medical treatment is prednisone (a cortisone-like drug) and other anti-inflammatory drugs. These, of course, have side effects, including peptic ulcers. Patients treated with prednisone often also take antacids or stomach acid-suppressing drugs such as ranitidine and cimetidine. Treatment is usually prescribed for life.

Many studies, however, support the use of natural anti-inflammatory supplements. Examples of these include cold-pressed flax seed oil, gamma linolenic acid (GLA found in evening primrose oil, black current seed oil and oil of borage) and omega-3-EPA (found in trout, cod, halibut, mackerel, salmon, shark, herring and other seafoods). Increasing these in the diet, or taking them in encapsulated supplement form, while decreasing the intake of saturated animal fats can have a remarkably good anti-inflammatory effect.

Optimizing the body's trace mineral balance may be crucial. It is therefore necessary to avoid foods known to interfere with mineral absorption, such as bran, coffee and tea. Minerals that may be involved include iron, zinc, copper, manganese, calcium, magnesium, boron, silicon and selenium. Excess lead and iron in the body can indeed cause a great deal of damage. If tests (blood, urine and hair) indicate that this is a problem, oral or intravenous chelation therapy may be necessary.

Vitamin A, B-complex vitamins, vitamin C, vitamin E, beta-carotene and bioflavonoids can be supplemented in higher than RDA doses as their antioxidant properties help prevent certain aspects of inflammation. The recommended intake doses for all these nutrients would have to be determined for the individual by a qualified health care practitioner based on appropriate biochemical tests. Tests that would be of particular value include blood, urine and hair mineral analysis.

Numerous clinical and anecdotal reports support the use of alfalfa as a natural anti-inflammatory substance. Other herbs that have been reported to have beneficial anti-inflammatory effects include devil's claw, white willow, white oak, yucca, chaparral, dandelion, hydrangea, kelp, aloe vera, Brigham tea, capsicum, dulse, garlic, parsley, red clover, comfrey, sassafras, licorice and ginseng. Like vitamin and mineral supplements, herbs are not without their side effects and are best administered and supervised by an experienced health care practitioner.

There are many ways to stimulate the body's natural production of cortisone. This is done by nutritional support of the adrenal glands with a high protein, low refined carbohydrate diet (i.e., no sugar and white flour products) and the following natural supplements:

Pantothenic acid (vitamin B5) . . . . *500 to 3000 mgs daily*
Vitamin C . . . . . . *6,000 mgs or more daily (depending on bowel tolerance)*
Magnesium citrate . . . . *400 mgs daily*
Potassium citrate . . . . *400 mgs daily*
Zinc citrate . . . . *90 mgs daily*
Raw adrenal concentrate . . . . *100 to 300 mgs daily*
Bioflavonoids . . . . *1,000 mgs daily*
Licorice root capsules or tincture . . . . *100 to 300 mgs daily*

Siberian ginseng and DHEA, astragalus and evening primrose oil (or borage or black currant oil) also provide adrenal support. Avoid sugar, white flour products, meats, processed foods, fried foods, dairy products and nightshade family foods (tobacco, tomatoes, potatoes, peppers, papri-ka, eggplant). Work out an individualized nutrition plan and supplement regime with your naturopath or health care practitioner.

There are a growing number of studies that demonstrate the relation-ship between food allergies (hypersensitivity) and connective tissue dis-eases. For those who find the rigors of fasting and food elimination diets too inconvenient or risky, the Elisa/Act blood test can pick up hidden allergies to any number of foods.

In some people who react adversely to all foods (pan-allergic), the possi-bility of an intestinal tract parasitic or fungal (candida) infection needs to be investigated and treated before starting on a food allergy elimination program. Although one cannot say that parasites or candida cause connec-tive tissue diseases, many nutrition-oriented physicians have reported suc-cesses when either the candida or parasitic infection was cleared first. Look into some of these possibilities with a health care practitioner.

Solutions for Osteoporosis

The porous bone disease osteoporosis affects 30 million North American women and increases their susceptibility to fractures. The role of calcium, estrogen and exercise in the prevention and treatment of osteoporosis is widely known, but there are many other aspects to consider, especially in cases that respond poorly to the conventional approach.

Magnesium, phosphorus, zinc, boron, copper, strontium, silicon and manganese all have important roles to play in the construction of healthy bones. High protein, high fat, processed or refined foods may lead to defi-ciencies in these essential trace minerals. Consuming more greens, whole grains, seeds and nuts is a good way of getting these nutrients.

Vitamins A, B6, C, D and K are the most essential to optimal bone health. Their importance is in the synthesis of connective tissue—the col-lagen matrix of cartilage and bone—or as co-catalysts for minerals and enzymes. Fruits, whole grains, legumes, seeds, nuts and vegetables are all good sources.

According to recently published work by Dr. John R. Lee (*Natural Progesterone: The Multiple Roles of a Remarkable Hormone*), "postmenopausal osteoporosis is a disease of inadequate osteoblast-mediated new bone forma-tion secondary to progesterone deficiency." Lee's research suggests that osteoporosis can be reversed with the use of natural progesterone cream from an extract of Mexican wild yam, applied daily for three out of four weeks each month. Unlike oral progesterone, the cream has no side effects.

A high protein diet increases the amount of calcium lost from the body through the kidneys. Diuretics (water pills) also stimulate bone loss and fracture risk by causing more urinary excretion of calcium and other minerals. Broad-spectrum antibiotics kill off the friendly intestinal bacteria that make vitamin K, an important bone-building factor. Fluoride is a strong enzyme inhibitor in the body and has been shown to directly boost fracture risk. Other factors that encourage osteoporosis are cigarette smoking, alcohol abuse and excessive thyroid hormone (L-thyroxin). See a doctor to discuss all these potential areas of prevention or intervention.

Sciatica

Sciatica is a condition that involves inflammation of the great sciatic nerve in the leg. It may be caused by many different conditions and produces acute or chronic pain down the back of the leg, originating in the buttock and extending to the foot. One of the most common causes of sciatica is degenerative disc disease, which can produce pain due to nerve root compression. Other causes of sciatica are gluteal muscle spasm, facet syndrome, piriformis muscle spasm, sacroiliac joint dysfunction due to short leg syndrome, sacroiliac sprain and lumbar strain/sprain. Conventional medical treatment involves analgesics, muscles relaxants and referral to physiotherapy. Many victims find more effective treatment with chiropractic, acupuncture, therapeutic massage, shiatsu or osteopathic treatments.

Sciatica is helped by changing from a meat-based to a more plant-based diet. Avoid meat, alcohol, hot sauces, spicy foods, fried foods, fatty foods, salty foods, coffee, tea, chocolate and other caffeine products, sweet foods and sugar. Eat more foods rich in B-complex vitamins like whole grains, brewer's yeast, olives, whole rye products, dark green leafy vegetables, yellow vegetables, raw seeds and nuts, lima beans, rice bran, bananas, sprouts, watercress and apples. Aloe vera juice (two to three ounces three times daily between meals) not only helps with sciatica, but also relieves ulcers. Other fresh juices that could be tried on a rotation or combination basis are the following:

Green drinks (spirulina, blue-green algae, chlorella, barley green, green kamut, etc.)
Potato
Dried olive tea
Nut milk and liquid chlorophyl
Carrot
Spinach
Beet
Cucumber
Celery
Parsley

Vitamins, Minerals & Other Factors:

Vitamin B complex
Vitamin B12 and B-complex injections
Biostrath elixir
Vitamin C
Bioflavonoids
Pycnogenol or pronogenol
Vitamin E
Calcium
Magnesium (Note: In severe or chronic cases, injections of magnesium sulfate are often very effective.)

Potassium
Silicon
Boron
Zinc
Copper
Manganese
Bromelain
Glucosamine sulfate
Evening primrose oil
Flax seed oil
Borage oil

Vitamins, Minerals & Other Factors:

Arnica oil or cream (topical application)
Black cohosh
Burdock
Camomile
Cinchona bark
Devil's claw (take with food or aloe vera juice to avoid hyperacidity)
Fenugreek
Ginger
Horseradish
Hypericum (St John's wort)
Juniper berries

Mugwort
Mullein
Natural progesterone cream (topical application)
Parsley
Rosemary
Skullcap
Stinging nettle
White willow
Wild yam extract
Valerina

Many of these herbs, vitamins and other natural supplements come in combination forms, thereby reducing the number of capsules, tablets or tinctures. A natural health care practitioner can recommend a personalized program of diet, supplements and other therapies for this sometimes troublesome condition. Dosages should be individualized.

Aside from standard physiotherapy, many sciatica sufferers are helped by chiropractic, acupuncture, shiatsu and massage therapy. Discuss these with your natural health care practitioner.

Bursitis Treatments

Bursae are thin-walled sacs lined with synovial fluid. They lubricate and ease the movement of the tendons and muscles over bony prominences, such as the elbow, the knee, the shoulder, the hip and other joints. Bursitis (inflammation of the bursa) occurs as a result of trauma, infection, diseases such as arthritis and gout as well as repetitive or excessive frictional force (sports).

In acute bursitis, pain and swelling can be helped by increasing fluids and by undertaking a short fruit or vegetable juice fast. The juices most often recommended include carrot, radish, watercress, spinach, black cherry, kale, celery and parsley.

Consider going vegetarian as a general principle. Strict vegetarian diets tend to ease inflammations of all types. Pineapples and papayas contain enzymes that have a special healing effect on bursitis. For chronic bursitis, testing for hidden food allergies may help lead to a permanent solution.

Short-term nutritional supplements with a beneficial effect on bursitis include:

Beta-carotene	Selenium
Bromelain	Vitamins A and D (cod or halibut liver oil capsules)
Curcumin (from tumeric)	Vitamin C and bioflavonoids
Omega-3 fatty acids	Vitamin E
Pycnogenol	Zinc chelate

Consult a doctor or naturopath familiar with food supplements and herbal remedies to help supervise progress and to monitor for potential side effects.

Some people claim a great benefit from drinking apple cider vinegar. Studies also indicate that a series of vitamin B12 injections alone can reverse bursitis. In comparison to cortisone shots, vitamin B12 is harmless. Side effects are 1,000 times more likely to happen with cortisone injections.

Some herbalists recommend bentonite clay, bryonia and comfrey as poultices. Bursitis also responds well to chiropractic manipulation, acupuncture, TENS (transcutaneous electrical nerve stimulation), ultrasound and homeopathy. Medical treatment is rarely necessary, and cortisone shots should be a last resort.

Gout

Gout is the name given to a condition that results from too much uric acid in the blood, joints, kidneys or other body tissues. When uric acid accumulates, it forms crystals and causes pain and swelling in the joints. If uric acid crystallizes in the kidney, stones may be produced. There are many causes of gout, including a long list of metabolic conditions (cancer, psoriasis, hemolytic anemia, specific enzyme defects like Lesch-Nyhan syndrome, etc.) and several kidney diseases. Some cytotoxic drugs, chronic lead poisoning, fungal or candida overgrowth and high sugar consumption can also lead to gout. Make sure a doctor determines the source of the problem before embarking on any natural therapy.

In uncomplicated cases, diet is very important in the prevention and treatment of gout. Weight reduction in obese individuals reduces uric acid levels significantly. Drink at least eight glasses of distilled water daily. For short-term relief, raw fruits, vegetables and their juices (especially celery, liquid chlorophyll, carrot, spinach and parsley) are recommended in large amounts. Whole grains, seeds and nuts should also be included in a diet aimed at reducing uric acid levels. Cherries and strawberries should be eaten in large amounts because of their ability to neutralize uric acid. One published study demonstrated that consuming half a pound of fresh or canned unsweetened cherries per day lowers uric acid and prevents gout attacks. When cherries are not in season, alternatives include hawthorn berries, blueberries, blackberries and raspberries.

Rich foods, coffee, sugar and white flour products aggravate gout. Avoidance of alcohol and purine-rich foods will help prevent the accumulation of uric acid. Purine-rich foods include red meats, sweetbreads, shellfish, anchovies, herring, sardines, meat gravies, consommé, mussels, all organ meats, asparagus and yeast products. Other foods that increase uric acid are fish, poultry, dried beans, lentils, peas, spinach, cauliflower, oatmeal and mushrooms.

These latter foods may be added back to the diet in small amounts once the acute attack is under control. Vitamin B3 (niacin) in large doses may also elevate uric acid and must be avoided in anything other than a B-complex supplement. Recent studies have also speculated that vitamin A toxicity and gout may be related. Supplementation with vitamin A should be questioned.

Supplements that help in the treatment of gout include vitamin B complex, folic acid, vitamin C, vitamin E and magnesium chelate. Folic acid inhibits the enzyme xanthine oxidase, which is responsible for producing uric acid. The prescription anti-gout drug allopurinol works because it inhibits this same enzyme.

Omega-3 and omega-6-EPA oils (flax seed oil, evening primrose oil borage oil) are important for their role in limiting inflammation. Another potent natural anti-inflammatory agent is bromelain. Bromelain is a proteolytic enzyme found in pineapples. The bioflavonoid quercetin is also helpful for gout because of its anti-inflammatory effect and its ability to inhibit xanthine oxidase. Studies also show that the amino acids alanine, aspartic acid, glutamic acid and glycine lower uric acid levels. One or more of these health food store supplements may be effective alternatives to prescription anti-inflammatory drugs.

Some traditional herbal remedies for gout include devil's claw, burdock and juniper. Devil's claw not only relieves joint pain but also reduces both serum cholesterol and uric acid levels. It can be used as a complement to other anti-gout remedies. See your health care practitioner for advice and supervision with these and all other natural remedies.

Dupuytren's Contracture

Dupuytren's contracture is an increase in fibrous tissue formation in the palmar fascia of the hand or the foot. This scar-like nodule in the palm or sole causes a flexion deformity leading to decreased function of the fingers or toes. The cause is unknown, but there is thought to be a genetic tendency. It is seen more often in connection with alcoholism, epilepsy, diabetes, tuberculosis, heart attacks and circulatory diseases. In some cases, a deficiency of vitamin B6 has been reported. Progression is variable and may occur over months to years. Conventional treatment is surgery, although this does nothing to alter the course of the deformity or to prevent recurrences. Cortisone injections only offer temporary relief.

Anything that improves oxygen supply to the tissues and the cardiovascular system or that contributes to the health of connective tissues will help Dupuytren's. Follow a vegan diet as much as possible. In other words, choose your diet from the four new food groups: whole grains, fruits, vegetables and legumes. Eat more olives, whole rye, lima beans, rice bran, bananas, sprouts, watercress and apples. Therapeutic juices to drink on a regular basis include combinations of carrot, celery, parsley, spinach, liquid chlorophyll and potato.

Natural supplements which complement conventional medical care in Dupuytren's are vitamin E, vitamin B6 and flax seed oil. The herb St. John's wort may be taken internally and topically, applied directly to the nodules on a regular basis. There are also many ways to stimulate the body's natural production of cortisone. This is done by nutritional support of the adrenal glands with the following natural supplements:

B-complex vitamins	Pantothenic acid (vitamin B5)
Bioflavoniods	Potassium citrate
Copper citrate	Vitamin C
Licorice root capsules or tincture	Zinc citrate
Magnesium citrate	

Siberian ginseng and DHEA (an extract of wild yam), astragalus and evening primrose oil also provide adrenal support. Work out an individualized dosage schedule and supplement regime with a naturopath or health care practitioner.

Heel Spurs, Plantar Fasciitis, Metatarsalgia and Burning Feet

Bone spurs are caused by calcium deposits and are most often seen in people who are overweight, have arthritis or have tendinitis.

Conventional medical treatment makes use of sponge-rubber cushion shoe inserts, short-wave diathermy, diapulse and other physiotherapy techniques. Alternating hot and cold foot baths may be helpful. Massage therapy, regular or laser acupuncture, chiropractic, podiatric and osteopathic treatments are also effective. In stubborn cases, cortisone injections are made directly into the heel. Surgery is rarely necessary.

Plantar fasciitis is an inflammatory condition located just in front of the heel. It is an inflammation of connective tissue, the cause of which is uncertain. The usual complaint is of pain beneath the heel on standing or walking. The pain may extend forward into the sole, and disability is sometimes severe. The abnormality does not usually show up on x-rays, but heel spurs may be seen in many cases. Metatarsalgia, neuritis and "burning foot syndrome" are similar types of nerve, muscle or ligament inflammation.

Natural treatment of these problems involves measures that enhance the health of the body's connective tissue. Healthy connective tissue requires many nutrients to function at an optimal level. These include the essential amino acids, vitamin A, vitamin E, vitamin C, vitamin D, calcium, magnesium, zinc, copper, manganese, silicon, selenium, boron, bioflavonoids, essential fatty acids and the mucopolysaccharides. A thorough nutritional evaluation for vitamins, minerals and amino acids would certainly help determine the nature of the micro-nutrient needs.

It's best to eliminate sugar, white flour products, coffee, tea, alcohol, beef and pork from the diet and eat a wide variety of seafoods as a protein source. Increasing the consumption of fresh raw fruits and vegetables is also recommended.

The mucopolysaccharides are also called the chondroitin sulfates. They are found in many different seafoods, especially mussels. If you are not a lover of seafoods, or prefer a vegetarian lifestyle, supplementation is an option. Natural anti-inflammatory supplements that may be of help are aloe vera juice (whole leaf, cold processed), glucosamine sulfate, shark cartilage, bromelain, licorice root extract, ginger root herbal tea, evening primrose oil, flax seed oil, kelp and green-lipped mussel.

In more difficult cases, megadose intramusclar injections of B-complex vitamins (especially vitamin B12) and magnesium sulfate are worth trying. So is vitamin C, pushed to bowel tolerance doses (e.g., just short of producing watery bowel movements). Several doctors have reported that burning foot syndrome can be successfully treated by megadoses of pantothenic acid (vitamin B5; 1,500 to 3,000 mgs daily for six weeks). Homeopathic injections with combination connective tissue remedies work in selected cases.

If the problem fails to improve with diet change or supplementation, one should also consider the possibility of food allergies, digestive enzyme insufficiencies (especially hydrochloric acid) and assimilation problems. A nutritional doctor or naturopath can order a comprehensive digestive and stool analysis, food allergy tests or other tests for nutritional status to find the source of the problem.

Tendinitis

Tendinitis is an acute or chronic inflammation of a tendon and the lining of a tendon sheath. Although the exact cause is unclear, tendinitis can occur after sudden, excessive pulling, strain or sprain of a limb. Repeated trauma from physically demanding sports can also result in tendinitis. The tendons most commonly affected are the Achilles (behind the ankle), the biceps (front of shoulder), the small tendons of the thumb, the upper patella (knee) and the rotator cuff (shoulder). Important preventive measures include stretching and warming-up before exercise.

First aid therapy begins with rest to avoid further injury, applying ice and cold compresses to the area to reduce swelling or bleeding and elevating the body part above the level of the heart to improve drainage. Effective physical treatments are TENS, ultrasound, massage therapy and acupuncture. Strengthening exercises for the affected area after inflammation subsides will help prevent reinjury.

Tendinitis heals more quickly if nutritional status is optimized. Vitamin A and beta-carotene are both required for collagen synthesis and wound healing. Vitamin C and bioflavonoids like quercetin and pycnogenol also play a major role in the maintenance of collagen and tendon repair. Double-blind, placebo-controlled studies suggest that bioflavonoids alone will cut healing time in half.

Vitamin E and the trace mineral selenium work synergistically as antioxidants, quenching the deleterious effects of free radicals produced in the inflammatory process. Zinc, copper and manganese also have potent anti-inflammatory effects. So do cod liver oil, flax seed oil and evening primrose oil. Other minerals with important roles to play are calcium, magnesium, silicon and boron. Vitamin B12 injections are also very effective.

Bromelain, an enzyme found in pineapple, is effective for virtually all inflammatory conditions and helps reduce pain, swelling, bruising and healing time after most injuries or surgical procedures. Botanical medicines like tumeric and curcumin have traditionally been used in Indian and Chinese systems of medicine for their analgesic and anti-inflammatory properties. Although all these complementary medicines are generally regarded as safe, severe pain, joint damage or loss of function demands immediate conventional medical or surgical intervention.

Ankylosing Spondylitis

Ankylosing spondylitis (AS) is also known as Marie Strumpell disease. It is a chronic, progressive inflammatory arthritic disease mainly affecting young men aged 10 to 30 years. The spinal joints and adjacent connective tissues are primarily affected. The cause is unknown, but there is some genetic susceptibility.

Onset is gradual and insidious over a period of years. Initially there may be low back pain in the sacroiliac and lumbar areas, sciatic pain, morning stiffness and low back pain. As the disease advances, the pain spreads up the spine into the mid-back and neck. In about one-third of the victims, the hips and shoulders may be involved. Other symptoms include fatigue, loss of appetite and weight loss, anemia, muscle stiffness, cramping, pain on breathing, decreased ability to take deep breaths and decreased mobility of the spine. A bent-over stance, waddling gait and chronic iritis are also features of AS. Diagnosis can be made by x-ray and blood tests.

Conventional medical treatment involves the prescription of various types of Acetyl Salicydic Acid (ASA). Another common practice is to prescribe nonsteroidal anti-inflammatory drugs such as indomethacin, cortisone-like drugs, antimalarials, gold salts, penicillamine and even experimental cytotoxic drugs. Stretching exercises, physiotherapy, chiropractic and massage therapy work on correct posturing and are important to optimize mobility. Surgery is sometimes necessary to replace a joint or to straighten the spine For more information, see the section Arthritis and Nutrition.

Carpal Tunnel Syndrome

Carpal tunnel syndrome is the name given to a condition produced by the entrapment of the median nerve at the wrist. It is most frequently seen in middle-aged women. Continuous pressure on the median nerve can bring about paresthesias in the thumb to ring fingers (numbness, tingling, pain), loss of muscle mass (atrophy) and weakness of the affected hand. Carpal tunnel syndrome may be associated with other diseases, such as rheumatoid arthritis, acromegaly and gout. It can also be secondary to a wrist fracture (Colle's fracture), premenstrual syndrome, pregnancy and the swelling that occurs with conditions such as hypothyroidism. High-dose lithium therapy for manic depressive illness can be associated with some cases.

When carpal tunnel syndrome occurs in the absence of diseases or health conditions, it is usually the end result of repeated wrist movements (sewing, typing, driving, playing video games, etc.). Nerve conduction tests verify the diagnosis. Conventional treatment is surgical release of the compression. Although surgery is usually effective, the syndrome can later develop in the other previously normal wrist. This suggests that carpal tunnel syndrome is a reflection of a systemic condition.

In early, reversible cases, effective non-invasive therapies include hot epsom soaks, range-of-motion exercises and strengthening exercises like squeezing a ball and working with small weights. Avoidance of repetitive motions is mandatory. Physiotherapy, acupuncture, chiropractic and massage therapy are all helpful, along with ultrasound and Galvanic nerve stimulation. If an underlying disease exists, this should be treated whenever possible (e.g., thyroid hormone for hypothyroidism).

Many cases of carpal tunnel syndrome benefit from essential fatty acid therapy. This includes the avoidance of saturated animal fats and supplementation with evening primrose oil, flax seed oil or borage oil. Avoidance of processed foods, caffeine and high protein animal products is useful.

Vitamin B6 in high doses, along with other B-complex vitamins (especially vitamin B2 and B3), has also been reported to be effective. In most cases, it takes six weeks or longer for B6 therapy to work. Magnesium, bromelain and bioflavonoids like pycnogenol, pronogenol, catechin, quercetin and hesperidin are also beneficial. White willow bark, devil's claw, St. John's wort and feverfew can be used for their anti-inflammatory and analgesic properties. A naturopath, nutritionist, herbalist or holistic doctor can recommend a personalized regime of diet and supplements.

9

Healing Foods for Healing Diets

by Jeanne Marie Martin

Certain foods are conducive to healing—and actually assist the body to heal—by providing nutrients that help to strengthen and boost the immune system. These nutrients give the body high quality fuel so it can function at its optimum best. They do not interfere with the healing process by putting poisons (chemical additives, pesticides and preservatives) into the body that will hinder digestion and healing and ultimately work against the body. Natural and organic foods are preferred for any health concern. Even some incurable diseases have been found to have a slower rate of degeneration when a more wholesome diet is employed. These special, wholesome foods are called healing foods.

Unlike refined sugars and white flours (which offer quick, temporary, unstable energy), healing foods are not overly easy to digest. But unlike red meats and hard cheeses (which require lots of extra body energy and long hours to process and assimilate), they are not hard to digest.

A well balanced diet has an abundance of vegetables and fruits as its main foundation—about 30 to 40 percent fruits and vegetables. A healing diet requires more vegetables (30 to 50 percent) and less fruit (five percent or less, depending on individual needs). Most North American diseases tend to be aggravated by excessive sugars and sweets, including fruit sugars. Therefore, it is better to limit (and sometimes even eliminate) fruit for specific ailments like food allergies, high or low blood sugar, candida albicans, parasites, etc., for short terms of several months and sometimes even for periods of a year or two. Fruit may, however, be helpful in the treatment of some ailments like cancer, for example. In such cases it may be beneficial to increase fruit consumption slightly, to about five to ten percent. Raw fruit is full of live enzymes and for maximum cleansing benefits it should be eaten alone or before other foods. (See Food Combining section for more information.)

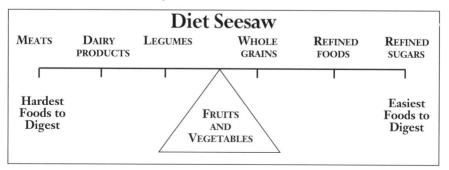

Diet Seesaw

| MEATS | DAIRY PRODUCTS | LEGUMES | WHOLE GRAINS | REFINED FOODS | REFINED SUGARS |

Hardest Foods to Digest

FRUITS AND VEGETABLES

Easiest Foods to Digest

When you go up and down on the diet seesaw by eating lots of meats and refined foods, your emotions and body energy go up and down too. When the foods you eat are closer to the centre of the seesaw, diet and lifestyle are more balanced. (See Diagram)

In order to speed healing, it is best to eliminate, or drastically reduce, refined foods and meats, which are at opposite ends of the energy seesaw. Sweets, refined foods and meat (including red meat, poultry and fish) should represent five percent or less of the diet. Shellfish like shrimp, crab, lobster and clams should be eliminated from healing diets, as they tend to be more toxic. However, one to two servings per month may be acceptable on some healing diets.

Dairy foods, which are mucous forming, difficult to digest and usually full of additives and preservatives, must also be reduced for optimum healing: they should represent about five percent or less of dietary intake. The best dairy products are natural, low-fat yogurt (which contains helpful enzymes that assist digestion); goat or sheep milk feta cheese; quark or other soft, natural and preferably organic cheeses and a small amount of butter (or Better Butter; see recipe) or clarified butter for some individuals. Eggs are included with dairy products, as they also contain cholesterol, fats and additives and are best if kept to a reasonable limit.

Tofu and soy products must also be kept to five percent or less, as they are difficult to digest and are easy to develop an allergy to. Some people try to replace dairy milk with large amounts of soy milk, which overburdens the system. When dairy milk is excluded, a variety of legumes and whole grains are the best replacement. Nuts and seeds must also be limited to five percent or less and should be eaten in their more digestive forms only. (See Healing Foods Guidelines below.)

The staples of a healing diet include 20 to 25 percent whole grains (mostly cooked, eaten warm); 15 to 20 percent tender legumes (beans, peas and lentils; cooked, eaten warm) and 30 to 50 percent fresh vegetables (raw and cooked). Individual needs may vary, so specific diet requirements should be personalized and discussed with a qualified health specialist.

A vegan diet (no animal products and no gelatin, dairy products, eggs, sugar and sometimes honey) or a macrobiotic diet (with reduced meat and dairy products and increased healing foods like whole grains, vegetables, burdock and herbs, etc.) are sometimes recommended for healing diets because they follow many of these guidelines and greatly support the immune system. However, it is not essential to stick dogmatically to these or other specific, exacting regimens in order to obtain the desired benefits. While an average, healthful diet should be comprised of 75 percent or more wholesome, high quality foods, a healing diet requires 90 to 100 percent wholesome foods. But unless the circumstances are severe (as in cases of AIDS or advanced cancer) or treatment requires a temporary, strict diet (as for candida albicans) it is not necessary to consume 100 percent "perfect" foods. For some, increasing good food intake by 20 percent or 50 percent and decreasing "agitating" foods may be enough to speed healing and dramatically improve overall health.

Healing Diets Food Ratios

30-50 percent	Vegetables (raw and cooked)
20-25 percent	Whole Grains (cooked, eaten warm)
15-20 percent	Legumes (beans, peas, lentils; cooked, eaten warm)
0-10 percent	Fruit (raw, cooked or dried)
0-5 percent	Red meats, poultry and fish
0-5 percent	Dairy products and eggs
0-5 percent	Seeds and nuts (ground or in butters)
0-5 percent	Tofu and soy products
0-5 percent	Oils, sweets and miscellaneous foods

Preparation of Healing Foods

How a food is prepared can have everything to do with how nutritious it is and how well it is digested and utilized by the body. A healthy individual can usually enjoy almost any food, while someone with health concerns must be more selective with their diet. The saying "One man's meat is another man's poison" is indeed an accurate statement. Each wholesome food can have a place in the diet at different times.

Note the use of the word wholesome: junk foods like fried foods, refined flours and sugars, heavily processed foods, low-nutrient foods and foods high in additives and preservatives are not wholesome. Essentially, all foods start out as healthful, but many become unwholesome after processing and cooking. Each food has unique properties, and each food has a unique combination of vitamins, minerals, proteins, carbohydrates, fats and water. Utilized correctly, each natural, whole food can be of benefit to the body at different times, unless that food has previously been abused, overused or the individual has a damaged digestive tract or impaired health.

One who is in a healing crisis must simplify diet and lifestyle. The less complicated the better. There should be a variety of foods in the overall diet, but each meal should be simple, without excessive variety or heavy fats, and without foods that are very difficult to digest, like meats, nuts and seeds and too many dry or raw foods.

The guidelines below lists foods to enjoy—foods that are in their most digestible and nutritious form. The foods to avoid indicate, in some cases, the same foods, but prepared in a different way that can actually be detrimental to healing and lower body energy levels. Following the guidelines, reasons are given as to why the foods to enjoy are better for you than the foods listed to avoid. Whenever possible, consume the recommended foods at least 75 percent or more of the time while on a healing diet. Consume these foods 90 percent or more of the time if a health situation is severe.

Remember: Individual needs will vary! Consult your health specialist for guidance.

Healing Foods Guidelines

Foods to Enjoy:
1. Leafy green lettuces; dark greens like spinach and wild greens; finely grated, fresh, raw beets and carrots; red bell peppers; English cucumbers; sliced or grated zucchini; avocado – for easier-to-digest salads.
2. Mock Tomato Sauce; orange yams; winter squash (especially butternut and buttercup); cauliflower; turnips; parsnips; shiitake mushrooms. (A little tomato is okay for candida, parasites and most diets.)
3. Shiitake mushrooms with no visible mold growth.
4. Basic or sub-acid fruits like apples, pears, peaches, all berries, firm kiwis, papayas, Japanese pear-apples, Chinese pears (and sometimes watermelon). Local fruit in season.
5. Grapefruits, lemons and limes.
6. Cooked whole grains, especially millet, quinoa, teff, wild and short-grain brown rice; very tender but not mushy, eaten warm.
7. Kamut and spelt flours.
8. Whole oats, oat groats, Scotch oats.
9. Cooked legumes blended into soups or mashed in casseroles or added to veggie burgers. More digestible eaten warm.
10. Ground nuts and seeds, nut and seed butters in warm, cooked foods. The best are almonds, cashews, filberts (or hazelnuts) and all seeds.
11. Natural, low-fat yogurt, goat or sheep feta cheese, quark or other natural, organic soft cheeses (and cooked cheeses).

12. Natural oils, either expeller pressed or cold pressed, especially raw flax and pumpkin. For cooking use: canola, sunflower, safflower, sesame and olive.
13. Maple syrup, natural/raw honey, fruit concentrate, rice syrup, real raw sugars, malt, molasses and other natural sweets.
14. Carob or carob powder (dark, roasted, not the raw powder).
15. Herbal seasonings like parsley, basil, oregano, thyme, rosemary, chives and mild seeds like cumin, celery, dill and fennel.
16. Sea salt and sea kelp.
17. Salt substitutes, herb blends and potassium chloride.
18. Herbal teas, especially mint, alfalfa, comfrey, raspberry or strawberry leaves, lemon grass, camomile, fennel or fenugreek.
19. Dandelion coffee substitutes and barley and grain coffees.
20. Club soda.

Foods to Avoid

1. Iceberg or head lettuce, cabbage, tomatoes, green bell peppers, regular cucumbers (unless organic), broccoli, cauliflower, grated potato or corn eaten raw in salads, as they are very hard on digestion.
2. Foods in the deadly nightshade family which include tomatoes, white potatoes, yellow sweet potatoes, peppers (except for the occasional red bell or cayenne pepper) and eggplant.
3. Button or regular white market mushrooms.
4. Sweet and tropical fruits like bananas, mangoes, pineapple, grapes, melons, dates, coconut and other dried fruits. (Occasional cooked, dried fruit is okay for some healing diets.) Avoid all fruit juices (except citrus).
5. Oranges.
6. White rices, all pastas, dry cereals, 9-grain and white breads and white or whole wheat crackers of any kind.
7. Whole wheat or white flours.
8. Rolled or flaked oats.
9. Cooked legumes served cold or marinated, sweet and sour, eaten hot or cold or with lots of sweetening added.
10. Raw or roasted nuts or seeds eaten alone or with other foods. Peanuts and peanut butter.
11. Milk, process cheeses, hard cheeses, cheeses with rennet and some uncooked cheeses.
12. All solvent-extracted oils: palm, corn, peanut, soy and coconut oils.
13. White and brown sugars, demerara or turbinado sugars, corn syrup, dextrose or artificial sweeteners/substitutes.

14. Chocolate or cocoa powder.
15. Spices (strong seeds, barks and roots) like cinnamon, nutmeg, mace, mustard, cardamom, coriander, tumeric, black pepper.
16. Regular table salt.
17. Excessive use of salt, tamari or other salty foods.
18. Red teas or spice teas with hibiscus, orange peel; red tea bags. Also caffeinated green, black and oriental teas.
19. Caffeinated and decaf coffee and coffee blends with sugars and additives.
20. Sparkling mineral waters.

Reasons:

1. Most people with severe ailments have impaired digestion. Some people who are ill cannot digest any raw vegetables except juices, while others tolerate the more nutritious, easier to digest veggies mentioned here. If raw veggies are a problem, drink 8–10 ounces of carrot juice with 20 percent beet juice and ¼–½ tsp "pure" barley green powder mixed in. Take 20 minutes to sip a glass and swish the juice in mouth to add helpful enzymes; use four to six times per week. Use organic veggies for juice. Eat raw salads at lunch and use organic veggies if there are digestive problems and/ or cancer. Eating lots of cooked vegetables, especially steamed, baked and broiled, will help the body heal and help prevent constipation.

2. For many ailments, nightshade family vegetables are toxic and interfere with healing. This book has a tomato sauce substitute. Orange yams, winter squash or white vegetables are the best substitutes for white or sweet potatoes. Orange veggies are high in vitamin A and great for cancer. Red bell pepper is more tolerable/digestible than green and is okay in small amounts. Cayenne aids the heart, helps circulation and helps keep arteries clear. Shiitake mushrooms may be used instead of eggplant in cooking.

3. Shiitake mushrooms are high in germanium and good for cancer. They also have less toxins and chemicals added during growing than button mushrooms. Use firm, non-moldy shiitakes in cooking.

4. Sweet and tropical fruits are for warm climates or summertime. The excessive sweets eaten by North Americans, including fruits, add problems for allergies, high/low blood sugar, candida albicans, parasites, etc. Local, non-sweet fruits are best for anyone living at a latitude above Los Angeles. Eat raw fruit alone. (See Food Combining.)

5. Oranges are alkaline and feed yeast and parasites. Almost every ailment is helped by exclusion of oranges and orange juice. Other citrus is

high in acid and helps kill yeast and parasites. Grapefruit, lemon and lime can assist healing and are rarely allergic.

6. White rices, breads, dry cereals and pastas have few nutrients, clog the digestive tract and feed parasites. They are essentially dead foods. Heavy multi-grain breads can burden or scratch intestines. Cooked, tender whole grains eaten warm are more digestible and are higher in nutrients. (Nutrients are more easily utilized in warm foods.) Keep soft whole grain breads to a minimum, a few servings a week. Brown rice must be cooked carefully and chewed well to be digestible. Although it is not necessary to totally exclude breads on a healing diet, it is best to keep bread consumption to a minimum.

7. Whole wheat and white flours come from devitalized grain with many cross-breedings and years of exposure to chemical sprays and pesticides. Kamut and spelt are a special strain of African and European wheat; they are less tampered with, less toxic, more digestible and higher in enzymes. Fifty percent of people with wheat allergies can eat kamut and/or spelt.

8. Oats are more nutritious and digestible when not rolled or flaked. Also, rolled and flaked oats tend to affect blood sugar levels, contribute to fatigue and feed yeast and parasites.

9. Most people who are not accustomed to eating and digesting beans have difficulty breaking them down without getting gas and indigestion. Well-cooked beans, blended or mashed, are easier to assimilate, especially when warm. Adding sweeteners to legumes is poor food combining and slows down digestion while making it more difficult. Excessive oils with cold beans hinders digestion. Get digestive enzymes if needed, as beans are essential healing foods. (See Special Cooking Guidelines for details on how to prevent gas.)

10. Nuts usually wreak havoc on most digestive tracts, whether raw or roasted in oil. Most store bought roasted nuts are rancid and will smell and taste that way to those with acute senses. Peanuts are high in mold content and hard to digest. Those in good health can eat whole nuts alone and should chew them to powder. Others should eat nuts ground or in butters or warmed in foods or sauces. Seeds are the same. Raw, ground sesame or flax seed is good mixed in hot foods. One teaspoon of ground flax seed, four to six times a week is good for most.

11. Yogurt is the only natural dairy food with helpful, digestive enzymes that assist in digesting it and other foods eaten with it. It is the easiest dairy product to digest. Not all yogurts contain live cultures. Plain yogurt is preferable. If you buy fruited varieties make sure the fruit is on the

bottom. Avoid cheeses made with rennet, as this enzyme, found in a calf's stomach, is hard for humans to digest. Avoid process cheeses as they are high in unhealthy additives and are hard to digest. Some hard cheeses, like imported varieties (mozzarella, Swiss, etc.) are high in rennet but may sometimes be eaten cooked as that helps break it down. These cheeses are mucous forming, high in fats and cholesterol, hard to digest and in raw form are high in mold content (feeds parasites).

12. The oil story is a complicated one. Choose natural oils and use in moderation. The healthful ones are given here. For more information on oils read *Fats that Heal Fats that Kill*, by Udo Erasmus.

13. Avoid all sweets on any healing diet. When using sweets, choose the natural ones suggested, in small amounts on rare occasions. Avoid all sweets for yeast/parasites. Refined sweets are more detrimental than natural. Some artificial sweets have been shown to contribute to brain tumors and cancer.

14. Carob contains ten times less fat than chocolate and has no caffeine or oxalic acid (which when mixed with calcium makes it unusable, as in chocolate milk). Carob is delicious when properly prepared.

15. Green herbs especially are full of minerals and enzymes which can assist healing (if not allergic). Spices can irritate the stomach lining and hinder digestion. Cooked black pepper is carcinogenic. Use cayenne pepper instead: one part cayenne per four to ten parts black pepper in recipes. (If cayenne is hot, use less.)

16. Many physicians now recommend sea salt instead of regular salt, as it is more digestible and beneficial and unlike table salt does not contain corn sugar (dextrose), artificial demoisterizers and whiteners. Sea salt has smaller crystals: ¼ tsp = 1 tsp table salt. Sea kelp adds iodine to the diet, which is not found in sea salt unless it is iodized. Sea kelp, like other seaweeds, is healing for the thyroid and may help expel heavy metals.

17. There are many blends of seasoning available in health stores for use instead of salt for those who need salt-reduced diets. Potassium chloride may also be experimented with as a substitute: use approximately ¼ of the amount indicated for salt. Like many foods, salt is not a problem unless abused. Those who eat more vegetables, grains and legumes can tolerate greater amounts of salt. That's why vegetarians can use more soy sauce and miso. Salt extends and flavors better when used in cooking rather than at the table. More hidden salt is found in prepackaged foods than one would use when cooking from scratch or at the table.

318

18. Almost all ailments require exclusion of caffeine for speedy healing. Most oriental teas are caffeinated. Red teas and rose hips that are crushed feed yeast and parasites. Be sure that loose/bulk green herbal teas are dried properly so they are not moldy.

19. Dandelion is great for the liver. Grain coffees can give you some of the flavor without the caffeine. Sometimes organic coffees that are naturally decaffeinated by water process can be enjoyed by coffee lovers. The caffeine in organic coffee tends not to be as detrimental as regular coffees. Many coffee blends may contain sugars, whiteners and other harmful additives.

20. Many people with health problems are constipated. Sparkling mineral waters add to this problem while club soda helps to loosen the bowels. Try club soda with a lemon or lime wedge. Be sure to brush teeth at night as club soda is acidic.

Food Combining

Food combining is a rather complex issue as there are many conflicting points of view. However, the most important food combining principles are:

1. Eat proteins separately from carbohydrate foods. This is a simple thing for most vegetarians to do, as it is okay to eat legumes and whole grains together. This means that all meats, eggs and most dairy products are best not eaten at the same meal with starches like breads, crackers, pasta, cereals or potatoes. Following this rule helps to speed digestion and healing and keeps one from absorbing as many calories from foods.

2. Eat raw fruit alone or before a meal so as not to hinder digestion. The enzymes in raw fruit make the foods easiest to digest. However, stomach upset, indigestion and fermentation of stomach foods may occur if raw fruit is eaten after a meal. Cooked fruit is like a carbohydrate food and is okay to eat during or after a meal. Dried fruit works the same way; cooked, it can be had with a meal. After eating raw fruit, try to wait 15 to 30 minutes before consuming other foods.

Other Special Food Combining Points:

1. Eat raw citrus fruit away from grains, as it makes them like lead in the system and increases absorption of calories. However, it is okay to cook citrus with grains. Don't eat raw fruit at night. Fruit sugar may keep you awake.

2. Eat desserts one hour or more after a full meal of other foods so as to lessen their effect on blood sugar levels and decrease calorie absorption. Don't eat desserts on an empty stomach.

3. Vegetarians especially should not overeat sweets. They create an imbalance in the system and a craving for non-vegetarian foods and alcohol. (A vegetarian or highly alkaline diet reduces the desire for alcohol and smoking!)

4. Eat raw vegetables first in a vegetarian meal to help stimulate and assist digestion. Meat should be eaten before salad in meat meals. Chew foods well to mix lots of saliva with them and assist the digestive process.

5. Eat "grounding foods" more often if your mental energy gets scattered easily: Enjoy lots of cooked vegetables, legumes and whole grains, eaten warm.

6. Avoid drinking liquids with meals. If desired, drink four to six ounces of water in small sips as needed.

7. Plain yogurt can sometimes be eaten with tart or sub-acid fruits. Yogurt may also be enjoyed with legumes to help digest.

8. A very healthy individual generally does not need to follow food combining if their digestion is in good shape and they are happy with their weight. For general maintenance, follow the food combining tips three to four days a week. For all special health concerns, or when under stress, follow food combining four to six days a week, seven days a week if digestion is greatly impaired.

9. Always follow the suggestions that work well for you and suit your individual needs. Certain body types and health problems require variations or omission of these tips. Consult your health specialist for diet changes as needed.

Meal Planning Guidelines

1. These menus need not be followed exactly; they are sample guidelines of nutritious meals. Using these suggestions, it is easy to plan meals and snacks that include most of the vitamins, minerals and nutrients that your body requires. Your health specialist will inform you of extra food requirements. Create your own menus in similar fashion. For more economical meals, serve the same dish 2–4 times per week, or freeze some leftovers for meals in later weeks.

2. Enjoy 2–3 meals per day, along with a few snacks if desired. Some people function better with two meals a day and some with three. If you wish to avoid breakfast or lunch, make sure to have at least one of these meals by noon.

3. Do not overeat any one type of food. No individual food should be eaten more than five or six days a week. It is better to have two servings of a food every other day than to have one serving every day. Rotate foods for better digestion and health and to avoid creating or aggravating allergies.

4. Weekly include: 5–12 servings of legumes; 7–12 servings of whole grains, eaten warm; 1–3 servings of tofu; 1–3 days a week enjoy nuts and seeds in cooked foods; different vegetables may be had every day. (Avoid any foods you are allergic to.)

5. Daily include: 4–8 servings of vegetables (at least two of green vegetables, one of orange vegetables); 2–5 servings of carbohydrates (cooked whole grains and starchy vegetables like squash and yams and white vegetables like cauliflower, parsnips and turnips; should be eaten warm); 1–2 servings of legumes; 1–2 servings bread or pancakes. Optional: 1 serving tofu or nuts/seeds. Fruit needs vary: usually 1–2 servings per day for most healing diets. (See Healing Foods for Healing Diets.)

6. A serving is: 1 piece or 1 cup fruit; ½–1 cup cooked vegetables; 1 cup raw vegetables; ½–1 cup cooked legumes or whole grains; 3–4 ounces (about 100 grams) tofu; 2–4 tbsp ground nuts or seeds or butters.

Remember: No rule must be followed all the time. These are safe, wholesome guidelines for better digestion and health. Follow these points most of the time.

Basic Rule: Follow the rules carefully and eat better when not feeling well. Splurge or break the rules (only occasionally) when you feel good. Individual needs will vary throughout the healing process. Consult a health specialist for more information. My books, *Vegan Delights, The All Natural Allergy Cookbook, For The Love Of Food* and *Hearty Vegetarian Soups and Stews*, contain more recipes. *Vegan Delights* has extra menus and is especially good for healing diets.

Sample Menus

Day 1

Pre-Breakfast Fruit: 2 kiwi fruits (high in potassium)

Breakfast:	Millet cereal*
Lunch:	Zesty Vegetable Sandwiches*
Supper:	Sunshine Green Salad* with Herbs and Oil Dressing*
	Lentil Soup* Parsley Rice Casserole*

Day 2
Pre-Breakfast Fruit: apple or pear

Breakfast:	Scrambled Tofu*
Lunch:	Spinach Salad with Avocado Dressing* Cream Bean and Tomato Soup* rye crackers
Supper:	Stuffed Red Peppers* with Mock Tomato Sauce* or Vegetarian Gravy*

Day 3 (weekend menu)
Pre-Breakfast Fruit: ½–1 grapefruit (or none, since cooked fruit is served with breakfast)

Breakfast:	Whole Grain Pancakes with cooked fruit*
Lunch:	Beet Treat Salad* with Yogurt Dill Dressing* or Cucumber Dill Dressing (vegan)* Spelt Vegetable Burgers with bun and toppings*
Supper:	short grain brown rice with Gomashio* (sesame salt) steamed vegetables Vegetable Casserole Supreme*

1 hour after supper: Raspberry Tofu Ice Cream* *(optional)*

* Recipes marked with an asterisk appear in the recipe section of this book.

Good Digestion Tips

1. Preparing and eating meals in a positive manner is good for digestion. Foods are harder to digest when one is under stress. Don't eat when upset, angry or tense. Or, if you must eat, eat lightly and chew foods carefully.

2. Eat in a calm, peaceful atmosphere. Pleasant, low music can also be a plus. Avoid watching TV or reading while eating. It takes concentration and energy away from digesting food.

3. Eat only when you are hungry and eat only enough to feel good. Never stuff yourself. It is better to let food spoil in the garbage than to let it spoil in your stomach. Excessive food clogs the system, robs body energy and, of course, adds inches to your waistline.

4. Chew your food well. Digestion begins in the mouth. If you eat slower, you generally eat less and absorb more nutrients.

5. Don't eat when overtired, restless, bored or upset.

6. Don't eat a big meal before sleeping or lying down. Digestion some-times takes twice as long while the body rests. Let your stomach rest with you. If you must have something before bedtime, try yogurt, crackers or a light, easy to digest snack.

7. Avoid fruit, sweets or vitamin C (especially chewable vitamin C) before bedtime or in the late evening—they may keep you awake.

8. After eating, get some mild exercise to help stimulate digestion—walking, bike riding or washing the dishes.

Miscellaneous Food and Healing Guidelines

1. A little sweetening (2–4 tsp or so) cooked 15 minutes or more into a sauce or big pot of soup will not feed candida yeast.

2. Although avocado is a fruit, it is neutral when digesting and can be eaten like, or with, vegetables or like, or with, fruit. There are about 160 calories in half a medium-sized avocado. Though an avocado is high in fats, it contains no cholesterol and the fat it does contain is easy to digest, assimilate and tolerate on a low-fat healing diet. Eat them in moderation though. About 1–2 whole avocados per week.

3. Other foods not yet mentioned that are especially good for most healing diets (unless allergic) are onions and garlic. They are espe-cially beneficial when cooked. Some will have trouble digesting them raw, especially the onions. Eat them according to tolerance. They help kill candida yeast. For those allergic, use 1–2 tsp prepared horseradish in a recipe in place of one small onion, 3–4 tsp prepared horseradish per one large onion. Other good healing foods include lecithin, flax seeds, seaweed, wild greens and edible flowers.

4. Other hard to digest foods to avoid include raw and cooked corn, corn chips, popcorn, salsa, potato chips, raw cauliflower, raw cab-bage, raw broccoli, pickled and fermented foods, alcohol and foods containing alcohol.

5. Avoid environmental poisons like tobacco smoke, bug sprays, pesti-cides, traffic fumes, strong paints, cleaning products or any artificial fabrics or substances that can be inhaled, ingested or rubbed against the skin. Get lots of fresh air and exercise.

6. Distilled water is the purest water available (if made with a stainless steel unit that has a carbon filter) for healing diets. Be sure to com-bine drinking good water with a high nutrient diet and include a daily mineral supplement as well.

7. To prevent early spoilage of foods (oil, mayonnaise, dressing, etc.), avoid contaminating them with saliva or perspiration, and avoid over exposing them to the air or excessive or prolonged heat. Avoid eating any part of fruits, vegetables, breads or other foods on which mold has begun to grow. Discard any food that may not be fresh. Always reheat leftovers on a stove or in the oven and discard any food not eaten after the second cooking.

8. Store foods covered in jars or reusable plastic bags or containers. Open foods spoil faster and grow bacteria more quickly. Improperly stored foods keep for shorter time periods. For longer storage life, produce should be kept in packages within the crisper sections of the refrigerator.

9. Learn to choose the freshest foods, wisely. Selecting good produce is an art. Shop for quality brand names and products that do not harm the environment. Check suppliers when you can. Check produce for softness/firmness, smell, texture, shape, color, bruises and blemishes. Make sure foods are fully ripe before using. Unripe produce lacks vitamins and flavor. Over-ripe fruit can have too high a sugar and/or mold content.

10. All of the ingredients found in this book are available at local markets, health food stores or ethnic shops. If you have trouble finding any specific items, or if you need more information about specific items or special ingredients called for in these recipes, check the glossary and buying guides in my book *The All Natural Allergy Cookbook*.

Special Cooking Guidelines

How to Cook Legumes Properly for Good Digestion (and No Gas!)

1. Measure the amount of beans required and sort through them to remove any damaged beans, gravel, dirt balls or foreign objects.

2. Soak 1 cup of dry beans in 3–4 cups of cool or room temperature water for eight or more hours, uncovered. Soak chick peas for 12 or more hours and soybeans for at least 24 hours.

3. Important: Throw away the water the beans soaked in! This water contains a gas released by the beans while soaking, which in turn gives you gas.

4. Rinse the beans several times and swish them around in fresh water.

5. Put the beans in a large pot so that beans only fill about half the pot and add fresh water until the beans are covered by one inch of water.

6. Bring the beans and water, uncovered, to a boil on high heat.

7. While the beans are boiling, a white foam or froth will generally form on top. Scoop this off and discard it. This part is what contributes to gas.

8. Add extra water if needed so the beans are still at least one inch under water. Cover them and turn the heat down to very low, just low enough to keep the beans barely bubbling.

9. Optional: Add 1 tsp ground fennel or, preferably, 1 tsp savory to the beans. This improves their digestibility.

10. Cook for 1¼ hours or more until the beans are very tender and a bean can easily be mashed with the tongue on the roof of your mouth.

11. Do not add any oil, salt or salty ingredients like seaweed or sea kelp to beans while they are cooking. These ingredients can actually toughen the beans so they stay hard. Add these ingredients when the beans are completely tender. When added after the beans are soft, oil and salt actually help them to become more digestible, and seaweed and sea kelp help to eliminate gas.

12. For those with excessive gas problems, bring dry beans to a boil when they are first added to their soaking water, then let them cool down, uncovered, for 6–8 hours (8–12 hours for chick peas/garbanzos; 12–24 hours for soybeans) before changing the water and cooking further. (In hot weather, beans must be refrigerated after the first few hours.) Another help for extreme cases is to sprout the beans before cooking, but this may alter the taste.

13. The beans that are easiest to digest are lentils, adzuki beans, pinto beans and chick peas. Those with sensitive digestion should try these first. People over age 60 who are not accustomed to beans should avoid all beans except lentils and adzukis, blended or mashed into recipes, unless or until they adjust to them.

14. Always chew beans slowly; never eat them quickly or when under excessive stress or fatigue.

15. Have some raw foods before eating the beans; this will aid in their digestion. Eating yogurt with beans is also helpful.

16. One cup dry beans makes about 2½ cups soaked or cooked beans.

Special Tips on Whole Grains

1. Grains are generally cooked in two or more cups of water per one cup of grain.

2. Cook grains until they are no longer crunchy, but not soggy or mushy. Grains should be tender and easy to chew. Improperly cooked grains are extremely hard to digest.

3. Very few grains need to be soaked before cooking, these include whole oats, rye, triticale, wheat kernels (berries) and wild rice (sometimes if the wild rice has been stored for a long time and appears overly dry, soaking would be helpful, generally it is not required).

4. Before cooking, check grains for dirt balls, gravel, husks and other foreign particles by spreading them out thinly and fingering through them.

5. Brown rice and quinoa are usually the only grains that need pre-washing, but you may wash any grain if you feel it needs it.

6. It makes little difference whether you start cooking a grain in cool or warm water. The exception is ground cereals, which get lumpy when put in warm water, unless mixed in carefully with a wire whisk.

7. To prevent grains from boiling over and to distribute heat evenly, water and grains together should never cover more than three-fourths of the cooking pot.

8. Do not add salt or oil to whole grains until the last 5–10 minutes of cooking; this will ensure that they cook properly and are more digestible.

9. Any grain in whole form will never burn during its first cooking process as long as the water does not run out and the grain does not become overcooked to the point that it falls apart (this usually takes over an hour). Also, they must be cooked on low heat.

10. Never stir whole grains while cooking or they will stick and burn. Keep grains covered while cooking.

11. When reheating cooked whole grains, add ¼–⅓ cup extra water per cup of grain. Cook the grain, covered, on very low heat until warmed (about 10–15 minutes). Brown rice can be reheated by steaming in a vegetable steamer.

12. One cup of dry whole grain or cereal makes about four servings.

13. The main dish grains can almost always be substituted one for the other in different recipes, except for wild rice, rye and buckwheat (kasha). Most grains are similar, but differ slightly in taste.

14. Wheat, rye, triticale, barley, oats, kamut and spelt contain gluten. Other grains contain minute amounts of gluten, but are not considered gluten grains and are not usually eliminated from gluten-free diets.

Preparing Main Dish Grains

Buckwheat and Pot Barley

Use about 2 cups water per 1 cup grain. Bring the grain to a boil, then turn down the heat to a low bubble. Cover and simmer 20–30 minutes, or until tender and no longer crunchy, adding extra water if needed. Cook onions with the grain, and add herbs and salt during the last 5 minutes of cooking time.

Kasha (toasted buckwheat; contains no wheat or gluten)

Cook the same as buckwheat, but use less water and reduce the cooking time to 15–20 minutes.

Whole Oats, Whole Triticale, Whole Rye, Whole Kamut, Whole Spelt (See Cooked Cereals under Breakfast recipes)

Short and Long Grain Brown Rice

Put rice in a pot and fill it with water. Rub the rice together with your fingers and swish it around to remove extra starches, dirt and stray husks. Discard all the water. If the water was very cloudy during the first washing, repeat the process once or twice until the water is relatively clear. Put 2–2½ cups water per 1 cup rice in the pot. Bring to a boil over medium heat then cover, turn down the heat and simmer 55–65 minutes. When the rice is no longer crunchy but easy to chew and tender (not soggy) it is done. Onions, herbs and spices can be added during the last 15–20 minutes of cooking time. Keep the pot tightly covered while cooking, but it won't hurt to peek!

Millet

Cook the same as rice, but use 2½ cups water per 1 cup dry millet. It usually does not need pre-washing. Simmer 45-60 minutes and use as a substitute for rice in rice dishes. This is one of the best grains, high in nutrients and very alkaline. It is especially good for delicate stomachs.

Quinoa (pronounced keen-wah)

Rinse thoroughly before cooking by rubbing the grains together in a pot of water and changing the water 2–3 times. This helps remove the saponin, which may irritate digestion and allergies. Use 2–3 cups water per 1 cup quinoa and bring the water and quinoa to a boil. Cover and simmer 20–25 minutes until tender. Add sea salt if desired. Use the cooked quinoa in place of rice or millet in main dishes. It is especially nice when finely chopped zucchini or broccoli are added on top and allowed to cook with the grain. It is delicious!

About Tofu

Tofu is a wonderful meat or dairy substitute made from soy. It is low in calories and contains no cholesterol. Eight ounces (about 225 grams) of tofu provides 164 calories, 17.6 grams protein, 292 mg calcium (the same as 8 ounces of milk), 286 mg phosphorus, 96 mg potassium and as much iron as 4–5 eggs.

Although tofu is bland by itself, it works wonders in recipes as it absorbs the flavors of the ingredients around it and actually extends and compliments the taste of sauces, gravies, herbs and spices. Used correctly, tofu is delicious and adds texture, protein and other nutrients to all types of dishes, dressings, sauces and desserts.

Store tofu completely covered by fresh water, preferably in a glass jar, in the refrigerator. Plain tofu is fresh as long as it retains its milky white color and has no scent or taste. If the tofu smells a bit, rinse it thoroughly. If no smell remains, it can be cooked but should not be eaten "raw." If the tofu still has an odor after rinsing, discard it!

Whenever the freshness of tofu is questionable, or to avoid any chance of bacteria growth, lightly steam it for 4–9 minutes before using. For most healing diets, it is best to pre-steam tofu used "raw" in recipes (e.g., Mock Egg Salad).

A variety of tofu is available: soft, medium, firm, regular, pressed and dessert. The dessert variety usually contains sugar and should be completely avoided. The soft tofu may be used in any dessert recipe for a less grainy texture. However, regular tofu may be used unless specified otherwise.

About Meat

It is best to totally avoid meats for most healing diets. However, some people can tolerate and even benefit by a little meat consumption on occasion, if it is particularly recommended by your health specialist.

Pork, in all forms, should be totally excluded as it greatly interferes with the healing process. Other red meats like veal, quality beef roasts and steaks and lamb roasts or chops may be eaten sparingly—one to four times per month total. If one is still in the process of cutting down on meat consumption, or if it is recommended, it could be eaten up to a couple of times per week.

Only organic, free-range chicken, turkey or other poultry should be consumed, if any, one to four times per month. The average chicken is full of hormones, toxins and fats that are as detrimental as pork for many individuals.

Salmon and white fish are the best of all seafoods to enjoy. Salmon is high in calcium, and both contain beneficial oils and nutrients. Obtain high quality, fresh fish whenever possible and never eat it fried. Avoid all shellfish (like lobster and shrimp) except for one to two servings per month if tolerated and recommended for you.

Avoid all processed meats, luncheon meats, meat spreads, ground meats, burgers, pâté, most organ meats, hot dogs and meat by-products.

Again, please note that meats may be tolerated on some healing diets, but they are usually best avoided. Meat can be replaced in the diet with legumes, whole grains and vegetables. Meat is not required for a healthful, nutritious diet—it is an indulgence, not a necessity.

Healing Foods Taste Terrific!

There is one more issue that needs to be discussed before proceeding—taste. Wholesome, healing foods are supposed to taste delicious. Digestion begins with taste: if we like a food, we salivate, preparing helpful digestive enzymes in the mouth that will continue into the intestines and help absorb food nutrients. It helps if food tastes wonderful—naturally wonderful that is. Artificial flavorings, colorings, preservatives and other additives actually dull the taste buds. Is it any wonder that the 7,000 or so taste buds we employ in our youth diminish to about 700 in old age? This ninety percent decrease is due to abusive foods and ill-health.

Eat fresh, naturally ripened vegetables and fruits as well as whole grains and legumes. Avoid artificial additives and heavily processed foods and you will find that your taste buds will resurrect. Simple foods will give you a burst of taste sensations that will thrill you and show you that you are alive! But give your taste buds time to alter. They will—and you will find that you love the taste of well-prepared natural foods. Remember also that when food is gobbled, it deadens the senses. Chew foods carefully to release their full flavors and help mix them with those digestive enzymes found in the mouth. Gandhi once said, "Chew your liquids and drink your foods." This is wise advice.

The basic healing diet for North Americans (it is different for other countries and climates) is a combination of foods that have heretofore been neglected because people didn't know any better. For instance, you may have thought vegetables were boring because:

1. Your taste buds were hibernating.
2. You had bad-tasting recipes.
3. You did not know how to prepare or cook them properly.
4. You were too tired (from lack of good nutrition) to prepare them.
5. You were not interested in them or curious about them.

You can prove to yourself that you love vegetables and other wholesome foods by learning about them and enjoying them in a well balanced diet. Anyone can easily see and experience the increase in energy and improvement of overall health that can occur when a proper healing diet is employed. Eating wholesome foods can make you feel wonderful!

There are no terrible tasting foods, only terrible recipes. Many people claim to dislike certain foods and then later find that it was the method of preparation and not the particular food that was distasteful. As with children, whose taste buds change frequently, adults need to try foods prepared in new ways on a regular basis and keep an open mind regarding unusual foods or unique ways of preparing familiar foods. You will most assuredly have some pleasant surprises, and you will probably live longer and better to enjoy more of these delicious, wholesome foods.

RECIPES

BREAKFASTS

Preparing Cereal Grains

Be sure to read Special Tips on Whole Grains before using any of the following recipes.

Cooked Cereals

Amaranth

Although amaranth can be cooked as a breakfast cereal, it is not that tasty. It is better to use the flour in recipes, or to cook the amaranth with another grain. If desired, cook it in 2 times as much water for a rice-like texture, and in 2½–3 times as much water for cereal or to add it to breads. Cook until tender, about 15–20 minutes. Serve plain or add flavorings as for millet.

Quinoa (pronounced keen-wah)

Rinse thoroughly before cooking by rubbing the grains together in a pot of water and changing the water 2–4 times. This helps to remove the saponin, which may irritate digestion or allergies. Once rinsed, this is a highly nutritious, very digestible healing grain. (Some say it is actually a seed, but there is no definite authoritative evidence of this at the present time.) Cook this like millet (see below), but use 2½–3½ cups water per 1 cup quinoa and cook until very tender and of a porridge-like consistency, 20–30 minutes.

Millet

For a soft, cereal-like texture, use 3–4 cups water per 1 cup millet. (Washing the grain is optional.) Bring water and millet to a boil together. Turn down the heat and simmer, covered, until the millet breaks down and is very soft and mushy, about 55–65 minutes. Add a bit of butter, salt and/or sweetening to flavor, or cook a few dates or chopped, dried apricots into the cereal during the cooking time and stir them around just before serving. To reheat millet, break it up gently with a fork and add a bit of extra water. Heat on low until hot throughout, about 10–15 minutes. Add flavorings. If one would like to avoid sweets, sauces or gravies can be used to flavor. Yes! Even for breakfast one can use a natural gravy.

Whole Oats, Whole Triticale, Whole Rye, Whole Kamut, Whole Spelt

These must be soaked in 2½ cups water per 1 cup grain for several hours or overnight. Then change the water and cook in 1½ cups water per 1 cup grain for 45–60 minutes. The grains are usually a little bit crunchy when done. Cook until fairly tender for the best digestion. Cook only one or two different grains together. Rye is rather heavy and is best mixed with another. Use the same flavorings as for millet.

Sweet Brown Rice

Cook and serve like millet cereal (above), but use 2½–3½ cups water per 1 cup rice. Cook until tender, 50–65 minutes.

Teff

Bring ½ cup teff seed and 2 cups water to a boil, then turn down heat and simmer for 15–20 minutes, or until all the water is absorbed. If desired, mix with another grain for added flavor and texture. Serve with the same flavorings as millet, or use a few currants or raisins cooked in to flavor it.

Whole Grain Pancakes (Serves 2)

Wet Ingredients:
- ¾–⅝ cup apple, peach or pear juice
- 4 tsp natural oil

Dry Ingredients:
- ½ cup flour: whole wheat, kamut, spelt, quinoa, millet, teff, amaranth or buckwheat
- ½ cup light flour: whole wheat pastry, unbleached white, kamut, spelt, tapioca or brown rice
- ⅓ cup arrowroot powder
- 4 tsp baking powder
- ¼ tsp sea salt

Mix the wet ingredients together. In a separate bowl, mix the dry ingredients together. Avoid using cinnamon in this recipe as it may hinder rising.

Oil a frying pan and bring it quickly to medium-high heat. Add the dry ingredients to the wet and mix well. Start making the pancakes immediately after the batter is mixed. Cook until the edges dry up a bit, about 1 minute. (Watch the heat or the pancakes will cook too fast and burn.) Turn over and cook another 15–30 seconds. Do not flatten the pancakes when turning them. Turn again to check for readiness, then flatten if desired. Re-oil the frying pan generously before starting each new batch.

Enjoy these pancakes with maple syrup, jam or a cooked fruit topping of raspberries, strawberries, blueberries or applesauce.

Millet Fruit Squares (Makes 9-16 squares)

Crust:
 1½ cups millet (wash first)
 3 ¾ cups water
 3–4 tbsp honey or maple syrup
 Optional: ¼–½ tsp sea salt
Fruit Filling:
 1 cup dried apricots, dates, figs, raisins or other fruit, chopped
 2–3 dried pineapple rings, chopped, or another ⅓ cup other dried fruit, chopped
 3–4 tsp grated lemon or lime rind (zest)
 4 tbsp lemon or lime juice
 ½ cup water
 Optional: ½–⅔ cup raw nuts or seeds, ground

Cook the millet with the water for about 45 minutes and let it cool. Gently stir in the sweetener and salt and spread half of the millet mixture on the bottom of an oiled 9" x 9" square baking pan. Sprinkle ¼–½ cup of nuts over the millet mixture in the baking pan and bake at 350° F for about 10 minutes. Allow to cool.

While the millet is cooking, heat the fruit filling ingredients in a saucepan on low to medium-low heat for 30–45 minutes, or until the fruit is tender and can be easily stirred into a mushy fruit spread. Allow to cool completely.

Use half or all of the fruit mixture (depending on how sweet you would like the squares to be), and spread it over the first layer of baked millet. Add the rest of the cooled millet mixture and spread it evenly on top of the fruit. Bake at 350 °F until firm and somewhat dryer, about 20 minutes. Cool completely and chill to help solidify. Serve at room temperature. Keeps 6–8 days refrigerated. Great for lunches and snacks, too.

Easy Millet Fruit Parfaits (Makes 8–14)

Use the Millet Fruit Square ingredients and prepare the hot millet and fruit filling. Layer a parfait glass with the millet mixture, then ground nuts or seeds, then fruit filling. Repeat the layering and top with a few raisins or ground nuts or seeds.

Chill and serve for breakfast or dessert. (For variation, substitute white quinoa for millet.)

Scrambled Tofu (Serves 2–3)

2 tbsp natural oil
2–3 green onions, diced
½ cup green pepper, finely chopped
7–9 mushrooms, chopped
14–16 ounces regular tofu, crumbled
2–3 tsp tamari soy sauce
½ tsp sea salt
½ tsp curry powder
Several dashes cayenne pepper

In a frying pan, heat the oil and sauté the onions, pepper and mushrooms for about 2 minutes. Add the tofu and remaining ingredients and sauté 3–6 minutes more, until the flavors mingle and the mixture is hot throughout. Serve immediately with toast or other accompaniments.

Special Breakfast Ideas

These may seem like unusual morning foods, but they are more nutritious, filling, sustaining and enjoyable than dry cereal or toast. Try these and other light supper foods for more sustaining, healing breakfasts.

1. Half a baked butternut or buttercup squash sprinkled with cinnamon.
2. Yam sauce on whole grains or on easy tamari tofu sauté.
3. Breakfast whole grains served with almost any of the sauces or gravies.
4. Steamed cauliflower with mock tomato sauce and raw, grated or ribboned zucchini.
5. Tofu rarebit, rice pudding, millet vegetable balls and other main dishes and sauces. Use your imagination for other hearty breakfast ideas.

SUPER SALADS

Garden Green Salad (Serves 2–4)

4–6 leaves of romaine, red or leaf lettuce
½ bunch spinach leaves
½ head of Boston or bibb lettuce
¼–½ cucumber or English cucumber, sliced in rounds or quarters
½–1 green, red, purple or yellow bell pepper, cut in strips
Optional: 1–2 tomatoes, cut in thin wedges

Wash and tear the greens into bite-sized pieces. Toss everything together and serve with an oil or creamy dressing.

Spinach Salad (Serves 2–4)

1 small bunch of spinach, stems removed
1 small zucchini, sliced in rounds or half rounds
1 large carrot or fresh, medium beet, grated
1 large avocado, cut in chunks, or 4 artichoke hearts, quartered

Combine all ingredients and toss together lightly. (If artichoke hearts are used, select the ones in water or rinse off the oil/marinade before using.)

Romaine Salad (Serves 2)

6–10 leaves romaine lettuce
2 stalks celery, chopped thin, or ½ small zucchini, chopped
1 small turnip or parsnip, grated very fine
1 red, yellow, purple or orange bell pepper, cut in thin strips
Optional: green onions or chives, chopped

Wash, dry, chop and mix all ingredients. Toss and serve with a favorite dressing.

Sunshine Green Salad

3 parts curly leaf or romaine lettuce
1 part spinach leaves (broad leafed variety)
Radishes, sliced paper thin
Carrots, grated
Small zucchini, grated, or alfalfa sprouts
Optional: red, purple or yellow bell pepper, cut in short strips

Wash, dry and tear the greens into bite-sized pieces. Toss them with the radishes and bell pepper, if any. After the salad is placed on a plate or in a bowl, top it with grated carrot in the center and zucchini, provided it is in season and is tender and white/light green in color. (The dark, yellow-toned zucchinis are bitter.) If fresh zucchini is not available, top the salad with well-rinsed alfalfa sprouts. Wash off the brown seed hulls as they are carcinogenic. Boston, bibb or red lettuce may be substituted if needed.

Super Sprout Salad (Serves 2–4)

1 cup alfalfa sprouts
1 cup other sprouts (mung, lentil, sunflower, etc.)
8–14 spinach leaves, torn
½ red, purple, yellow or orange bell pepper, cut in strips, or 4–6 radishes, sliced in thin rounds
Optional: 1 avocado, chopped or sliced
Optional: 1–2 tomatoes, cut in thin wedges or chopped

Be sure to choose very fresh sprouts for the best flavor and digestibility. To make them more digestible and to avoid their carcinogenic properties, rinse them very thoroughly to remove all the brown hulls. Toss gently with all the other ingredients and serve with your favorite dressing.

Wild Green Salad (Serves 2)

I cup wild or mixed special greens (arugula, sorrel, cress, lamb's quarters, red oak, young dandelions and /or mint leaves, etc.)

½–I small boston or bibb lettuce, torn

4 artichoke hearts, quartered, or 8–16 olives, whole or sliced

I tomato, cut in chunks, or I red, purple or yellow bell pepper, cut in strips

Optional: small handful of edible, mixed wild flower heads

Toss everything together and serve with a favorite dressing.

Wild Zucchini Rice Salad (Serves 2–4)

I–2 small zucchini, grated

4–6 radishes, sliced thin, or I tomato, sliced in wedges or chunks

I red, yellow, orange or purple bell pepper, cut in strips

½ or less bunch of spinach, torn small

½–I avocado, cut in chunks, or 4–6 artichoke hearts, quartered

½ cup dry wild rice and brown rice mixed, cooked

The ½ cup dry rice makes about 1 cup cooked. Cool or chill the cooked rice before using in the salad. Mix all the ingredients together and toss in a favorite dressing. This makes a great meal for two or a prelude to a meal for four. (If artichoke hearts are used, select the ones in water or rinse off the oil/marinade before using.)

Millet or Quinoa Salad

Choose any leafy green salad as a base for this recipe. Add ½–1 cup pre-cooked millet or quinoa. Toss all the ingredients in an oil or creamy dressing and enjoy.

Greek Salad (Serves 2)

I–2 tomatoes, cut in chunks

½ organic cucumber (or English cucumber), cut in quarters, then chopped

I yellow, purple or orange bell pepper, cut in I inch chunks

½ cup black olives, cut in half lengthwise

Optional: ¼–½ red onion, chopped small

Optional: I–3 tbsp feta cheese, crumbled

Mix everything and toss in an oil based dressing, preferably one with olive oil. If possible, let the salad and dressing marinate together in the fridge for 15–30 minutes before the meal. Stir once while marinating.

Beet Treat Salad (Serves 2–4)

2–4 beets, grated
1 avocado, chopped
6–8 large lettuce leaves (leaf, red, romaine, bibb or Boston), torn
1 purple, yellow or orange bell pepper, sliced in rings
¼–½ cup lentil, mung, alfalfa or other sprouts (hulls removed)

Prepare and toss all the ingredients together except for the beets. Dish out the salad and spread the beets over the top. Use lemon juice or Lemon Herb Dressing for the best flavor.

SALAD DRESSINGS

Herbs and Oil Dressing

1¼ cups canola, safflower or sunflower oil
1 tbsp dried parsley flakes, crushed
1 tsp each: sea salt, paprika and tamari soy sauce
½ tsp basil
¼ tsp each: sea kelp, marjoram and thyme
Several dashes cayenne pepper
Optional: ½–1 tsp vegetable broth powder
Optional: flax seed oil (see below)

Mix or beat the ingredients together well and refrigerate for a couple of hours so the flavors can mingle. Beat or shake the mixture a few times as it chills. Serve chilled on all kinds of leafy green and sprout salads. Keeps refrigerated for up to one month or more. (Flax oil can be added to individual servings of dressing for added omega-3 and omega-6, but do not add to entire recipe as it only keeps a few days mixed with other ingredients.)

Lemon Herb Dressing

Use the Herbs and Oil Dressing but eliminate the vinegar and tamari soy sauce. Instead, add 2–4 tbsp freshly squeezed lemon juice and increase the sea salt to 1¼ tsp if desired. For added flavor, blend in 2 green onions or 1–2 cloves garlic, or according to taste.

Cucumber Dill Dressing

I large cucumber, peeled and seeded
2 tsp dill weed
¼ cup natural oil
¼ cup water
Several dashes of cayenne pepper and sea kelp
Sea salt to taste
Optional: 1–2 cloves garlic, crushed

Blend all ingredients well, chill and serve. Best used within five days. Great dressing for low-fat diets if some water is used. Use ¼–½ cup flax oil for extra nutrients and a surprisingly nice flavor.

Tahini Tofu Dressing

6 ounces tofu, crumbled
½ cup sesame tahini
5–6 tbsp water
3–4 tbsp flax or pumpkin oil
½–⅔ cup lemon juice, freshly squeezed
2 tbsp fresh, chopped parsley, or 1 tbsp dried parsley, crushed
1 tsp prepared horseradish, or 1–3 green onions, chopped
½ tsp each: paprika and sea salt
⅛ tsp sea kelp
Cayenne pepper to taste
Optional: 1 tsp toasted sesame oil

Use a food processor or blender to combine all ingredients well. Serve immediately, or chill before using as a salad dressing or vegetable dip. Keeps 2–4 days refrigerated.

Avocado Dressing

2 ripe, medium avocados
3–4 tsp fresh parsley, chopped
½ cup canola, safflower or sunflower oil
¼ tsp onion or horseradish powder or to taste
⅛–¼ tsp sea salt
Few dashes sea kelp
Cayenne pepper to taste
Optional: 1 tsp toasted sesame oil

Blend all ingredients well and correct seasonings according to taste. Chill and serve on salads or vegetables. Keeps refrigerated for up to three days.

Yogurt Garlic Dressing

1 cup plain low-fat yogurt
1–2 cloves garlic, pressed
1–2 tbsp fresh lemon juice
Optional: few dashes cayenne pepper
Optional: few dashes sea salt

Mix together very well with a fork. Do not use a blender to mix. Chill before serving.

Yogurt Dill Dressing

1 cup plain, low-fat yogurt
2–3 tsp dill weed
1–3 tsp fresh lemon juice
Optional: ¼ cup or less chives or green onion tops, finely chopped
Optional: dash or two of cayenne pepper

Mix (don't blend) all ingredients well. Serve at room temperature or chilled if desired.

Yogurt Green Onion Dressing

1 cup plain, low-fat yogurt
½ cup green onions (white and green parts), chopped
2–3 tsp fresh parsley, chopped
1–2 tsp tamari soy sauce
¼ tsp each: paprika and basil
Optional: sea salt to taste

Mix all ingredients thoroughly in a blender. Serve chilled.

HEALING SOUPS

Garlic and Greens Soup (Serves 4)

    10–12 medium-large garlic cloves, sliced
    2 tbsp butter or natural oil
    4 large cloves garlic, pressed
    4 cups water or stock
    4–5 green onions (green part only), finely chopped
    I bunch spinach leaves
    ¼ cup tomato juice
    I–2 tbsp parsley
    I tsp vegetized sea salt
    ½ tsp dark miso

Sauté the garlic slices in the oil or butter on low to medium heat until thoroughly browned (more than 10 minutes), stirring frequently. Remove and discard the garlic. Add the water and the remaining ingredients except the miso. Simmer 20–25 minutes. Remove 1 cup of liquid from the soup and stir the miso into it until it is completely dissolved, then re-add the liquid to the soup and stir. This robust yet light soup is very healing and strengthening. It is especially good for flus, colds and infections. Best eaten within 3–5 days. Do not freeze.

Healing Greens Soup (Serves 2–3)

    3–5 bunches mixed greens: spinach, beet greens, chard, kale and/or
        mustard greens (about 3–3½ cups cooked)
    4–6 green onions (green parts only), chopped
    I cup nut, rice or soy milk
    I–2 tsp maple syrup or rice syrup
    I–1½ tsp vegetable sea salt
    I tsp vegetable broth powder, or I vegetable bouillon cube
    2–3 dashes powdered ginger, or a bit of freshly squeezed ginger juice

Choose firm, bright or dark green leaves. Remove any blemishes. Wash the greens and chop lightly. Steam the greens until tender. Blend the cooked greens with the remaining ingredients. Simmer on medium-low heat until hot throughout, about 15–20 minutes. Enjoy this hearty soup, rich in iron and minerals.

Creamy Carrot Soup (can be dairy-free) (Serves 4)

    4 cups carrots, slivered and steamed until tender
    1⅔ cups steaming water or vegetable stock
    2–3 tbsp butter, or I–2 tbsp unrefined, cold-pressed oil (optional)
    2 tbsp tamari soy sauce

2 tsp parsley
2 tsp dill weed or tarragon, crushed
½ tsp sea salt
Several dashes sea kelp
Cayenne pepper to taste
Optional: I tsp fresh onion or garlic, or ¼ tsp onion or garlic powder, or a
  few dried mint leaves, crushed

Liquefy all ingredients until smooth in a blender or food processor. Then heat the soup in a saucepan on low to medium heat just up to boiling. Do not boil. Serve hot, garnished with chopped chives, green onions or chopped fresh parsley. Will keep 3–5 days refrigerated. Do not freeze.

Seaweed Soup (Serves 4–6)

6 cups water, stock or broth
I–2 ounces dried seaweed, or 4 ounces fresh (wakame or kombu
  are best), rinsed or sliced
I large onion, chopped
2 carrots, thinly sliced
3–4 stalks celery, chopped
I–2 vegetable bouillon cubes, or I–2 tsp vegetable broth powder
2 tbsp natural oil
2–3 tsp parsley
½ tsp sea salt
Several dashes sea kelp
⅓ cup dark miso (brown rice or soy miso are good), keep separate

Sauté the onions and vegetables in the hot oil in a pot big enough to hold all the soup. When the vegetables are tender and the onions are slightly transparent, add the water, seaweed and the rest of the ingredients (except the miso). Let the soup cook, covered, for about 25–35 minutes.

Remove the soup from the heat, take 1 cup of broth from the soup and stir the miso into it. When the miso is dissolved into the broth, mix it with the rest of the soup and leave covered, away from heat, for about 5–10 minutes so the flavors can mingle. Do not cook the miso; this destroys valuable vitamins and enzymes. Serve the soup immediately. Leftover soup can be reheated slightly, but never let it boil. Keeps refrigerated 5–6 days. Do not freeze.

Adzuki or Pinto Bean Soup (Serves 10–12)

2 cups dry adzuki or pinto beans, soaked and cooked (2 cups dry
   bean makes 5 cups cooked)
10–12 cups water, stock or broth
1 large onion (about 2 cups), finely chopped
2–3 tbsp tamari soy sauce
12 tbsp parsley
2 tbsp natural oil
4 tsp vegetable broth powder
2 vegetable bouillon cubes
½–1 tsp sea salt or vegetable salt
½–¾ tsp sea kelp
Cayenne pepper to taste
Optional: 1–2 tsp sweetening (to balance flavors)
3–4 tbsp dark miso (keep separate)

Cook the adzuki or pinto beans until very tender. After cooking, add
enough water or stock to total 10 cups of liquid. Add the onion and cook
on low to medium heat for 20 minutes. Then add the remaining ingredients (except the miso) and cook another 20 minutes on medium heat.

Take 2–4 cups of beans and liquid from the soup, blend or process into
liquid, and re-add it to the soup. Next, take out 1 more cup of the liquid
from the soup and mix the miso into it, stirring it carefully to break down
any lumps before adding the miso liquid to the soup. Add 1–2 cups extra
(hot) water to the soup if a thinner, milder soup is desired. Serve hot and
enjoy. Keeps well 7–8 days refrigerated and freezes wonderfully. An easy
to digest and highly nutritious soup.

Hearty Vegetable Soup (without tomatoes or mushrooms) (Serves 6–8)

6 cups water or vegetable stock
1–2 cups chopped cauliflower, small turnips or Jerusalem artichokes,
   unpeeled and cut into small chunks
2–3 stalks celery, chopped, or 1 large bell pepper (not green), chopped
3 carrots, thinly sliced
1 large onion, chopped small
1 small zucchini, thinly sliced or chopped
1 large stalk broccoli, chopped small
1 cup fresh or frozen peas or chopped green beans
Optional: 1 cup fresh or frozen corn (may be sliced off the cob)
1–2 tbsp natural oil
1 tbsp tamari soy sauce
3–4 tsp vegetable broth powder or 3–4 vegetable bouillon cubes

2–3 tsp parsley
1½ tsp sea salt
½ tsp each: basil, oregano and sea kelp
Several dashes cayenne pepper
Optional: bit of honey
Optional: 1-2 tbsp dark miso (keep separate)

Steam the white vegetables and carrots for 10 minutes before making the soup. In a large pot, sauté the onions in the oil until slightly transparent. Add the water, steamed vegetables and the rest of the ingredients (except the miso).

Cook the soup on low to medium heat until the vegetables are tender but not soggy and the flavors develop, about 40–60 minutes. Take 2–3 cups of the soup's liquid, along with some vegetables, and blend it. Add it back to the soup. This adds flavor and depth and gives the soup a natural thickness. Correct the soup's spices according to personal taste and add a bit of honey to balance the flavors if desired. Extra water can be added to thin the soup. For more taste and nutritional value, blend 1–2 tbsp miso with one cup of the broth and then add back to the soup after it has been cooked. Keeps refrigerated for 6–7 days. Do not freeze.

Lentil Soup (Serves 5–6)

4½–5 cups water or stock
1 cup dry brown (green) lentils
4–6 stalks celery, chopped, or 2–3 stalks broccoli, chopped
2 carrots, sliced
1 large onion, chopped
1–2 cloves garlic, minced
2 tbsp butter or natural oil
2 tbsp tamari soy sauce
3 tsp parsley
1 tsp each: sea salt and vegetable broth powder
½ tsp each: basil, oregano and thyme
⅛ tsp cayenne pepper
Several dashes of sea kelp
Optional: ½ tsp dill weed

Bring the dry lentils, vegetables and water or stock to a boil on high heat, then simmer on low heat for 1 hour, or until the lentils are very tender. Add the remaining ingredients and simmer another 15–20 minutes, stirring occasionally. Serve hot and enjoy. Keeps 7 days in the refrigerator or may be frozen for later use.

Broccoli or Zucchini Soup (Serves 3–4)

    3–4 stalks broccoli (about 4 cups), chopped for steaming, or 3–4 small
      zucchini (about 4 cups), chopped
    1½ cups nut milk or rice milk
    2–3 tsp parsley
    ½ tsp basil
    ¼–½ tsp sea salt
    ¼ tsp each: thyme and paprika
    Several dashes cayenne pepper
    Optional: 1–3 tsp tamari soy sauce
    Optional: for Zucchini Soup only, add a few spinach leaves, or
      ¼ to ½ tsp dill weed or tarragon

Use good quality broccoli or zucchini, as it is very important to the flavor of the soup. Steam the vegetables until tender, then blend with the nut milk and herbs. Put the soup in a saucepan and heat to almost boiling on medium heat. Do not boil or overheat. Serve immediately.

This is a wonderful, creamy soup, more flavorful than some soups made with cow's milk (the dairy milk actually detracts from the flavor of the vegetables). Keeps 3–5 days refrigerated. Do not freeze.

Broccoli Squash Soup (Serves 4–6)

    2 cups pre-cooked spaghetti or acorn squash
    5 cups broccoli, chopped and steamed
    3 cups water or stock
    1 vegetable bouillon, cube or 1 tbsp tamari soy sauce
    2 tbsp parsley
    2 tsp chopped raw onion or prepared horseradish
    1 tsp each: basil and paprika
    ½–¾ tsp sea salt or vegetable salt
    Optional: 1–2 tsp liquid sweetener to balance flavors

Combine all ingredients in a blender until smooth and then simmer in a covered pot until all the flavors blend and mingle, about 15–25 minutes. Serve hot. Garnish with chopped chives, green onion tops or fresh parsley. Keeps 4–6 days. Best if not frozen.

Parsley Cauliflower Soup (Serves 4–6)

    4 cups cauliflower, chopped
    1 cup water or stock
    1 bunch spinach leaves
    1½ cups nut milk
    1 cup fresh parsley, coarsely chopped
    1–2 tbsp natural oil or butter

I vegetable bouillon cube
I tsp vegetable broth powder
2–3 tbsp tamari soy sauce
2–3 tsp white or yellow onion, chopped
I tsp each: paprika and basil
Vegetable sea salt to taste
I cup parsley, very finely chopped

In a covered pot, simmer the cauliflower in the water for 4 minutes. Add the washed spinach leaves and continue cooking until both are tender, about 6–8 minutes. Blend the simmered vegetables and cooking water with the other ingredients, except the cup of finely chopped parsley. Put the blended soup mixture in a medium saucepan and stir in the finely chopped parsley. Bring the mixture just up to a boil and let it simmer on low heat so the flavors can mingle, about 12–18 minutes. Correct the seasonings as desired. Serve garnished with extra sprigs of parsley or chopped green onion. Keeps for 3–6 days if refrigerated. Do not freeze.

Mud Soup (vegan black bean soup) (Serves 8–10)

2–2¼ cups dry black beans
1½–2½ cups water
I large onion, chopped*
1–2 cloves garlic, or I tsp garlic powder*
3 vegetable bouillon cubes
2 tbsp parsley
I tsp sea salt
I tsp paprika
½ tsp basil
¼ tsp sea kelp
Cayenne pepper to taste
Optional: Gomashio (sesame salt, see recipes)

This soup is hearty, healing and nourishing for those who enjoy basic flavors. Cook the pre-soaked beans in 8 or more cups of water, so that the beans are always covered by at least ½ inch of water. Start cooking on high heat and turn down to a simmer after boiling. After 1½ hours of cooking, or when the beans are tender, add the fresh onion and garlic and cook another 15–20 minutes. Add the extra water and remaining ingredients and mix in a blender until smooth. Use just enough water to make the blender work easily. Simmer the blended soup on medium-low heat for 20–25 minutes so the flavors can mingle. Serve hot. Keeps 7–8 days refrigerated or may be frozen for up to three months.

As a substitute for onions and garlic, use 3–4 tsp of prepared horseradish, added in the blender.

Cream Bean and Tomato Soup (dairy-free, can be vegan) (Serves 8–12)

  2 cups brown or black beans (pinto, kidney, black bean or adzuki)
  6–7 cups water or stock
  4–6 large ripe tomatoes, or 1 large can tomatoes (28oz/796ml),
    cored and chopped
  1 cup shiitake mushrooms, sliced or chopped
  1 large onion, chopped (about 1 cup or more)
  4 tsp dried parsley, or ¼ cup fresh parsley, chopped
  2–3 vegetable bouillon cubes
  2–3 tsp vegetable broth powder
  1–2 tbsp natural oil (or butter)
  1–2 tbsp tamari soy sauce or vegetable bouillon
  1 tsp each: dill weed, basil and sea salt
  ½ tsp oregano
  ¼ tsp sea kelp
  Cayenne pepper to taste

Soak the 2 cups dry beans in 6–8 cups water for 8 hours or more, then drain and rinse thoroughly. Cover the beans with 1 inch of water and bring to a boil on high heat. Scoop off any froth and discard. Continue to cook on low heat (just bubbling) for 1½–2 hours, or until very tender. Then measure the liquid and add or subtract water or stock as necessary to bring it to the 6–7 cups required. Add the remaining ingredients and cook on low heat until everything is tender, about 25–35 minutes. If desired, the mushrooms may be sautéed separately in the oil (or butter) before adding them to the soup. Blend the soup bit by bit until thoroughly liquefied. Return the soup to the pot and simmer for about 10 minutes, or until the flavors have mingled. Serve hot and garnish with chopped parsley, chives or green onion tops. This is a very thick, rich soup. Do not eat more than two bowls at a sitting, and include salad, vegetables or other light foods to round off the meal.

Green and Orange Harvest Vegetable Soup (vegan "GO" soup) (Serves 8–12)

  10 cups water or stock
  1 cup red lentils
  2½–3 cups yam (1 very large or 2 medium), chopped
  3 large carrots, chopped
  3–4 stalks celery, chopped
  1 medium to large stalk broccoli, chopped
  2 small zucchini, cut in half moon slices
  1 large onion, chopped*

2 tbsp natural oil*
2–3 tbsp tamari soy sauce or vegetable bouillon
3 tbsp parsley
2–3 vegetable bouillon cubes
1 tbsp liquid sweetening
1½–2 tsp sea salt
1 tsp each: paprika, basil, and oregano
¼ tsp sea kelp
8–10 dashes cayenne pepper, or to taste
2 tbsp light or dark miso

Chop and rinse the yams and steam them with the carrots until semi-tender. Bring the water to a boil with all the remaining vegetables in it. Sauté the onion in the oil. After 30–45 minutes, add the steamed vegetables, onion and all the remaining ingredients (except the miso) to the soup pot. Simmer for 20–25 minutes more so that flavors can mingle.

After the soup is done, remove ½ cup or so and mix the miso into it. Re-add the miso liquid to the soup, stir and enjoy. Make sure the soup never boils when being reheated so as to preserve the healing enzymes in the miso. Keeps 6–8 day refrigerated. May be frozen, but is better fresh.

As a substitute for the onions and oil, use 3–4 tsp prepared horseradish added to the soup with last ingredients.

APPETIZERS, SNACKS AND SANDWICHES

Easy Nut or Seed Pâté (Serves 6–8)

I cup almonds or sunflower seeds, ground

I cup cornmeal, kamut flour or amaranth flour

I tbsp arrowroot powder or soy flour

3–4 tsp parsley flakes, crushed

I ½ tsp basil, crushed

I tsp thyme, crushed

¾–I tsp sea salt

½ tsp sage leaves, finely crushed, or ⅓ tsp ground sage

¼ tsp sea kelp

Several dashes cayenne pepper

I ½ cups water

¼ cup sunflower or other natural oil

2 tbsp tamari soy sauce

3-4 tsp prepared horseradish

I cup cauliflower, parsnip, carrot or small turnip, finely grated

Mix the first group of dry ingredients together in a bowl. Grate the vegetable. Add the remaining ingredients in the order given, stirring in the vegetable last. Mix well. Preheat an oven to 400° F. Generously oil a 9 inch glass pie plate and scoop in the pâté mixture. Put in the oven and immediately turn the heat down to 350° F. Bake for 50–60 minutes until well browned.

Let the pâté cool 1–2 hours and then chill thoroughly to set before serving. It may be warmed or re-heated later if desired. It is tastiest when served at room temperature. Enjoy the pâté as an appetizer or main protein dish, by itself or with crackers or bread. Keeps up to 7 days refrigerated or may be frozen in pie wedges. Great for picnics, lunches or parties.

Easy Veggie Nut Dip (Makes 2 cups)

2 ½ cups broccoli or carrots, chopped, or 3 cups spinach

½ cup sesame tahini or other nut butter

2 tsp parsley

¼ tsp or to taste of vegetable sea salt

Several dashes of powdered sea kelp or dulse

Several dashes cayenne pepper

Steam the vegetable until tender. Combine with the other ingredients and mix in a food processor until smooth. Serve with veggie sticks, rice cakes, rye crackers or light whole grain bread.

Tahini Yogurt Dip or Spread (Makes 2 ½ cups)

1½ cups plain, low-fat yogurt

1 cup sesame tahini (or sunflower butter)

½–⅓ cup fresh lemon juice

¼ cup parsley, finely minced, or 1 tbsp dried parsley, crushed

1–2 cloves garlic, crushed

½–1 tsp ground cumin

½ tsp paprika

Sea salt and cayenne pepper to taste

Mix all ingredients together well with a large spoon, or mix gently with a wire whisk. Chill thoroughly. Serve with veggie sticks, pita bread wedges or other soft, whole grain bread. Makes a great appetizer or snack. Keeps 5–6 days refrigerated.

Middle Eastern Falafel Spread (Makes 3 cups)

1 cup dry chick peas (garbanzos), soaked and cooked

⅓ – ½ cup sesame tahini

2–3 tsp onion, grated or chopped very fine

2–3 cloves garlic, pressed

2–3 tsp tamari soy sauce

2 tsp parsley, crushed

1 tsp chili powder

1 tsp whole cumin seeds

¾–1 tsp sea salt

¼–½ tsp ground cumin

¼ tsp sea kelp

¼ tsp celery seed

Several dashes cayenne pepper

Cook the chick peas until very tender, then drain and save the liquid. Combine with the other ingredients, and while the chick peas are still very hot, mash them until totally smooth (or use a food processor to blend them). Keeps refrigerated for 7–8 days or may be frozen for up to 3 months with no loss of flavor. (To make a thinner spread, add extra bean liquid.)

Falafel Sandwich (hot or cold)
(Serves 3 – Makes 6 large ½ pita sandwiches)

3 large pita breads, cut in half
1½ cups falafel spread
2 medium tomatoes, sliced in thin wedges
1 large bell pepper (not green), cut in thin strips
½ small zucchini, cut in thin rounds
3–4 shiitake mushrooms, cut in thin slices
Optional: 1 large avocado, cut in thin wedges
Optional: ½ lb or more tofu cheese (cheddar or "amber" style), grated

Cut the pita breads in half and open their pockets. Spread a layer of falafel spread (about 4 tbsp) along the inside of one of the sides of the pocket. Layer the vegetables inside the pita pocket and top with the grated tofu cheese. Serve the sandwich cold or, for even more superb flavor, bake the pockets on a flat baking tray at 350° F for 10–14 minutes, or until the cheese is melted, the vegetables are tender and the pita is lightly toasted.

Zesty Vegetable Sandwiches
(Makes 2–4 small sandwiches)

2–4 pita breads, cut into half moons, or 4–8 slices of bread
3–4 shiitake mushrooms, chopped
2–3 green onions, chopped
1 red, purple, yellow or orange bell pepper, cut into strips and each strip cut into thirds
¼ small zucchini, sliced and quartered
2–3 tbsp mung bean sprouts or sliced water chestnuts
Optional: 1 clove garlic, minced
2–3 tsp oil
1–2 tsp fresh chopped parsley
⅛ tsp each: oregano, basil and thyme
Sea salt and cayenne pepper to taste

Heat the oil in a skillet and sauté the vegetables until nearly tender. Add the herbs and seasonings and stir until everything is tender, yet still a bit firm. Spread butter, mayonnaise, mustard or other spread on the inside of the pita or on the bread. Spoon on the cooked veggies and spread evenly in the sandwich. Serve hot or cold for a special taste treat with less calories than many sandwiches.

Curried Rice Sandwiches (Makes 3–4 sandwiches)

3 cups hot, cooked brown rice or basmati brown rice (about 1 cup dry)
1–2 red, green, purple or yellow bell peppers
1 Spanish onion, chopped

1 small clove garlic, pressed

3 tsp curry powder

½ tsp curry paste

½ tsp ground coriander

½ cup bouillon or pineapple juice

2–3 tsp olive oil

Sea salt and cayenne pepper to taste

2–3 pita breads, cut in half moons

⅓ English cucumber, sliced

Plain, low-fat yogurt

Cook the rice until tender. In a large skillet, sauté the onion in olive oil until semi-tender. Add the pepper, garlic and seasonings and sauté until tender and the mixture emits a smokey aroma. Turn the heat down, stir in the rice and continue stirring until thoroughly blended. Pour the bouillon or juice into the mixture and stir for another minute. Add sea salt and cayenne to taste. Remove from heat and serve hot, or chill for serving cold later. Fill a half pita bread with the rice and top with cucumber slices and plain, low-fat yogurt. Keep the sandwich fillings and pita breads separate until ready to serve so they won't get soggy. A delicious, savory, yet mildly-spiced sandwich or meal. Rice keeps for 5–7 days.

Mock Egg Salad

12–14 ounces (350–400grams) tofu, crumbled

2 stalks celery, very finely chopped

½–1 red pepper, very finely chopped

5–7 green onions (green parts only) or handful or chives, very finely chopped

½ tsp garlic powder

¼ tsp paprika

Vegetable sea salt to taste

Several dashes sea kelp or dulse

Several dashes to taste cayenne pepper

Optional: 1–2 tsp fresh or ¼ tsp dried parsley

Combine all ingredients in a bowl with a spoon. Mix well, but gently. Serve stuffed in celery sticks, bell peppers or pita bread wedges, or on crackers. Keeps 2–3 days refrigerated.

Perfect Hard Boiled Eggs

Place the eggs in a pan and add enough water to cover them by at least one inch. Bring them to a rolling boil on medium heat. Cover pan and remove from heat immediately. Let sit about 20 minutes or more in the hot water. Then plunge the eggs in cold water and peel under cold water as well. Use the eggs in recipes or enjoy them as they are. This cooking method also helps avoid the blue or gray color around the yolk that denotes overcooking. It is almost impossible to overcook these, even if they are forgotten an extra half hour or so in the hot water.

Egg Salad (Serves 2)

4 hard boiled eggs
2–4 tbsp low fat mayonnaise or tofu mayonnaise
1 small stalk of celery or ¼ red pepper, minced very fine
⅛ tsp paprika
Several dashes each: cayenne pepper and sea kelp
Vegetable sea salt to taste
Optional: 1 tsp fresh parsley, chopped, or ⅛ tsp dill weed

Mash the hard boiled eggs with the mayonnaise and seasonings until very fine. Add the finely chopped vegetable, mix and chill for later use. Stuff into celery sticks or eat in a sandwich or with vegetable dippers. Keeps 1–3 days refrigerated.

MARVELOUS MAIN DISHES

Spelt Vegetable Burgers (Serves 8)

1¼ cups spelt flour
1 cup ground sunflower seeds or nuts
2 tbsp arrowroot powder or soy flour
½ cup parsnips or small turnips, chopped small
½ cup bell pepper (not green), chopped small
½ cup shiitake mushrooms, chopped small
½–¾ cup onion, chopped fine
1–2 cloves garlic, minced
½ cup water
3–4 tbsp olive oil
3 tsp dried parsley or 3 tbsp fresh parsley, chopped small
½ tsp each: sea salt, basil, oregano and dill weed
Optional: 2–4 tsp tamari soy sauce

Steam the vegetables until tender, (except for the onions and garlic; keep them raw) then mash them and add the remaining ingredients. Use a fork to mix well. Form the mixture into 8–12 burgers and lightly coat each one with extra flour. Oil a frying pan or flat grill and cook on medium-low heat until nicely browned on each side. Serve on a bun, if desired, with mustard, ketchup or a sauce of some kind.

Lentil Burgers (Serves 6)

    2 cups dry brown lentils, cooked until tender and drained
    ¾ cup bread or cracker crumbs
    1 cup onion, finely diced
    2 tbsp arrowroot powder or unbleached white or kamut flour
    2 tbsp miso (tamari as a second choice) or 2 vegetable bouillon cubes
    3 tsp parsley
    1 tsp dill weed
    ½ tsp vegetable sea salt
    Several dashes each: cayenne pepper and sea kelp
    Tomato juice
    Optional: ½–1 cup celery, chopped

Mix the warm lentils with the other ingredients and use just enough tomato juice to hold the mixture together. Shape into burgers. Add extra flour if needed. Oil a frying pan or griddle and heat to medium-hot. Fry burgers for 12–18 minutes on the first side and 6–12 minutes on the second side, or until nicely browned and warm throughout. These are best served without a bun, with ketchup or a sauce or gravy. Try Arrowroot Sauce, Mock Tomato Sauce or Vegetarian Gravy.

Broiled Tofu Burgers (marinated) (Serves 4–6)

    14–16 ounces regular, plain tofu (in one square block)
    Marinade:
    1½ cups water
    ¼–⅓ cup tamari soy sauce
    ½ tsp curry powder
    ¼ tsp cumin powder
    ⅛ tsp or less cayenne pepper
    Several dashes sea kelp

Freeze the block of tofu (packaged or in a plastic bag) overnight or until it is frozen solid. This helps to texturize the tofu. Defrost it by putting the package of tofu in hot water. When it is defrosted, remove the package, rinse the tofu and gently press out all the excess water. Slice the tofu into slabs about ½ inch thick. Simmer the tofu slices in the marinade for 15–20 minutes. Then drain the tofu slices and broil them for 2–3 minutes on each side. Serve with mustard, ketchup, mayonnaise or other toppings, and a bun if tolerated.

Easy Tamari Tofu Sauté (Serves 2)

8 ounces (225grams) regular tofu, cut into french fry size strips or ½ inch cubes
Tamari soy sauce
Optional: several dashes cayenne pepper

Rinse and cut the tofu. Put a few tablespoons of tamari in a frying pan and heat on high heat. When the tamari starts to sizzle, add the tofu chunks and stir constantly over high heat for several minutes until most or all of the tamari is absorbed into the tofu and the tofu has a rich, brown, seared coating. Serve at once as a side or main dish, by itself or with an added sauce like Mushroom Gravy, Yam Sauce, Creamy Cashew Sauce, Sweet Onion Sauce or your own favorite. It tastes delicious all by itself, as the sauté process adds exceptional flavor. (Note: The pan will look hard to clean but wipes clean if soaked in water for a few minutes.)

Tofu Rarebit (Serves 4)

14–16 ounces (400–450grams) regular tofu
2 cups Mock Tomato Sauce or Vegetarian Gravy
1–2 tsp tamari soy sauce or miso, or 1 vegetable bouillon cube
½ tsp sea salt
½ tsp paprika
Several dashes cayenne pepper
2–3 tbsp natural oil
1 small onion, chopped
2 stalks celery, chopped
1 cup shiitake mushrooms, sliced
Optional: 10–14 black or green olives
4–8 pieces light whole grain toast or whole grain pancakes
Garnishes: ½ cup or more chopped fresh parsley, extra olives and/or other
    chopped, fresh vegetables

Blend the tofu, sauce and all the seasonings until fairly smooth. Heat the mixture on medium-low heat until bubbling hot. While the sauce is heating, prepare the vegetables and toast. Heat the oil and sauté the onion and celery until semi-tender. Then add the mushrooms and olives, if any, and continue to sauté until everything is as tender as you like it. Place the warm toast on a dinner plate and cover with the sautéed vegetables and sauce. Garnish with chopped, fresh parsley, extra olives and/or other chopped, fresh vegetables. Use a knife to cut the toast and enjoy! Whole Grain Pancakes also work well instead of toast. The sauce and sautéed veggies keep 2–3 days refrigerated.

Wonderful Millet Vegetable Balls (Serves 3–4)

2 cups cooked millet, cold (about ¾ cup uncooked millet)
½ cup hazelnut flour or ground almonds or other nuts
2 tbsp arrowroot powder or unbleached white or kamut flour
2–3 tbsp natural oil
1 cup large onion, chopped
1 cup shiitake mushrooms, chopped
1 cup broccoli or asparagus, chopped small
1 cup carrots, chopped small
1 cup celery or bell pepper, chopped small
½ cup black or green olives, chopped
2 cloves garlic, minced
2 vegetable bouillon cubes
2–3 tsp tamari soy sauce or miso
3–4 tsp dried parsley, or 2–3 tbsp fresh parsley, chopped
1 tsp dill weed
1 tsp paprika
½ tsp marjoram
½ tsp thyme
Optional: ¼–½ tsp sea salt (if unsalted bouillon cubes are used)
Optional: ½ cup nuts or seeds, ground or chopped

Keep the first three ingredients separate. Heat the oil and sauté the onions, broccoli and carrots until semi-tender. Add the other vegetables and sauté 1–2 minutes more. Add all the remaining ingredients and sauté a couple minutes more. Break up the bouillon cubes in the stir-fry and mix them in well. Remove the sauté from the heat and combine with the millet-flour mixture. Form the mixture into ⅛–¼ cup balls. The smaller balls can be stir-fried in a lightly oiled frying pan and used as "meat balls" with spaghetti squash and Mock Tomato Sauce, or they can be eaten plain or served with a gravy or sauce (try Arrowroot Sauce, Vegetarian Gravy or Toasted Sesame Sauce). The balls can also be baked at 400° F until hot and toasted, about 18–22 minutes. Will keep 4–6 days refrigerated. Makes about 5 cups. Leftover balls are terrific for lunches and snacks—a wonderful protein and vitamin lift. Eat them at room temperature or hot.

Rice or Quinoa Vegetable Balls

Substitute brown rice or quinoa for millet in the preceding recipe. Cook ⅞ cup of rice in 2¼ cups water until the rice is tender and soft. If using quinoa instead of millet, cook 1–1⅛ cups quinoa in 2 cups water so that the grain will be less tender than usual. Be sure to measure the cooked grain to ensure that you have the right amount for the recipe. Other grains may also be used. Experiment with buckwheat, pot barley, bulgur and other whole grains.

Millet, Rice or Quinoa Vegetable Burgers

Prepare the Millet Vegetable Balls recipe and use ½–¾ cup of the mixture for each burger. Lightly coat the burger with whole wheat, kamut or spelt flour. Cook 4–5 minutes on each side over medium-high heat. Serve with natural ketchup, mustard, pickle and a bun if desired.

Tofu Vegetable Balls or Burgers

Prepare the Millet Vegetable Balls recipe, substituting 16 ounces (about 450 grams) of regular tofu, crumbled, for the millet. Cook the recipe the same as the Millet Vegetable Balls or Burgers.

Cabbage Rolls (Serves 4–6)

  2 cups kasha or buckwheat
  1 medium onion, chopped
  2 tbsp natural oil
  1½–2 cups (about ⅓ lb) mushrooms, sliced
  10–16 large cabbage leaves, whole
  2–4 tbsp sunflower seeds or nuts, ground
  2 tsp parsley
  1 tsp sea salt
  ½ tsp each: basil, paprika and dill weed
  ¼ tsp sea kelp
  ⅛ tsp or less each: marjoram and savory
  Several dashes cayenne pepper
  2–3 cups Mock Tomato Sauce (or Vegetarian Gravy), heated

Cook the grain until tender. In a large frying pan, sauté the onion in the oil until semi-tender, about 2 minutes. Add the mushrooms, nuts, herbs and spices and sauté for another 5 minutes or so, until the onions are tender and transparent.

While the other ingredients are cooking, steam the separate cabbage leaves for 5 minutes or more until they are slightly tender but still a little crisp. When the grains are finished cooking and the vegetables are sautéed, mix them all together. Fill each cabbage leaf with a little of the grain and vegetable mixture while everything is still hot. Fold up the cabbage leaves and tuck them, folded side down, into a large, low sided, lightly oiled baking dish. (A 9" x 13" glass pan with 1–1½ inch sides works best.) If the leaves won't stay folded, use toothpicks to keep them in place. Be careful to count the toothpicks and remove them all before serving the cabbage rolls.

Cover the cabbage rolls with hot Mock Tomato Sauce and bake at 325–350° F for 15–20 minutes until everything is totally hot and the sauce flavors the cabbage. Serve immediately, using sauce from the bottom of the baking pan as gravy.

Parsley and Rice Casserole (Serves 4–6)

- 8 cups cooked brown rice (2 1/2 cups rice cooked in 5 1/2 cups water
- 1 small or medium onion, finely chopped
- 2–3 cloves garlic, minced
- 2 tbsp natural oil
- ½ cup water
- ¼ cup raw ground nuts
- 2 tbsp whole wheat, kamut or spelt flour or arrowroot powder
- 2 vegetable bouillon cubes
- ¾–1 cup dried parsley flakes or 1–1½ cups fresh parsley, finely chopped
- 1 tsp each: dill weed, sea salt and paprika
- Optional: 1 cup shiitake mushrooms, chopped
- Optional: ½ cup pine nuts (grinding is optional with these)

While the rice is cooking, sauté the onions and garlic in the hot oil until almost tender. Add the mushrooms and pine nuts, if using, and sauté 1–2 minutes more. Soften the bouillon cubes in the hot rice, then mix thoroughly. Add the sautéed mixture and all the remaining ingredients to the rice. Combine carefully so as not to mash the rice. Place the mixture in a lightly oiled 9 or 10 inch baking dish and smooth the top. Sprinkle on extra paprika for added eye appeal. Bake in a pre-heated oven at 350° F for about 30 minutes until hot and somewhat firm throughout. Serve immediately. Keeps refrigerated for 5–7 days. Best if not frozen.

Vegetable Casserole Supreme (Serves 4–6)

I cup dry chick peas, soaked, cooked and mashed (makes 2 1/2 cups)
2–3 tbsp natural oil
I cup onion, chopped (I medium-sized)
2 cloves garlic, minced
2½ cups carrots, grated (4–5 medium)
I red, purple, yellow or orange pepper, finely chopped
I cup broccoli or green beans, finely chopped
6–8 cups celery, chopped
I cup shiitake mushrooms, sliced
I–1½ cups water or broth
2 tbsp tamari soy sauce
½ cup cornmeal, amaranth or teff flour
2 tbsp ground sesame seeds or nuts
2 vegetable bouillon cubes or I tbsp vegetable broth powder
I tbsp parsley
I tsp each: basil, paprika and thyme
½ tsp sea salt
¼ tsp sea kelp
Several dashes cayenne pepper

Cook the chick peas and discard all but 2–3 cups of the cooking water. (The water can be used for making broth or for mashing the chick peas.)

In a large skillet or pot, sauté the onion in hot oil for a minute or two before adding the vegetables, one by one, beginning with the carrots. Sauté until the vegetables are slightly tender. Mix the vegetables with the remaining ingredients, including the mashed chick peas. Spread the mixture into a 9" x 9" baking dish and top with an extra sprinkling of ground seeds or nuts and generous sprinklings of paprika. Bake for 30–40 minutes at 350° F until browned and cooked throughout. Keeps 5–7 days refrigerated and may be frozen if necessary.

Soy-Carrot Loaf (Serves 8–10)

1½ cups soybeans (or chick peas), soaked and pre-cooked
1½–2 cups nut or rice milk
2 cups carrots, finely grated
I cup celery or broccoli, chopped
2 large eggs, beaten (or 2 tbsp dry egg replacer with ½ cup liquid)
I large onion, chopped
1–2 cloves garlic, minced or pressed
⅓ cup cornmeal, teff or amaranth flour
2 tbsp natural oil
I tbsp tamari soy sauce or 1–2 vegetable bouillon cubes

2 tsp each: basil and paprika
Several dashes each: sea kelp and cayenne pepper
Optional: bread crumbs

Grind the tender, precooked soybeans or chick peas in a hand grinder or food processor. Mix all the ingredients together well, except for the bread crumbs. Spread the mixture into a lightly oiled casserole and press the bread crumbs onto the top of the loaf. Bake the loaf at 375° F for 40–50 minutes or until browned and cooked throughout. Serve hot. Keeps 4–6 days refrigerated and may be frozen.

Stir-Fried Vegetables with Horseradish on Whole Grains (Serves 2–4)

Brown rice, millet, quinoa, buckwheat or kasha grain
2-3 tbsp toasted sesame oil
¼–½ cup peeled ginger root, sliced or chopped
Hard Vegetables:
2 carrots, sliced on a long slant about 1/8 inch thick
1 stalk broccoli, chopped in long, thin pieces
2–4 stalks celery, sliced on a long slant about 1/3 inch thick
1–2 cups bok choy, Chinese cabbage or kale, chopped
Optional: 1 red bell pepper, cut in strips
Other Ingredients:
4–8 shiitake mushrooms, sliced or chopped
½–1 cup mung bean sprouts or snow peas (deveined)
2–5 tbsp tamari soy sauce
1–2 tbsp ginger, grated fine
2–5 tsp prepared horseradish
Optional: 1 small can water chestnuts, sliced
Optional: 4 ounces plain or marinated tofu, cut in small cubes
Optional: several dashes each: cumin powder, coriander, cayenne pepper
Optional: ½ cup or more black bean sauce, bouillon broth or another
    Oriental sauce

Cook the whole grain until tender. While the grain is cooking, heat a wok, iron skillet or frying pan with the oil until hot and sizzling (but not smoking). Add the ginger and sauté for 2–3 minutes, then add the hard vegetables and sauté another 3–6 minutes until fairly tender. The heat should be just high enough to keep the vegetables sizzling the entire cooking time. Keep stirring.

Add the remaining ingredients except for the sauce and sauté a few more minutes. (Some prefer to remove the ginger pieces after the flavor has cooked into the dish.) Serve hot and enjoy over fresh, cooked whole grains. The vegetables keep 1–2 days refrigerated after cooking.

Stir-Fried Vegetables with Onions and Garlic on Whole Grains

Follow the directions for Stir-Fried Vegetables with Horseradish (above), but omit the horseradish. Instead, along with the ginger, but before adding the hard vegetables, sauté one medium to large white or yellow onion, chopped, and 2–4 cloves chopped garlic.

Stuffed Red Peppers (Serves 4–6)

I cup dry brown rice, millet or quinoa
4–6 medium red bell peppers, cut in half lengthwise and seeded
2 very large or 3–4 medium carrots,
   finely minced or grated
I very large onion, finely chopped
2–3 tsp parsley
I tsp sea salt
½ tsp each: basil, oregano, and paprika
⅛ tsp each: marjoram, thyme and sea kelp
I–2 tbsp ground sesame seeds or sunflower seeds
Several dashes cayenne pepper
I–2 tbsp natural oil

Cook the brown rice or other grain until tender and fairly dry. In a large skillet heat 1–2 tbsp oil and sauté the onions, carrots and herbs until the vegetables are slightly tender. Add the cooked grain to the skillet and sauté for 5 minutes more so the flavors can mingle. Place the raw red peppers in a large, uncovered baking dish, (about 9" x 13" x 1½"), and fill them with the grain-vegetable mixture. Fill the bottom of the baking dish with about ½ inch of water. Bake the peppers at 350° F for 15–25 minutes, until the grain is lightly browned and the peppers are tender but still a little crisp. Serve covered with hot Vegetarian Gravy, Arrowroot Sauce or Mock Tomato Sauce. Keeps 2–4 days refrigerated.

Tofu-Stuffed Zucchini (Serves 4–6)

4–6 small zucchini, ends removed, cut in half lengthwise
14–16 ounces of regular tofu (not soft)
½ cup red pepper, finely chopped
2 green onions, diced
4–8 shiitake mushrooms, chopped
2 tbsp butter or natural oil
I–2 tsp tamari soy sauce
½ tsp sea salt
½ tsp curry powder
Several dashes cayenne

Steam the zucchini for 4–7 minutes until slightly tender. In a frying pan, melt the butter and sauté the onions, pepper and mushrooms for a minute or two. Add the tofu and remaining ingredients and sauté for a few minutes until the flavors mingle.

Place the strips of zucchini, cut side up, in a low baking dish with about ¼ inch or more of water on the bottom. Cover the zucchini with the tofu mixture and bake for 10–15 minutes until everything is hot and tender throughout. Serve immediately.

Greek Vegetable Briam (Serves 6–8)

    I large cauliflower (about 3–4 cups), chopped in chunks
    1–2 cups shiitake mushrooms, chopped
    2 medium zucchini, sliced in ¼ inch rounds or chopped
    I medium or large onion, finely chopped
    4–5 large tomatoes, chopped, or I large can tomatoes,
       drained and chopped
    ½ cup tomato juice
    I lb feta cheese, crumbled or chopped into small bits
    2 tbsp olive oil (another may be used in a pinch)
    2 tbsp parsley
    I tsp oregano
    ½ tsp basil
    ½ tsp sea salt
    Optional: several dashes cayenne pepper

Steam the cauliflower until tender. Heat the oil in a large skillet and sauté the onion a minute or two. Add the zucchini and mushrooms and sauté for a few minutes more until semi-tender. Add the tomatoes and herbs and continue to sauté for another 2–3 minutes. Remove from heat and add the tomato juice and cauliflower to the vegetable mix. Place the vegetable mixture in a lightly oiled 9" x 13" baking dish or into small individual baking dishes and cover with the feta cheese. Bake in a pre-heated oven at 400° F until fully tender and the cheese is melted and browned, about 30 minutes or more. Can be enjoyed as a side or main dish. Best served with other protein dishes.

Kidney Bean Stew (Serves 12–14)

2½ cups dry kidney beans, soaked and cooked

7–8 medium carrots, sliced in ⅓ to ½ inch chunks

1–2 cups shiitake mushrooms, chopped into small chunks

8–10 stalks celery, sliced in 1 inch chunks

6 medium turnips or parsnips, chopped in one inch chunks, or 1 very large cauliflower (about 4 cups), chopped the same

3–4 medium onions, chopped

2–3 red peppers, cut in chunks

2 small zucchini, cut in chunks

1–2 cups broccoli, chopped

Optional: 1–2 cups fresh peas or green beans, chopped

Optional: 6–10 Jerusalem artichokes, unpeeled and chopped.
   (These are especially good for high or low blood sugar.)

2–3 tbsp tamari soy sauce*

2 tbsp vegetable broth powder, or 3–4 vegetable bouillon cubes

2–3 tbsp parsley

1½ tsp sea salt

1 tsp each: sea kelp and basil

½ tsp paprika

⅛ tsp or less of cayenne pepper

Optional: 1/8 tsp each: cumin powder and thyme

Cook the beans until tender. Steam the hard vegetables (turnips or parsnips, carrots, cauliflower, broccoli and artichokes, if using) for 10–15 minutes. When the beans are done, drain off all except 2 cups of cooking water. Then add the precooked and other vegetables along with the herbs and remaining ingredients.

Simmer everything together on low to medium heat for 20–25 minutes until the flavors mingle. Serve hot along with a crusty bread. Will keep about 7 days refrigerated and freezes well. Hearty and delicious!

If soy products are not tolerated in a diet, obtain chick pea miso or use vegetable bouillon (2-3 tsp) and sea kelp (¼ tsp) in place of 1 tbsp tamari or soy miso.

SAUCES AND GRAVIES

Tahini Sauce

I small or medium onion, chopped
2–3 tbsp natural oil
1–1½ cup water
I cup sesame tahini
2–3 tbsp tamari soy sauce
3 tsp finely grated ginger
I tbsp maple syrup or other liquid sweetener
I tsp sea salt
Several dashes nutmeg
Cayenne pepper to taste

Sauté the onion in hot oil until tender. Add the remaining ingredients and simmer everything on low heat for about 30 minutes. Serve hot over steamed vegetables and grains.

Toasted Sesame Sauce (Makes about 3 ½ cups)

I cup sesame tahini
I cup hulled, white sesame seeds
2 cups water or milk substitute
2 tbsp arrowroot powder (or other thickener)
1–2 tbsp white or yellow onion, chopped
I clove garlic, crushed
I tbsp tamari soy sauce
I vegetable bouillon cube
2–3 tsp lemon peel, grated (zest)
Sea salt to taste
Few dashes cayenne pepper to taste

Spread the sesame seeds thinly on a flat baking pan or pie dish and bake at 300° F for 12–18 minutes. Stir once or twice and remove from oven when lightly browned and toasted. Blend the toasted seeds, ¼ cup at a time, until finely ground. Place the seeds and all the remaining ingredients in the blender and liquefy. Heat in a saucepan on medium-low heat, stirring regularly, until thickened and hot throughout. Serve on vegetables, grain, burgers, casseroles or pasta. Keeps 6–8 days refrigerated.

Arrowroot Sauce

  2 tbsp arrowroot powder
  1½ cups cool water
  2–3 tbsp tamari soy sauce
  1–2 vegetable bouillon cubes or 1–2 tsp vegetable broth powder
  Several dashes each cayenne pepper and sea kelp
  Optional: dash of sweetening if desired to balance flavors

Mix the arrowroot thoroughly with the water in a saucepan, using a wire whisk. Add the remaining ingredients and mix well. Cook over medium heat, stirring constantly, until thickened. Keep warm over low heat. Serve over hot vegetables, whole grains or stir-frys. Keeps up to 7 days refrigerated, or may be frozen.

Vegetarian Gravy (Makes 2½ cups)

  2 cups kidney, pinto or adzuki bean cooking juice
  2–3 tbsp tamari soy sauce or dark miso
  1 tbsp natural oil
  ⅓ cup whole wheat, kamut, millet or quinoa flour
  ¼–½ tsp chili powder, vegetable broth powder or curry powder
  ¼ tsp sea salt or vegetable sea salt
  ¼ tsp sea kelp
  Several dashes cayenne pepper

Use previously frozen bean juice, or cook ½–1 lb of one of the beans listed above until very tender; drain off and save 2 cups of the liquid. Use the muddiest part of the liquid for this recipe. Use the beans in another recipe, or freeze them for later use.

Combine all the remaining ingredients with the cooled bean juice and stir over medium-low heat until thickened. Use a wire whisk or blender to mix well. Correct the seasonings to taste, and serve the gravy on potatoes, rice, whole grains, vegetables, mock meatloafs, burgers and other dishes.

Avocado Tofu Sauce

  14–16 ounces (400–450grams) soft or regular tofu
  2 medium or large avocados, ripe, peeled and pitted
  ¼–½ cup water, broth or stock
  1–2 tsp tamari soy sauce or miso
  1 vegetable bouillon cube
  Few dashes cayenne pepper and sea kelp
  Vegetable sea salt to taste

Use a food processor or homogenizing juicer to mix everything thoroughly. Heat on very low heat, just until hot. Stir regularly. Serve hot over vegetables, legumes, pasta or whole grains. Add a bit of lemon or pineapple juice if desired. Keeps 1–2 days refrigerated.

Yam Sauce (Makes about 5 cups)

7½–8 cups peeled yams, chopped (3–4 large yams)
¾ cup milk substitute
1 tbsp tamari soy sauce
2–3 tsp white onion, minced or put through a garlic press
1–1½ tsp curry powder
½–¾ tsp sea salt
Several dashes of cayenne pepper, to taste
Optional: several dashes sea kelp

Steam the yam until tender. Use a food processor or masher to mix all the ingredients until smooth. Reheat the sauce on low heat in a saucepan or double-boiler. Serve hot on vegetables, over whole grains or on pasta noodles. Serves 4–6. Keeps 3–5 days refrigerated.

Sweet Onion Sauce (Serves 4–6)

4 cups onions, finely chopped
1 tbsp cold-pressed oil
⅓–½ cup water or broth
2–4 tbsp tamari soy sauce*

Sauté the onions in the oil and water on high heat, stirring constantly, until tender. Add the tamari and turn the heat to medium-low and cover the pan. Simmer for one hour. Serve hot or cold over whole grains and/or vegetables, as a bread spread, gravy or topping for loaves, casseroles or burgers. Keeps 7–10 days refrigerated.

Miso may be used instead of tamari: Mix 2–4 tbsp dark miso with part of the water. Add to onion mixture after it has simmered.

Garlic Sauce (Makes 1½ cups)

1 cup water, stock or broth
1/2 cup natural oil
8–10 cloves garlic, pressed
1–2 tbsp tamari soy sauce
1 tsp paprika
1/2 tsp each: basil and thyme
1/4–1/2 tsp sea salt
Several dashes each of cayenne pepper and sea kelp

Beat the ingredients together with a wire whisk in a saucepan. Bring to a low boil on medium heat, stirring regularly. Then cover, turn down to low and simmer for 15–20 minutes until the flavors mingle and the sharp edge is off the garlic. Stir and serve. Keeps 1–2 weeks refrigerated.

Creamy Garlic Sauce

Grind 5 tbsp raw cashew pieces or blanched almonds to make 4 tbsp ground nuts. Blend the ground nuts with Garlic Sauce, either before or after heating, to make a smoother, creamier garlic sauce with added flavor.

Mock Tomato Sauce (Serves 6)

7 cups orange yams, peeled and chopped, or butternut or buttercup squash, peeled and chopped
1 cup beets, chopped
1 cup white or yellow onion, chopped
2 cloves garlic, minced
2–3 tsp natural oil, or 2–3 tbsp water
6 cups water or stock
2–3 tbsp tamari soy sauce
1 strip of wakame or kombu seaweed, washed and minced
3 tsp dried parsley
1 tsp basil
½ tsp oregano
¼ tsp each: sea kelp, marjoram, thyme
⅛–¼ tsp rosemary, crushed
1–2 bay leaves (remove later)
2 tsp liquid sweetening
2 tsp apple cider vinegar

Steam the yams or squash and the beets until tender. Sauté the onions until transparent. Blend all the ingredients until smooth and heat in a sauce pan until hot throughout and the flavors mingled, about 20 minutes or more. Serve hot in place of tomato sauce over vegetables, steamed cauliflower, spaghetti squash, whole grains, veggie burgers and casseroles.

VEGETABLE SIDE DISHES

Mashed Yams or Squash

Bake, or preferably steam, yams or cut squash pieces until tender. Peel off the skins or leave them on. Mash the very tender vegetables with a small-holed hand masher. If skins are left on, use a food grinder or processor to blend the skins in. Add a milk substitute and sea salt, cinnamon or other seasonings to add flavor. Whip the vegetables just like mashed potatoes and serve hot. Children especially love this easy-to-eat treat.

Baked Turnips (Serves 2)

2–3 fresh, small white (or purple) turnips

Choose firm, bright colored turnips. Clean them with a good scrub brush and cut off the root and the stem end. Slice in ¼ inch rounds and bake on a lightly oiled baking sheet about ¼ inch apart. Bake at 400° F for 9–14 minutes until very tender but not dry. Delicious plain (or see below).

Herb Baked Turnips (Serves 2–3)

3–4 medium turnips, unpeeled, sliced 1/4 inch thick

¼ cup natural oil

I tsp dried parsley flakes, crushed

½ tsp dried basil flakes, crushed

⅛–¼ tsp sea salt

Few dashes each: cayenne pepper and sea kelp

Mix oil, herbs and spices together well. Dip the turnip slices in the mixture and bake as above.

Baked Turnip Fries (Serves 4)

6–8 medium-sized white turnips, peeled or unpeeled

Natural oil

Sea salt

Chop the turnip into french-fry size strips and use a brush to lightly coat with oil. Place on a flat baking sheet and lightly salt if desired. Bake at 350–375° F for 20 minutes or more until the baked fries are very tender. Serve hot and enjoy.

Artichokes (Serves 2)

1–2 globe artichokes

Dipping Sauces: Tofu Mayonnaise or Veggie Butter

Selection and Preparation: Choose firm, dark green (with no purple or fuzz), unwrinkled globe artichokes. Wash and cut off all the stalk except for about ¼ inch. Pull off and discard the first row of leaves around the stalk. With a sharp, serrated knife, cut ¾–1 inch off the tip end of the artichoke and discard. Snip ¼–½ inch off the tips of each remaining leaf with scissors or knife. Place the artichokes upside down (top down, stalk up) in a vegetable steamer over mildly boiling water and steam for 40–50 minutes until very tender. When a knife pokes in and out easily, they should be done.

How to Eat an Artichoke: Starting with the bottom row of leaves nearest the stalk, pull off one leaf at a time and dip the part that was attached to the artichoke in the sauce or dip. With the inner part of the leaf facing upwards, pull the base of the leaf between your teeth, pulling off all the tender, easy-to-chew parts. (The easy parts are the edible parts.) Discard the rest of each leaf. As you get closer to the center, you can eat more of each leaf, as it gets more tender until you reach the "choke," which is a stringy and kind of prickly part that you scrape off with a spoon and discard. What's left is entirely edible! Dip it in the sauce and enjoy the best part—the "heart." A delectable treat. Savor the delicious, stimulating aftertaste of the artichoke in your mouth. This is a wonderful healing food for the liver.

Beet Treat (Serves 2)

1–3 beets, grated
1–2 fresh lemons, juiced

Mix the beets and lemon juice together and serve on lettuce or spinach leaves, or in or around an avocado half. Delicious! The lemon juice makes the beets taste sweet. Beets are a wonderful treat for the liver.

Marinated Vegetables (Serves 4 or more)

¼ cup sunflower or safflower oil
¼ cup flax seed oil
2½ tbsp apple cider vinegar
4 tsp parsley flakes, crushed
2 tsp tamari soy sauce
½–¾ tsp sea salt
½ tsp basil
½ tsp oregano
Several dashes each: sea kelp, vegetable salt and cayenne pepper
3–4 cups of one or more chopped vegetables, about 1 inch or smaller pieces:

> *Include one or more of the following:*
> English cucumber or organic cucumber
> Zucchini, sliced and quartered
> Shiitake mushroom chunks or slices
> Red bell pepper chunks
> Tomato chunks

Beat together all the ingredients except for the vegetables. Add the vegetables and toss to coat in oil and herbs. Let the mixture sit in the refrigerator for 1–2 hours, tossing occasionally, until the flavors mingle and the vegetables soften. Drain the vegetables and let them sit at room temperature for 5–8 minutes before serving; this way the flavors will be more distinct. Save the leftover oil and herb mixture to make a new batch within 2 days, or store any leftover marinated vegetables in this mixture to preserve them for up to 3 or 4 days in the refrigerator.

Serve these vegetables all by themselves with toothpicks as a party appetizer or snack. They also make a nice salad when served over an avocado half, or on a bed of spinach leaves or chopped lettuce.

SPECIAL RECIPES

Gomashio (Sesame Salt)

1–2 cups hulled (white) sesame seeds
3 tbsp–½ cup sea salt
Optional: 1–2 tsp sea kelp

In a dry, heavy iron skillet, place 1 cup of the sesame seeds. Cook over low to medium heat, stirring regularly, until the seeds are lightly toasted. (Sesame seeds can also be toasted in the oven in a low pan at 300° F, stirring often.) Do not use brown, unhulled seeds as they pop and jump out of the pan when toasting. Grind the toasted seeds in a blender (¼ cup at a time) or food processor (all at once) or use a mortar and pestle. Grind until most of the seeds are crushed fine and then mix them with sea salt: about ⅒–¼ part sea salt to ⁹⁄₁₀–¾ parts ground sesame. Add sea kelp for added iodine. Use this seasoning to enhance flavor while cooking or at the table. Add about ¼–½ tsp kelp per 1 cup gomashio.

Natural Ketchup

12 ounces tomato paste or sauce
2–3 tbsp apple cider vinegar
1–3 tbsp liquid sweetening
1 tsp parsley
⅛ tsp each: basil, paprika and tamari soy sauce
Few dashes each: cayenne pepper and sea kelp
Sea salt to taste

Simmer ingredients on low heat for 15 minutes or more. Add a little water to thin if desired. Cool and refrigerate. Keeps 1–3 weeks refrigerated, depending on how well you keep it bacteria-free.

Veggie Butter

½ lb (225 grams) lecithin spread (6 ounces regular tofu can be used as a second
    choice along with 2 ounces natural oil)

½ small red pepper or 1 small stalk celery, chopped fine

5 tbsp tomato paste or 6 tbsp mashed, steamed carrot

1–2 tbsp white or yellow onion, minced

1 tbsp dried parsley flakes

1 tsp each: garlic powder, oregano and dill weed

½ tsp basil

Optional: sea salt or vegetable sea salt to taste

Combine all ingredients in a food processor or homogenizing juicer. Chill well before using. Keeps refrigerated for 1–2 weeks if the lecithin spread is used, or may be frozen. Keeps 4–7 days refrigerated if tofu is used. A food mill may also be used.

Tofu Mayonnaise

1 lb (450 grams) regular tofu

½ cup raw cashew pieces or blanched almonds, ground

½ cup water

¼–⅓ cup fresh lemon juice

1 tbsp honey, maple syrup or fruit concentrate

2–3 tsp arrowroot powder or ½ tsp guar gum or xanthan gum

1 tsp sea salt

Optional: ½–1 tsp white miso and/or onion powder

Blend or use a food processor to combine all ingredients thoroughly. Chill completely and use like regular mayonnaise in recipes. Keeps 5–7 days refrigerated.

Better Butter (Makes 4 cups)

1 lb (2 cups) butter

2 cups natural oil (canola, sunflower or safflower are best)

Optional: Several dashes sea salt

Optional: 1–4 tbsp flax seed oil

Leave the butter in a large bowl at room temperature until it is very soft. Use a hand mixer to slowly mix in the oil, about ¼ cup at a time. Only use the flax oil if the butter will be eaten within a week, or just make ¼ or ½ the recipe with the flax oil for extra nutrients. Once the oil is completely blended, put into covered containers and refrigerate. Without flax oil, it keeps 1–3 weeks refrigerated, depending on how well you keep it bacteria-free. Unlike butter, this blend cannot be left out of the refrigerator all day or it may become rancid. This recipe reduces cholesterol amounts and is better for you than margarine—it costs less too! Herbs and flavorings may also be added to this blend for specialty butters. Once refrigerated it re-solidifies just like butter.

Clarified Butter

Many people who are allergic to dairy products are unable to enjoy butter, but many can tolerate clarified butter. It adds flavor to many dishes, and when liquid or softened it can be used in place of oil in many main dishes.

Heat 1 lb of butter in a heavy saucepan on very low heat for 1 hour until the butter is melted and has separated. Skim off the foamy white milk solids from the top of the liquid. Save the yellow liquid below it, but be careful not to include the whey and milk solids on the bottom of the pan. Store in a covered container and refrigerate. It stays fresh for many weeks.

BEVERAGES

Dairy-Free Milks

Note: These dairy-free drinks are not dietary substitutes for milk, but are intended to be used as a milk substitute in cooking. The nutrients found in milk are also available from legumes, whole grains and green leafy vegetables.

Cashew Nut Milk

1 cup water
2–3 tbsp raw cashew pieces, ground or whole

Mix ingredients thoroughly in a blender for several minutes until the water becomes white. Strain if necessary and stir well before using. Keeps several days in the refrigerator or may be frozen for later use.

Note: Technically speaking, all cashews must be slightly cooked before being sold. Buy the ones called "raw."

Thick Cashew Nut Milk

Follow the Cashew Milk recipe but use 3–4 tbsp cashews.

Blanched Almond Nut Milk

Follow the directions for either of the Cashew Milks but use blanched almonds instead of the cashew pieces.

Alfalfa Milk
    I cup alfalfa sprouts
    Water

Rinse the sprouts thoroughly to remove all brown hulls, or cut off the brown seed hulls if necessary. Process the sprouts in a blender with just enough water to keep the blades turning well and to create a "milk." Add extra water if necessary to create the desired consistency. Straining is optional. Use with or without sweetening in recipes.

Zucchini Milk
    I cup grated zucchini
    Water

Choose firm, fresh, bright green/white colored zucchini. The dark or yellowish ones are bitter. Peel zucchini if desired. Blend the grated zucchini in the blender with just enough water to keep the blades turning well and to create a thick, white "milk." Add extra water or strain if desired. Use with or without sweetening in recipes.

Other Milk Substitutes

Soy milks, rice milks, powdered milks, coconut and other liquid milks can be purchased in your local health food store and some supermarkets. Use these in recipes from this book or in place of dairy milk in other cookbooks. There will be some change in flavor.

How to Make Herb Teas

Leaf or Flower Tea (and powdered rose hips)

Use one teaspoon of loose tea per cup. Steep only. Boiling makes the tea bitter and also kills valuable vitamins and enzymes. To steep: Boil the water. When it comes to a bubbling boil, remove the water from the heat, pour into a teapot if desired, add the tea and cover the pot. Then let it steep (sit) for 8–12 minutes. Strain and drink. A tea ball may be used for leaf and flower teas that require steeping.

Seed or Twig Teas (and crushed and broken rose hips)

One-half to one-quarter teaspoon loose tea per cup. Bring water and tea to a boil together and let boil on a low bubble for 5–10 minutes. Then let it steep for another 10 minutes off the heat. Strain and drink.

Root or Bark Tea (and whole rose hips)

One-quarter teaspoon root or bark, broken or chopped into small pieces. Make sure tea is broken up as much as possible. Prepare the same as seed and twig tea except that it should be on a low bubble for 15–20 minutes. Follow with steeping for 10 minutes. Strain and drink.

Powdered Root or Powdered Bark Tea

One-tenth to one-sixteenth teaspoon powdered tea per cup. Mix the tea well in the water before heating. Then bring to a boil and keep it on a low bubble for 20–30 minutes. No need to strain.

Herb Tea Bags

Each herb tea bag can be used to make two to three cups of herb tea. For the first cup of tea, add the tea bag to the hot water so the flavor will not be too strong or too bitter. For extra cups from the same bag, pour hot water over tea bag for full flavor. If the tea bag is fragile, don't pour the hot water directly onto the bag but rather off to the side so the bag does not break and spoil the tea. If the bag should break, strain the tea with a small bamboo or stainless steel strainer. For tea pots, use one tea bag per 2 cups water, add the bag to the water and cover pot while tea steeps.

How to Make Herb Tea Combinations

When making herb tea combinations, special care must be taken not to overcook the teas. For example, when making a combination of twig and leaf tea, one cannot boil the leaf tea with the twig tea or the tea would become bitter and lose vitamins. Leaf tea should never be boiled! The twig tea should be low boiled by itself and the leaf tea should be added to the boiled twig tea during the steeping time only. For orange and lemon peels, use only unsprayed, organic fruit rinds and prepare like twig tea. Cinnamon sticks will add flavor if used to stir teas.

Sample Herb Tea Combinations

Peppermint, alfalfa, camomile
Spearmint and strawberry leaves
Peppermint, comfrey, lemon grass
Raspberry leaves and comfrey poured over lemon rounds
Rose hips, strawberry or raspberry leaves (high in vitamin C)
Fennel seeds and alfalfa leaves
Fenugreek seeds and mint leaves
Rose hips, peppermint and slippery elm powder (for colds)
Create your own combinations!

CAUTION: Stick with the bulk (loose) teas mentioned here and a few other flower teas for pleasure drinking. Some bulk teas have strong medicinal powers and can cause stomach upset, headaches or nausea if used incorrectly. Check with your health specialist regarding which teas are appropriate for your particular health concerns.

DELICIOUS DESSERTS

Blueberry or Blackberry Tofu Ice Cream (Makes 4 cups)

2½–3 cups sliced blueberries or blackberries (fresh or frozen)
600 grams soft tofu
⅓–½ cup maple syrup, fruit concentrate or other liquid sweetener
2 tsp real vanilla extract or flavoring
1 tsp slippery elm powder or guar gum powder
Optional: couple dashes sea salt

Mix everything together in a food processor, or mix and put through a homogenizing juicer. Freeze solid. Process again or put through juicer once more. Freeze a second time and enjoy. Keeps frozen many weeks. Remove from freezer several minutes before serving to soften slightly. Delicious and high in calcium and protein too! Try raspberries or other berries as well.

Peach or Apricot Tofu Ice Cream

Follow the recipe for Blueberry or Blackberry Tofu Ice Cream only use 2½–3 cups sliced fresh, sweet peaches or apricots instead of the berries. Instead of vanilla, use 2–3 tsp grated lemon rind. For a special flavor, try 8–12 drops real lemon flavoring.

Creamy Vanilla Tofu Ice Cream (Makes 2½–3 cups)

300 grams (10 ounces) soft tofu
½–¾ cup maple syrup (For a sweeter version, use an extra ¼ cup of maple
 syrup or fruit juice, preferably peach, pear, apple or apricot.)
2 tbsp arrowroot powder
4–6 tsp real vanilla
1 tsp guar gum or slippery elm powder
Few dashes sea salt
Optional: for added richness add ¼ cup ground, raw, cashews or blanched
 almonds

Combine all the ingredients in a food processor (or blender) and freeze solid. Defrost for 5–10 minutes or so and use a food processor or homogenizing juicer to soften the mixture and mix it again. Freeze a second time and enjoy. Remove from freezer a few minutes before serving. Add fruit or carob topping, granola or nuts if desired.

Carob Mint Tofu Ice Cream

Follow the recipe for Creamy Vanilla Tofu Ice Cream. Use the extra maple syrup or fruit juice and add ⅓–½ cup carob powder along with ¼–½ tsp (or more) peppermint extract. Do not add the extra ground nuts.

Frozen Fruit Slushes and Ices

Choose one or two fruits and freeze them solid. Try berries, papaya, kiwi, pears, peaches, apricots, citrus fruits, cherries, avocados, or other fruits suitable for freezing. Add just enough liquid sweetener or fruit juice to the frozen fruit so that it will blend or process easily and taste sweet enough for a dessert. Add a few dashes of sea salt, vanilla, rum, maple or other flavoring if desired. Freeze the mixture solid. Break the frozen mixture into chunks and soften with a food processor or homogenizing juicer. Re-freeze the mixture until it is totally solid, then process the mixture again and enjoy as a fruit "slushie," or keep frozen and enjoy as an ice. Remove the ice from the freezer a few minutes before eating to soften.

Delectable Carob Fudge

1–1¼ cups honey, maple syrup or fruit concentrate
1 cup sesame tahini or nut butter
1–1¼ cups sifted carob powder
½–1 cup sesame seeds or shredded coconut
8–14 drops peppermint extract
2 tbsp arrowroot powder
1–2 tsp real vanilla

Heat the nut butter and liquid sweetening on low to medium heat until hot and soft. Remove from heat and stir in the remaining ingredients. Press the mixture into a lightly oiled 9 or 10 inch glass pie plate or similar pan and press extra coconut or sesame seeds on top. Chill thoroughly. Cut and serve. Keeps up to 3 months refrigerated.

Lemon Rice Pudding

2 cups pre-cooked brown rice, cold
⅔ cup thick nut milk or sweet fruit juice (apple, pear, peach or apricot are good)
½–⅔ cup maple syrup or fruit concentrate
2 tbsp arrowroot powder
2–3 tsp grated lemon rind
2 tsp real vanilla
1–1½ tsp cinnamon
1 tsp guar gum or xanthan gum
⅛ tsp sea salt
Optional: ½–⅔ cup raisins or currants

Three-quarters of a cup of dry brown rice makes about 2 cups of cooked brown rice. However, be sure to measure after cooking, as rice varieties expand differently. Use sweet brown rice if available.

Preheat the oven to 375° F. Combine all ingredients carefully with a fork so as not to mash the rice. Mix thoroughly. Spread the mixture in a lightly oiled 9" x 9" casserole dish and bake 35–45 minutes, uncovered, until "set" and somewhat firm. Serve this tasty, nutritious dessert hot or cold.

Happiness Cake (Makes one 9" x 9" cake)

    2 cups sprouted wheat kernels (berries), ground
    1 cup honey, maple syrup or fruit concentrate
    1 tsp real vanilla
    ⅔ cup whole wheat flour
    ⅓ cup whole wheat pastry or unbleached white flour
    1 tbsp baking powder
    1 tsp cinnamon
    ½ tsp sea salt
    ¼ tsp each: ginger and nutmeg
    Few dashes allspice

Mix the sweetener, ground wheat berries and vanilla together (use a blender, grinder or food processor). Sift the remaining ingredients in a separate bowl. Gradually stir the dry ingredients into the wet and mix well. Lightly oil and flour a 9" x 9" square pan. Press the mixture into the pan. Preheat oven to 325° F and bake for 35–50 minutes or until lightly browned. The cake may be topped with Tapioca Maple Frosting.

Tapioca Maple Frosting (Makes 2 cups)

    2 cups tapioca flour
    1–1¼ cup maple syrup
    3–4 tsp real vanilla
    4 tbsp arrowroot powder
    Few dashes sea salt

Combine all the ingredients in a food processor. Chill only slightly before spreading on a cool cake. This is a thick, rich frosting, a bit like a glaze. Keeps refrigerated up to 8 days or more.

Tofu Cheesecake (Makes one 9 or 10 inch round cake)

    1½ lbs (750 grams) soft tofu (or regular tofu if soft is unavailable; soft will not
      be gritty)
    1 cup maple syrup or fruit concentrate
    ¼ cup natural raw sugar or other natural granular sugar
    3 tbsp natural light oil
    4 tbsp arrowroot powder
    3 tbsp grated lemon rind
    2 tsp guar gum or xanthan gum
    1 tsp vanilla extract

¼–½ tsp sea salt
Optional: 8–14 drops natural lemon flavoring
Optional: 1 pie crust shell

Mix all the ingredients, except the pie crust, in a food processor or homogenizing juicer. Line a 10 inch pie plate with a pie crust or if no crust is used, oil a 9 inch pie plate. Preheat the oven to 350° F. Spread the tofu mixture evenly in the crust or the oiled pie plate, and smooth out the top so the "cheesecake" will be even. Bake for about 45 minutes, or until the cake is set and turns a medium-golden color. Chill thoroughly and serve with Raspberry Topping or other fruit topping. To add a fruit layer to the cheesecake, the topping can be spread over a cool cheesecake and chilled, or the topping can be spooned on before serving each piece.

Fruit Topping

½ lb (1½–2 cups) fresh or frozen raspberries or strawberries, blueberries, sliced
peaches or apricots, etc.
¾–1 cup water
2–3 tbsp arrowroot powder
2–6 tbsp liquid sweetener

Heat the fruit in half the water and mash as it heats (or slice before heating). Mix the remaining water thoroughly with the arrowroot powder, making sure there are no lumps. Add the arrowroot mixture and sweetener to the fruit and stir constantly over medium heat until the sauce becomes brightly colored and thickens. Chill and serve with Tofu Cheesecake or use as a topping on ice cream and cakes.

Tofu Whipped Cream

6–8 ounces (½ lb) very fresh soft or regular, plain tofu (Do not use pressed,
flavored or Japanese varieties, or previously frozen tofu.)
4–6 tbsp maple syrup or fruit concentrate
1–2 tsp real vanilla flavoring
Optional: 2 tsp arrowroot or tapioca flour or ½ tsp guar gum or xanthan (corn)
gum (to thicken)
Optional: 1–2 dashes cinnamon

Rinse the tofu in cold water and press between several layers of paper or clean cloth towels to squeeze out all water possible. Break the tofu into small pieces and put it in the blender or food processor. Add the remaining ingredients and blend. Taste and adjust flavoring as desired, then blend again if necessary. Add an optional thickener if desired. Chill and serve.

Appendix 1

Associations, Educational Institutions and Support Groups

alive, CANADIAN JOURNAL OF HEALTH AND NUTRITION, Box 80055 Burnaby, BC V5H 3X1; 604-438-1919; fax: 604-435-4888; *mail and messages received here for Dr. Z. Rona, alive Advisor.*

ALIVE ACADEMY OF NUTRITION, 7436 Fraser Park Dr., Burnaby, BC V5J 5B9; 604-435-1919; fax: 604-435-4888; *home study nutrition course and other educational opportunities.*

ALLERGY AND ENVIRONMENTAL HEALTH ASSOCIATION, 85 Walmsley Blvd., Toronto, ON M4V 1X7; *quarterly newsletter and support for environmental illness.*

AMERICAN BIOLOGICS, Mexico S.A. Medical Center, 15 Azucenas St., Tijuana, Mexico; 619-429-8200; *Live Cell Therapy and Metabolic /Nutritional Treatment for Degenerative Diseases (Cancer, AIDS).*

AMERICAN BOARD OF CHELATION THERAPY, 70 West Huron St., Chicago, Illinois 60610; 312-266-7246; *established the protocol for chealtion therapy and certifies physicians in chelation; call or write for names of physicians practicing chealtion therapy.*

AMERICAN COLLEGE OF ADVANCEMENT IN MEDICINE, 23121 Verdugo Dr., Suite 204, Laguna Hills CA 92653, USA, 714-583-7666; *certifies physicians in chelation; call or write for names of physicians practicing chealtion therapy.*

AMERICAN COLLEGE OF NUTRITION, 722 Robert E. Lee Drive, Wilmington, NC 28480; 919-452-1222; *produces a journal and newsletter; provides lectures on nutrition research.*

AMERICAN HOLISTIC MEDICAL ASSOCIATION AND AMERICAN HOLISTIC NURSES ASSOCIATION, 4101 Lake Boone Trail, Suite 201, Raleigh, NC 27607; 800-878-3373; 919-787-5146.

AMERICAN ACADEMY OF BIOLOGICAL DENTISTRY, P.O. Box 856, Carmel Valley, California 93924; 408-659-5385; fax: 408-659-2417; *promotes non-toxic diagnostic and therapeutic approaches to clinical dentistry.*

AMERICAN ACADEMY OF ENVIRONMENTAL MEDICINE, P.O. Box 16106, Denver, CO 80216; 303-622-9755.

AMERICAN ASSOCIATION OF NATUROPATHIC PHYSICIANS, P.O. Box 20386, Seattle, WA 98102; 800-235-5800.

AMERICAN NATURAL HYGIENE SOCIETY, P.O. Box 30630, Tampa, FL 33630; 813-855-6608.

APLASTIC ANEMIA FOUNDATION OF AMERICA, P.O. Box 22689, Baltimore, MD 21203; 301-955-2803.

ASSOCIATION FOR VACCINE DAMAGED CHILDREN, contact Mary James, 67 Shier, Winnipeg, MB R3R 2H2; 204-895-9192; or contact Leona Rew, 22 Malone St., Winnipeg, MB R3R 1L4; 204-895-4015; *information on the damaging effects of vaccinations, book lists, etc.*

BASTYR COLLEGE OF NATUROPATHIC MEDICINE, 144 NE 54th St., Seattle, WA 98105; 206-523-9585; *courses and training in naturopathic medicine.*

BRITISH COLUMBIA NATUROPATHIC ASSOCIATION. #204 - 2786 West 16th Ave., Vancouver, BC V6K 3C4; 604-732-7070.

COALITION FOR ACCESS TO PREVENTIVE MEDICINE (CAPM), 128 Queen St. South, Box 42264, Mississauga, ON L5M 4Z0; 416-636-3960.

CPR-MD (COALITION OF PHYSICIANS FOR RESPONSIBLE MEDICAL DEMOCRACY) - P.O. Box 42256, 128 Queen St. S., Mississauga, ON L5M 4Z0.

CANADIAN COLLEGE OF NATUROPATHIC MEDICINE, 60 Berl Ave., Etobicoke, ON M8Y 3C7; 416-251-5261; *offers a diploma program in naturopathic medicine.*

CANADIAN COLLEGE OF OSTEOPATHY, 21 - 2601 Matheson Blvd. E., Mississauga, ON L4W 5A8; 416-629-7688.

CANADIAN NATUROPATHIC ASSOCIATION, Box 4520, Station C, Calgary, Alberta T2T 5N3; 403-244-4487.

CANADIAN SCHIZOPHRENIA FOUNDATION, 7375 Kingsway, Burnaby, BC V3N 3B5, 604-521-1728.

CANCER CONTROL SOCIETY, 2043 N. Berendo St., Los Angeles, CA 90027; 213-663-7801; *information available through memberships, Cancer Control Journal, Clinic Directory, Patient List, Cancer Book House, Movies, Conventions and Clinic Tours.*

CFIDS ASSOCIATION, FOR INFORMATION ON THE CHRONIC FATIGUE SYNDROME; P.O. Box 220398, Charlotte, North Carolina 28222-0398; 800-442-3437; 900-988-2343 (information line); fax: 704-365-9755; *largest organization for information, etc. on CFS and immune dysfunction syndrome.*

THE CHOICE, COMMITTEE FOR FREEDOM OF CHOICE IN MEDICINE, INC., 1180 Walnut Ave., Chula Vista, CA 92011.

CONSUMER HEALTH ORGANIZATION OF CANADA, 280 Sheppard Ave. E., #207, P.O. Box 248, Willowdale, ON, M2N 5S9; 416-222-6517. CURE AIDS NOW: *information on ozone, hydrogen peroxide and other oxidative therapies and their use in the treatment of AIDS; newsletter and practitioner list* - P.O. Box 4184, Salisbury, NC 28144-0102.

DAMS (DENTAL AMALGAM MERCURY SYNDROME) - 725-9 Tramway Lane NE, Albuquerque, NM 87122; 505-291-8239; fax:505-294-3339; *newsletter and other information dedicated to informing the public about the potential risks of mercury in dental amalgam fillings.*

ECLECTIC INSTITUTE INC., 11231 S.E. Marlet St., Portland, Oregon 97216; 503-256-4330; *natural alternatives for the optimization of health.*

EDTA CHELATION LOBBY ASSOCIATION OF BC, P.O. Box 67514, Station O, Vancouver, BC V5W 3T9; 604-327-3889.

ENVIRONMENTAL DENTAL ASSOCIATION, 9974 Scripps Ranch Blvd., Suite #36, San Diego, CA, 92131; 619-586-1208; fax: 619-693-0724; *educational, research, referral and other resources for non-toxic dentistry.*

FOUNDATION FOR TOXIC-FREE DENTISTRY, P.O. Box 608010, Orlando, FL 32860-8010; 407-299-4149; *information and referrals to biologic dentists.*

FREEDOM OF CHOICE IN HEALTH CARE, P.O. Box 92225, 2900 Warden Ave., Scarborough, ON M1W 3Y9; 416-282-1016; *a group devoted to obtaining a just and equalized system in which every individual can freely choose their preferred method of treatment in maintaining their health.*

GEORGIAN BAY NLP CENTRE; P.O. Box 1210, Meaford, ON, N0H 1Y0; 519-538-1194; fax: 519-538-1063; *free catalogue of books, tapes and videos on NLP, Stress Management,Education, Hypnosis, Personal Development, Health Care, etc.*

GREAT LAKES CLINICAL MEDICINE ASSOCIATION, 70 W. Haron, Chicago, Il 60610; 312-266-7246.

HERB RESEARCH FOUNDATION, 1007 Pearl St., Suite 200, Boulder, CO 80302; 303-449-2265; *listing of practitioners knowledgeable about herbs. Members receive HERBAL-GRAM, a quarterly which presents research reviews from the scientific literature, follows legal issues, market trends and media coverage of herbs.*

INTERNATIONAL BIO-OXIDATIVE MEDICINE FOUNDATION, P.O, Box 13205 Oklahoma City, OK 73113-1205; 405-478-4266; *information on chelation therapy, H2O2, ozone and other oxygen related therapies.*

INTERNATIONAL HEALTH FOUNDATION, INC. Box 3494, Jackson, TN 38303; *provides international roster of physicians interested in candida-related disorders; helps children with repeated ear infections, hyperactivity, attention deficits and related behavior and learning problems.*

THE LIFE EXTENSION FOUNDATION, P.O. Box 229120 Hollywood, Florida 33022-9120; 305-966-4886; 800-841-LIFE; *newsletter, books, supplements for life extension.*

LIFE SCIENCE INSTITUTE, 1108 Regal Row, Austin, TX 78748; 800-889-9989.

THE M.E. (CHRONIC FATIGUE SYNDROME) ASSOCIATION OF CANADA, 400 - 246 Queen St., Ottawa, ON K1P 5E4; 613-563-1565; fax: 613-567-0614.

NATIONAL ASSOCIATION FOR RARE DISORDERS P.O. Box 8923, New Fairfield, CT 06812; 203-746-6518.

NATIONAL COLLEGE OF NATUROPATHIC MEDICINE, 11231 Southeast Market St., Portland, OR 97216; 503-255-4860; *for referrals to naturopathic doctors in your area.*

NATIONAL HEALTH FEDERATION, P.O. Box 688, Monrovia, CA 91016, U.S.A.

NATIONAL INSTITUTE OF FITNESS, 202 N. Snow Canyon Rd., Box #380938, Ivins, UT 84738; 801-673-4905.

NATIONAL INSTITUTE OF NEUROLOGICAL DISORDERS AND STROKES (NINDS), 9000 Rockville Pike, Bethesda, MD 20892; 301-496-5751.

NATIONAL ORGANIZATION FOR RARE DISORDERS (NORD), P.O. Box 8923, New Fairfield, CT 06812; 203-746-6518.

NATIONAL VACCINE INFORMATION CENTER, 512 W. Maple Ave., Suite 206, Vienna, Virginia 22180; 703-938-0342; fax: 703-938-5768; *information on vaccines and the prevention of vaccine damage.*

NIGHTINGALE RESEARCH FOUNDATION, 383 Danforth Ave., Ottawa, ON K2A 0E1; 613-728-9643; fax: 613-729-0825; *information and support groups for Chronic Fatigue Syndrome/ME.*

ONTARIO HERBALISTS' ASSOCIATION, 7 Alpine Ave., Toronto, ON M6P 3R6.

PATIENT INFORMATION ON CHRONIC ILLNESS, 41 Green Valley Court, Kleinburg, ON L0J 1C0; 416-832-5340.

PRINCETON BIO CENTER, 862 RT 518, Skillman, NJ 08558; 609-924-9423; *information on treatment of schizophrenia and other mental illnesses with orthomolecular medicine.*

SOUTHWEST COLLEGE, 6535 E. Osborn Rd., Scottsdale, AZ 85251; 602-990-7424; *offers a degree program in naturopathic medicine.*

SUPPLEMENTS PLUS, 451 Church St., Toronto, ON M4Y 2C5; 416-962-8369; 800-387-4761; fax: 416-961-4033; *informa-*

tion and sales of nutritional, herbal and homeopathic remedies.

TOURETTE'S SYNDROME ASSOCIATION, 42-40 Bell Blvd., Bayside, NY 11361; 718-224-2999.

THE TOWNSEND LETTER FOR DOCTORS, 911 Tyler St., Port Townsend, WA 98368-6541; *publishes monthly newsletter for natural health care practitioners; highly recommended for its political and editorial content.*

VITAMIN INFORMATION PROGRAM, *Hoffmann-La Roche Ltd.*, 2455 Meadowpine Blvd., Mississauga, ON L5N 6L7; 905-542-5615; Fax: 905-542-7130; *free literature and copies of research studies on vitamins, antioxidants for health professionals.*

WORLD RESEARCH FOUNDATION, 15300 Ventura Blvd., Suite 405, Sherman Oaks, CA 91403 USA; 818-907-5483; fax: 818-907-6044; *information on therapies inside and outside mainstream medicine for any health condition.*

Appendix 2
Laboratories and Testing Information

ANAMOL LABORATORIES
P.O. Box 96
Concord, ON L4K 1B2
905-660-1225
Fingernail, mineral analysis

BALCO
1520 Gilbreth Rd.
Burlingame, CA 94010
800-777-7122

DOCTOR'S DATA INC.,
P.O. 111
30 W. 101 Roosevelt Rd.
West Chicago, IL 60185
800-323-2784

GREAT SMOKIES DIAGNOSTIC LABORATORY
18A Regent Park Blvd.
Asheville, NC 28806
704-253-0621
Comprehensive stool and digestive analysis

MERIDIAN VALLEY CLINICAL LABORATORY
24030 132nd Ave. SE
Kent, WA 98042
206-631-8922; 800-234-6825
Comprehensive stool and digestive analysis

METAMATRIX MEDICAL LABORATORY
5000 Peachtree St. Industrial Blvd.
Suite 110
Norcross, GA 30071
800-221-4640 (for doctors only)
404-446-5483
Amino acid analysis

NATIONAL BIOTECH LABORATORY
3212 NE 125th St.
Seattle, WA 98125
800-846-6285

IMMUNO LABS, INC.
1620 West Oakland
Park Boulevard
Fort Lauderdale,FL 33311
800-231-9197

SERAMMUNE PHYSICIANS LABORATORIES
1890 Preston White Dr.,
Suite 201
Reston, VA 22091
800-553-5472
Allergy testing; Elisa/Act test

TRACE MINERALS INTERNATIONAL
2618 Valmont Rd.
Boulder, CO 80304-2904
303-442-1082

Appendix 3
Vitamin, Mineral and Herb Suppliers

ADVANCED NUTRITIONAL RESEARCH
One Washington St.
P.O. Box 807
Ellicottville, NY 14731
800-836-0644

ALLERGY RESEARCH GROUP
400 Preda St.
San Leandro, CA 94577
800-545-9960

AMNI (ADVANCED MEDICAL NUTRITION INC.)
2247 National Ave.,

P.O. Box 5012
Hayward, CA 94540
800-437-8888

BIO-THERAPEUTICS/PHYTO-PHARMICA
P.O. Box 1745
Green Bay, WI 54305
800-553-2370

BIOTICS RESEARCH CORP.
Probiologic, Inc.
14714 NE 87th St.
Redmond, WA 98052
800-678-8218

BHI (BIOLOGICAL HOMEOPATHIC
INDUSTRIES, INC.)
11600 Cochiti S.E.
Albuquerque, NM 87123
800-621-7644

BOERICKE & TAFEL, INC.
2381 Circadian Way
Santa Rosa, CA 95407

J. R. CARLSON LABORATORIES INC.
15 College Dr.
Arlington Hts., IL 60004-1985
800-323-4141

DAVINCI LABORATORIES
20 New England Dr.
Essex Jct., VT 05453
800-325-1776

DOLISOS AMERICA INC.
3014 Rigel Ave.
Las Vegas, NV 89102
800-365-4767

DOUGLAS LABORATORIES
Wabash & Main, P.O. Box 8583
Pittsburgh, PA 15220
412-937-0122

EMERSON ECOLOGICS INC.
436 Great Rd.
Acton, MA 01720
800-654-4432

ENZYME PROCESS LABORATORIES, INC.
1 Commercial Ave.
Garden City, NY 11530
800-521-8669

FOR YOUR HEALTH PHARMACY
13215 SE 240th St.
Kent, WA 98042
800-456-4325

GREENS PLUS
Orange Peel Ent., Inc.
730 14th St.
Vero Beach, FL 32960
800-643-1210 (USA)
800-387-4761 (Canada)

JO MAR LABORATORIES
251 East Hacienda Ave.
Campbell, CA 95008
800-538-4545

KLABIN MARKETING
115 Central Park West
New York, NY 10023
212-877-3632 (in NY)
800-933-9440 (outside NY)

KLAIRE LABORATORIES
1573 W. Seminole St.
San Marcos, CA 92069
619-744-9680 (in CA)
800-533-7255 (outside CA)

LIFE EXTENSION FOUNDATION
P.O. Box 229120
Hollywood, FL33022-9120
305-966-4886
800-841-LIFE

MURDOCK PHARMACEUTICALS
1400 Mountain Springs Park
Springville, UT 84663
800-962-8873

NATREN
3105 Willow Lane
Westlake Village, CA 91361
800-992-3323 (CA)
800-992-9393

NUTRIPHARM INC.
Birmingham, AL 35243
800-88-OMEGA
(800-886-6342)

NUTRISOURCE CORPORATION
1550 Rancho Del Hambre
Lafayette, CA 94549
800-544-4542

PATHWAY APOTHECARY PHARMACY
5415 Cedar Lane
Bethesda, MD 20814
301-530-1112

PROBIOLOGIC INC.
West Willows Technology Ctr.
14714 NE 87th St.

Redmond, WA 98052
800-678-8218

PROFESSIONAL HEALTH PRODUCTS
4307-49 St.
Innisfail, AB T4G 1P3
800-661-1366

SCANDINAVIAN NATURAL HEALTH & BEAUTY PRODUCTS INC.
13 North 7th St.
Perkasie, PA 18944
215-453-2505

STANDARD HOMEOPATHIC CO.
210 210W. 131st St. Box 61067
Los Angeles, CA 90061
213-321-4284

THORNE RESEARCH PRODUCTS
Sandpoint, ID 83864
800-228-1966

UAS LABORATORIES
9201 Penn Ave. S. #10
Minneapolis, MN 55431
800-422-3371

Bibliography

ADA Reports. Position of the american dietetic association: vegetarian diets. *Journal of the American Dietetic Association* 93 (no. 11): 1317–1319.

Abraham, G.E. et al. 1981 Effect of vitamin B6 on plasma and red blood cell magnesium levels in premenopausal women. *Ann. Clin. Lab. Sci* 11(4): 333-336.

Ahmed, F. E. 1991. Effect of diet on progression of renal disease. *American Dietetic Association* 10:1266–1269.

Airola, P. 1974. *How to get well*. Phoenix: Health Plus Publishers.

Airola, P. 1979. *Every woman's book*. Phoenix: Health Plus Publishers.

Allard, J. 1993. The antioxidant vitamins: Their role in chronic and smoking related diseases affecting women. Paper presented at Nutrition and Women's Health: New Perspectives. Symposium sponsored by Hoffmann-La Roche Ltd.

Alter, M. J., and R. E. Sampliner. 1989. Hepatitis C and miles to go before we sleep. *The New England Journal of Medicine* 321 (no. 22): 1538–1539.

American Academy of Allergy and Immunology Committee on Adverse Reactions to Foods. July 1984. Adverse reactions to foods. *U.S. National Institute of Allergy and Infectious Diseases*. NIH publication no. 84-2442.

Aparicio, M. et al. 1991. Low protein diet and renal osteodystrophy. *Nephron* 58: 250–252.

Associated Press. October 28, 1988. Studies suggest ozone fights AIDS. *Los Angeles Times*.

Associated Press. April 14, 1994. Beta carotene cancer study a big surprise. *Toronto Star*.

Astrup, A. 1986. Thermogenesis in human brown adipose tissue and skeletal muscle induced by sympathomimetic stimulation. *Acta Endocrinologica* 112, supp. 278.

Astrup, A. et al. 1991. Thermogenic synergism between ephedrine and caffeine in healthy volunteers: a double-blind, placebo-controlled study. *Metabolism* 40 (no. 3): 323–329.

The Alpha-Tocopherol, Beta Carotene Cancer Prevention Study Group. 1994. The effect of vitamin E and beta carotene on the incidence of lung cancer and other cancers in male smokers. *The New England Journal of Medicine* 330 (no. 15): 1029–1035.

Augsburger, A. 1991. Macular degeneration: medical treatment may help slow progression. *Geriatrics* 46 (no. 10):17.

Avorn, J. et al. 1994. Reduction of bacteriuria and pyuria after ingestion of cranberry juice. *JAMA* 271: 751–4.

Ayres, S. et al. 1973. Raynaud's phenomenon, scleroderma and calcinosis cutis: response to vitamin E. *Cutis* 11: 54–62.

Ayres, S. 1978. Is vitamin E involved in the autoimmune mechanism? *Cutis* 21: 321-325.

Babb, R. R., and S. Wagener. 1989. Blastocystis hominis: a potential intestinal pathogen. *West J. Med.* 151: 518–519.

Badgley, Laurence. 1987. *Healing AIDS naturally.* Foster City, CA : Healing Energy Press.

Balch, James F., and Phyllis A. Balch. 1990. *Prescription for nutritional healing.* Garden City Park, New York: Avery Publishing Group Inc.

Ballweg, Mary Lou, and the Endometriosis Association. 1987. *Overcoming endometriosis.* New York: Congdon & Weed.

Baltin, H. 25–26 May, 1983. Oxygen partial pressure measurements in arterial and venal blood: before, during and after ozone treatment. Paper presented at Sixth Ozone World Congress of the International Ozone Association, Washington, DC.

Barnard, Neal D. May/June 1991. The need for new food recommendations. *PCRM Update.*

Barnes, Broda O. 1976. *Hypothyroidism: the unsuspected illness.* New York: Harper and Row.

Bassett, I. B. et al. 1990. A comparative study of tea-tree oil versus benzoyl peroxide in the treatment of acne. *Medical Journal of Australia* 153: 455–458.

Bauer, H., and H. Staub. 1954. Treatment of hepatitis with infusions of ascorbic acid: comparison with other therapies. *Journal of the American Medical Association* 156 (no. 5): 565.

Bauernfeind, J. C. 1980. The safe use of vitamin A: A report of the international vitamin A consultative group. Washington, DC: The Nutrition Foundation.

Behan, P. O. 1991. Myalgic encephalomyelitis: Post viral fatigue syndrome: Diagnostic and clinical guidelines for doctors. *M.E.* (Canada Ottawa, ON; 613-563-1565.)

Beilin, L. J., and I. B. Puddey. 1992. Alcohol and hypertension. *Clinical and Experimental Hypertensive Theory and Practice.* A14 (no. 1 & 2): 119–138.

Belch J. J. F. et al. 1986. Evening primrose oil (Efamol) as a treatment for cold-induced vasospasm (Raynaud's phenomenon). *Prog. Lipid Res.* 25: 335–40.

Belch J. J. F. et al. 1985. Evening primrose oil (Efamol) in the treatment of Raynaud's phenomenon: a double-blind study. *Thromb. Haemost.* 54 (no. 2): 490–94.

Bell, Iris R. et al. 1990. Vitamin B12 and folate status in acute geropsychiatric inpatients: affective and cognitive characteristics of a vitamin nondeficient population. *Biological Psychiatry* 27 (no. 2): 125–37.

Bell, Iris R. 1991. B complex vitamin patterns in geriatric and young adult patients with major depression. *Journal of the American Geriatric Society* 39 (no. 3): 252-257.

Bendich, A., and L. Langseth. 1989. Safety of vitamin A. *American Journal of Clinical Nutrition* 49: 358–71.

Benton, David. 1991. *Vitamin and mineral intake and cognitive function, micronutrients in health and disease prevention.* New York: Adrianne and Butterworth, C.E., Marcelle Dekker Inc.

Bernstein, J., and S. Alpert, et al. 1977. Depression of lymphocyte transformation following oral glucose ingestion. *Am. J. Clin. Nutr.* 30: 613.

Bethel, May. 1977. *The healing power of herbs.* Hollywood, CA : Melvin Powers, Wilshire Book Company.

Bhutani, L. K., and S. M. Bhate. 1979. Vitamin A in the treatment of lichen planus pigmentosus. *British Journal of Dermatology* 100: 473.

Bieler, H. G. 1965. *Food is your best medicine.* New York: Random House.

Bills, T,. and L. Spatz. 1977. Neutrophilic hypersegmentation as an indicator of incipient folic acid deficiency. *American Journal of Clinical Pathology* 68 (no. 2): 263.

Bjarmason, I., et al. Nov. 1984. Intestinal permeability and inflammation in rheumatoid arthritis: effects of sonsteroidal anti-inflammatory drugs. *Lancet:* 1186–1192.

Bland, Jeffrey. 1983. *Nutraerobics.* San Francisco: Harper & Rowe.

Bland, Jeffrey. 1983. Medical applications of clinical nutrition. New Canaan, CT: Keats.

Blake, Steve. 1994. *Globalherb: herb software program and database for Macintosh and IBM compatible computers.* Felton CA: FALCOR.

Blakeslee, Sandra. Nov 1990. The lead-calcium time bomb. *American Health* 68–72.

Blot, W. J., and J. Y. Li, P. R. Taylor, et al. 1993. Nutrition intervention trials in Linxian, China: supplementation with specific vitamin/mineral combinations, cancer incidence and disease-specific mortality in the general population. *J. Natl. Cancer Inst.* 85 (no. 18): 1483-1492.

Botez, M., et al. 1976. Neurologic disorders responsive to folic acid therapy. *Canadian Medical Association Journal* 115: 217–23.

Bower, B. D., and E. A. Newsholme. March 18, 1978. Treatment of idiopathic polyneuritis by polyunsaturated fatty acid diet. *Lancet :* 583–85.

Braly, James. 1992. *Dr. Braly's food allergy and nutrition revolution.* New Canaan, CT: Keats Publishing, Inc.

Braly, James. 1993. Insulin-dependent diabetes: an IgG-mediated cow's milk allergy? *The Immuno Review* 1 (no. 2). (Available from Immuno Laboratories Inc., 1620 West Oakland Park Blvd., Fort Lauderdale, FL 33311; phone 800-231-9197 or 305-486-4500.)

Brennan, Richard. Feb 9, 1994. Poor food, bad hygiene plague hospitals, MPPs told. *The Toronto Star.*

Bruckheim, Allan. 1992. *The family doctor.* Portland: Creative Multimedia Corporation. (A textbook on CD-ROM.)

Braverman, Eric R., and Carl C. Pfeiffer. 1987. *The healing nutrients within.* New Canaan, CT: Keats Publishing Inc.

Breneman, J. C. 1978. *Basics of food allergy.* Springfield, IL: Charles C. Thomas.

Buck, A. C., and R.W. M. Rees, L. Ebeling. 1989. Treatment of chronic prostatitis and prostadynia with pollen extract. *British Journal of Urology* 64: 496–499.

Bunday, Sally, and Vicky Colquhoun. 1990. Why the lack of treatment for hyperactive children? *Journal of Nutritional Medicine* 1: 361–363.

Buist, Robert. 1984. *Food intolerance: what it is and how to cope with it.* Sydney, Australia: Harper & Row.

Buist, R. A. 1984. Vitamin toxicities, side effects and contraindications. *International Clinical Nutrition Review* 4 (no. 4): 159–71.

Bukowlecki, L., et al. 1982. Ephedrine: a potential slimming drug, directly stimulates thermogenesis in brown adipocytes via beta-adrenoreceptors. *International Journal of Obesity* 6: 343–50.

Burton Goldberg Group. 1993. *Alternative medicine: the definitive guide.* Puyallup, Washington: Future Medicine Publishing, Inc.

Burleson, G. H., and T. M. Murray, M. Pollard. 1975. Inactivation of viruses and bacteria by ozone, with and without sonication. *Applied Microbiology* 37: 340–344.

Butterworth, C .E., et al. 1982. Improvement in cervical dysplasia associated with folic acid therapy in users of oral contraceptives. *American Journal of Clinical Nutrition* 35: 73.

Campbell R. E., and F. W. Pruitt. 1952. Vitamin B12 in the treatment of viral hepatitis. *American Journal of Medical Science* 224: 252.

Campbell R.E., and F. W. Pruitt. 1955. The effect of vitamin B12 and folic acid in the treatment of viral hepatitis. *American Journal of Medical Science* 229: 8.

Canadian Organic Growers Inc. 1994. *Toronto and Region Directory.* Toronto, ON: Rooftop Communications. (For a copy, send $6 payable to Jeff Johnston: Organic Directory 65, Scadding Ave., Suite 1016, Toronto, ON M5A 4L1; 416-466-2841.)

Cantekin, Erdem I. 1993. Antimicrobial therapy for otitis media with effusion. *JAMA* 270 (no. 4): 449–451.

Carter, James P. 1993. *Racketeering in medicine: the suppression of alternatives.* Norfolk, Virginia: Hampton Roads Publishing Company, Inc.

Ceriello, A., et al. 1991. Vitamin E reduction of protein glycosylation in diabetes. *Diabetes Care* 14: 68–72.

Chaitman B. R., and T. J. Ryan, R. A. Kronmal, et al. 1990. Coronary artery surgery study (CASS): comparability of 10 year survival in randomized and randomizable patients. *J Am Coll Cardiol.* 16: 1071.

Chaitow, Leon. 1988. *Vaccination and immunization: dangers, delusions and alternatives.* Essex, England: The C.W. Daniel Company Ltd.

Chaitow, Leon. 1988. *Amino acids in therapy.* Healing Arts Press.

Chaitow, Leon. and N. Trenev. 1990. *Probiotics.* New York: Harper Collins.

Champault, G., et al. 1984. Medical treatment of prostatic adenoma: a controlled trial. *Ann. Urol.* 18: 407–10.

Christensen, Larry. 1991. The role of caffeine and sugar in depression. *The Nutrition Report* 9 (no. 3): 17–24.

Cimons, Marlene. Feb 22, 1991. U.S. Offers plan to reduce lead risk to children, *The Los Angeles Times* A1 & A34.

Cohen, Jeffrey A., and Karl Gross. Peripheral neuropathy: Causes and management in the elderly. *Geriatrics* 45 (no. 2): 21–34.

Cohen, L., et al. 1990. Dietary antioxidants and blood pressure. *American Journal of Clinical Nutrition* 512: abstract 18.

Cohen, M. L. 1992. Epidemiology of drug resistance: Implications for a post-antimicrobial era. *Science* 257:1050–1055.

Collins, W. P. 1989. Biochemical indices of potential fertility. *International Journal of Gynecology and Obstetrics* 1: 35–43.

Collins, W. P. 1985. Hormonal indices of ovulation and the fertile period. *Advances in Contraception* 1: 279–294.

Costello, C. H., and E. V. Lynn. 1950. Estrogenic substances from plants: I. glycyrrhiza. *J. Am. Pharm. Soc.* 39: 177–80.

Coulter, Harris L., and Barbara Loe Fisher. 1991. *A shot in the dark.* New York: Avery Publishing Group.

Cox, I. M., and M. J. Campbell, D. Dowson. 1991. Red blood cell magnesium and chronic fatigue syndrome. *Lancet* 337: 757–760.

Cramer, D. W., and E. Wilson et al. 1986. The relation of endometriosis to menstrual characteristics, smoking and exercise. *Journal of the American Medical Association* 255 (no. 14): 1904–8.

Cranton, Elmer. 1990. *Bypassing bypass.* Troutdale, VA: Hampton Roads.

Crayton, J. W., et al. 1981. Epilepsy precipitated by food sensitivity: Report of a case with double-blind placebo-controlled assessment. *Clin. Electroencephalo* 12 (no. 4): 192–8.

Creasy, Rosalind. 1986. *The gardener's handbook of edible plants.* San Francisco, CA: Sierra Club.

Crook, William G. 1987. *The yeast connection.* New York: Random House.

Crook, William G. 1988. *Detecting your hidden allergies.* Jackson, TN: Professional Books.

Crook, William G. 1991. *Help for the hyperactive child.* Jackson, TN: Professional Books.

Crook, William G. 1992. *Chronic fatigue syndrome and the yeast connection.* Jackson, TN: Professional Books.

Daling, J. R., et al. 1994. Risk of breast cancer among young women: relationship to induced abortion. *Journal of the National Cancer Institute* 86 (no. 21).

D'ambrosio, E., et al. 1991. Glucosamine sulfate: A controlled clinical investigation in arthritis. *Pharmatherapeutics* 2:504–508.

Davis, G. L., et al. 1989. Treatment of chronic hepatitis C with recombinant interferon alfa. *The New England Journal of Medicine* 321 (no. 22): 1501–1505.

Davies, Stephen, and Alan Stewart. 1987. *Nutritional Medicine.* London: Pan Books.

Day, Charlene A. 1991. *The Immune system handbook: Your owner's manual.* Toronto: Potentials Within.

Deahl, M. P. Lithium-induced carpal tunnel syndrome. *Br. J. Psychiatry* 153: 250–1.1988.

Debrand, J. 1974. *Magnesium deficiency and platelet aggreability.* Bescanon: These de Medicine.

Deitch, Eswin, et al. 1991. Bacterial translocation from the gut impairs systemic immunity. *Surgery* 109 (no. 3) 269–276.

Delva, Dianne. 1991. Vitamin B12 deficiency without anemia. *Canadian Family Physician* 37: 1493–1497.

Demarco, Carolyn. 1994. *Take charge of your body: A woman's guide to health.* 6th ed. Winlaw, BC: The Well Woman Press.

Demarco, Carolyn. 1994. Witches for the burning: Surviving a modern day medical inquisition. *Wellness MD 4* (no. 1): 10–13.

Demitrack, Mark A., et al. 1991. Evidence for impaired activation of hypothalamic-pituitary-adrenal axis in patients with chronic fatigue syndrome. *Journal of Endocrinology and Metabolism* 73 (no. 6): 1224–1234.

Diamond, Harvey. 1995. *Leave my breasts alone!: How to prevent breast cancer.* In press.

Di Bisceglie, A. M., et al. 1989. Recombinant interferon alfa therapy for chronic hepatitis C. *The New England Journal of Medicine* 321 (no. 22): 1506–1510.

Dickerson, J. W. I., and H. A. Lee, eds. 1978. *Nutrition and disorders of the nervous system: Nutrition in the clinical management of disease.* London: Edward Arnold.

Digiesi, V., and F. Cantini, B. Brodbeck. 1990. Effect of coenzyme Q10 on essential arterial hypertension. *Current Therapeutic Research* 47: 841–845.

Dixon, Hamilton S. 1992. Allergy and laryngeal disease. *Otolaryngologic Clinics of North America* 25 (no. 1): 239–250.

Dobbins, John P. Feb.1992. AIDS cured by hyper-oxidation. *Health Freedom News.*

Dohan, F. C., and J. C. Grasberger et al. 1969. Relapsed schizophrenics: more rapid movement on a milk-and-cereal-free diet. *British Journal of Psychiatry* 115.

Dore, P., et al. 1989. Lipoid nephrosis secondary to food allergy: Report of two cases. *Rev. Fr. Allergol* 29 (no. 3): 133–137.

Duke, J. A. 1985. *Handbook of medicinal herbs.* Boca Raton, FL: CRC Press.

Dulloo, A. G., and D. S. Miller. 1987. Aspirin as a promoter of ephedrine-induced thermogenesis:potential use in the treatment of obesity. *American Journal of Clinical Nutrition* 45: 564–9.

Dunne, Lavon J. 1990. *Nutrition Almanac, 3rd ed.* New York: McGraw-Hill.

Dysken, M. A. 1987. A review of recent clinical trials in the treatment of alzheimer's dementia. *Psychiatric Annals* 17 (no. 3): 178.

Eaton, K. K. and A. Hunnisett. 1991. Abnormalities in essential amino acids in patients with chronic fatigue syndrome. *Journal of Nutritional Medicine* 2: 369–375.

Edwin, E., et al. 1965. Vitamin B12 hypovitaminosis in mental diseases. *Acta Med. Scand.* 177: 689–99.

Egger, J., et al. 1989. Oligoantigenic diet treatment of children with epilepsy and migraine. *The Journal of Pediatrics* 114: 51–8.

Egger, J., et al. 1992. Effect of diet treatment on enuresis in children with migraine or hyperkinetic behavior. *Clin. Pediatr.* 31: 302–307.

Eisenberg, D. M., et al. 1993. Unconventional medicine in the united states. *New England Journal of Medicine* 328: 246–252.

* Elghamry and Shihata IM. 1965. Biological activity of phytoestrogens. *Planta Medica* 13: 352–7.

Ellis, J. M., and J. Presley. 1973. *Vitamin B6: The doctor's report.* New York: Harper & Row.

Embon, O. M., et al. 1990. Chronic dehydration stone disease. *British Journal of Urology* 66: 357–362.

Empey, Lonnie R. 1991. Fish oil-enriched diet is mucosal protective against acetic acid-induced colitis in rats. *Canadian Journal of Physiological Pharmacology* 69: 480–488.

Engler, Marguerite M., and Sandra K. Erickson. 1992. Dietary gamma-linolenic acid lowers blood pressure and alters aortic reactivity and cholesterol metabolism in hypertension. *Journal of Hypertension* 10: 1197–1204.

Erasmus, Udo. 1986. *Fats And Oils.* Vancouver: Alive Books.

Erasmus, Udo. 1993. *Fats that Heal Fats that Kill.* Vancouver: Alive Books.

Ewertz, M. 1992. Oral contraceptives and breast cancer risk in Denmark. *European Journal of Cancer* 28a (nos. 6/7): 1176–1181.

Faccinetti, et al. 1991. Magnesium prophylaxis of menstrual migraine: effects on intracellular magnesium. *Headache* 31:298–304.

Fagard, F. 1991. Physical exercise and the management of hypertension. *Bulletin of the World Health Organization* 62 (no. 2): 149–153.

Fahmy, Z. 25–26 May, 1983. The treatment of rheumatoid arthritis with ozone. Sixth Ozone World Congress of the International Ozone Association, Washington, DC

Fast, Julius. 1987. *The omega-3 breakthrough.* Tuscon, AZ.: The Body Press.

Ferenci, P., et al. 1989. Randomized controlled trial of silymarin treatment in patients with cirrhosis of the liver. *Journal of Hepatology* 9: 105–113.

Finnegan, John. 1992. *The facts about fats: A consumer's guide to good oils.* Malibu, CA: Elysian Arts.

Finnegan, John. 1992. *Fats and oils: A consumer's guide.* Malibu, CA: Elysian Arts.

Fischer, William L. 1988. *How to fight cancer and win.* Vancouver: Alive Books.

Fisher-Rasmussen, W., et al. 1990. Ginger treatment of hyperemesis gravidarum. *European Journal of Obstetrics, Gynecology and Reproductive Biology* 38: 19–24.

Flier, J. S., and L. H. Underhill. 1984. Thermogenesis in brown adipose tissue as an energy buffer. *New England Journal of Medicine* 311 (no. 24): 1549–58.

Folin, M., and E. Contiero, M. Vaselli. 1991. Trace element determination in humans. *Biological Trace Element Research* 31.

Folkers, K., et al. 1984. Enzymology of the response of the carpal tunnel syndrome to riboflavin and pyridoxine. *Proc. Natl. Acad. Sci. USA* 81 (no. 22): 7076–8.

Food processor II: Nutrition and diet analysis system, The. Salem, OR: ESHA Research. (Available for Macintosh and IBM-compatible personal computers from ESHA Research, PO Box 13028, Salem, OR 97309; 503-585-6242.)

Fortune, F., and J. A. G. 1993. Buchanana. Oral lichen planus and coeliac disease. *Lancet* 341: 1154–1155.

Friedman, Burton. May 1990. B vitamin for burning feet. Cortlandt Forum: 27–19.

Friedman, Howard S. 1990. Coronary Bypass Graft Surgery: re-examining the assumptions. *Journal of General Internal Medicine* 5:80–83.

Fromberg, M. 1992. Diet and calcium stones. *Canadian Medical Association Journal* 146 (no. 11):1894.

Frydl, V., and H. Zavodska. 1989. Diabetic polyneuropathy and vitamin B1. *Medwelt* 40: 1484–6.

Fuhr, J. E., et al. 1989. Vitamin B6 levels in patients with carpal tunnel syndrome. *Arch. Surg.* 124: 1329–30.

Gaby, Alan. 1993. *Preventing and reversing osteoporosis.* Roseville, CA : Prima Publishing.

Galland, L., and D. D. Buchman. 1988. *Superimmunity for kids.* New York: E.P. Dutton.

Galland, Leo, et al. 1990. Giardia lLamblia infection as a cause of chronic fatigue. *Journal of Nutritional Medicine* 1: 27–31.

Garcia-Belenguer, S., et al. 1992. Nutritional muscular dystrophy from deficiencies of selenium and vitamin E in ruminants. *Med. Vet.* 9 (no 2): 84–92.

Gardner, Joy. 1987. *Healing yourself during pregnancy.* Freedom, CA: The Crossing Press.

Garewal, Harinder S. 1991. Precancerous lesions: role of antioxidant nutrients in preventing malignant transformation of cells. *Vitamin Nutrition Information Service.* Hoffmann-La Roche Ltd.

Garrow, J. G. 1988. Exercise, diet and thermogenesis. *Current Concepts in Nutrition* 15:51–65.

Gerster, Helga 1991. Review: Antioxidant protection of the ageing macula. *Age and Ageing* 20: 60–69.

Gerstein, H. C. 1994. Cow's milk exposure and type I diabetes mellitus. *Diabetes Care* 17 (no. 1): 13–19.

Ghent, William R. 1993. Iodine replacement in fibrocystic disease of the breast. *CJS* 36 (no. 5).

Gillespie, Larrian. 1986. *You don't have to live with cystitis!* New York: Rawson Associates.

Gislason, Stephen J. 1989. *Core diet for kids.* Vancouver: PerSona Publications.

Gislason, Stephen J. 1991. *Nutritional therapy.* Vancouver: PerSona Publications.

Gittleman, Ann Louise. 1993. *Guess what came to dinner: Parasites and your health.* New York: Avery Publishing Group Inc.

Gittelman, R., and B. Eskenazi. 1983. Lead and hyperactivity revisited: An investigation of nondisadvantaged children. *Archives of General Psychiatry* 40: 827–33.

Glassman, Mark S., et al. 1990. Cow's milk protein sensitivity during infancy in patients with inflammatory bowel disease. *The American Journal of Gastroenterology* 85 (no. 7): 838–840.

Glick, J. Leslie. 1990. Dementias: the role of magnesium deficiency and hypothesis concerning the pathogenesis of Alzheimer's disease. *Medical Hypothesis* 31: 211–225.

Gluck, Joan. Feb 1991. Asthma from aspartame. *Cortlandt Forum* 116: 36–49.

Glum, Gary. 1988. *Calling of an angel.* Silent Walker Publishing.

Goldenberg, D.L. 1989. Treatment of fibromyalgia syndrome. *Rheum. Dis. Clin. North. Am.* 15: 61.

Goldstrich, Joe D. 1994. *The cardiologist's painless prescription for a healthy heart and a longer life.* Dallas: 9-HEART-9 Publishing.

Goode, Helen F., et al. 1991. Evidence of cellular zinc depletion in hospitalized but not in healthy elderly subjects. *Age and Aging* 20: 345–348.

Gorbach, S. L. 1990. Lactic acid bacteria and human health. *Annals of Medicine* 22: 37–41.

Gottschall, Elaine. 1987. *Food and the gut reaction.* London, ON: The Kirkton Press.

Graham, Judy. 1989. *Multiple sclerosis: A self-help guide to its management.* Rochester, VT: Healing Arts Press.

Greenberg, S., and W. Frishman. 1990. Coenzyme Q10: A new drug for cardiovascular disease. *Journal of Clinical Pharmacology* 30: 596–608.

Gregory, Scott J. 1992. *A holistic protocol for the immune system.* California: Tree of Life Publications.

Grimes, D.S. 1976. Refined carbohydrate, smooth-muscle spasm and disease of the colon. *Lancet* 1: 395–97.

Gursche, Siegfried. 1993. *Healing with herbal juices.* Vancouver: Alive Books.

Haanen, H. C. 1991. Hypnotherapy relieves refractory fibromyalgia. *Journal of Rheumatology* 18: 72–75.

Haas, Elson M. 1992. *Staying healthy with nutrition: The complete guide to diet and nutritional medicine.* Berkeley, CA: Celestial Arts.

Haase, Gunter R., et al. May 15, 1990. Neuropathy: Diabetic? nutritional? *Patient Care*: 112-134.

Hamilton, Kirk. 1990. *Clinical pearls in nutrition and preventive medicine,* Sacramento, CA: IT Services.
(For subscriptions contact IT Services, 3301 Alta Arden #3, Sacramento, CA 95825 USA; 800-422-9887; 916-489-4400.)

Hamilton, Kirk. 1991. *CP Currents.* Sacramento, CA: IT Services.
(For subscriptions, contact IT Services, 3301 Alta Arden #3, Sacramento, CA 95825 USA; 800-422-9887; 916-489-4400.)

Hands, Elizabeth S. 1990. *Food finder, food sources vitamin and minerals.* Salem, OR: ESHA Research.

Harvey, Jean. 1990. Superior calcium absorption from calcium citrate than calcium carbonate using external forearm counting. *Journal of the American College of Nutrition* 9 (no. 6): 583–587.

Hathcock, John, N., et al. Evaluation of vitamin A toxicity. *American Journal of Clinical Nutrition* 52: 183–202. 1990.

Hathcock, John, N. 1992. Safety of vitamin supplements. *Vitamin Information* 7 (no. 2).

Hauser, W. E., and J. S. Remington. 1982. Effect of antibiotics on the immune response. *Am. J. Med.* 72: 711–16.

Heimlich, Jane. 1990. *What your doctor won't tell you.* New York: Harper Collins.

Hemila, H. 1992. Vitamin C and plasma cholesterol. *Critical Review in Food Science and Nutrition* 32 (no. 1): 33–57.

Hemila, H. 1991. Vitamin C and lowering blood pressure: need for intervention trials. *Journal of Hypertension* 9 (no. 11): 1076–1077.

Hendler, Sheldon Saul. 1991. *The purification prescription.* New York: William Morrow and Company.

Henken, Y., et al. Sept. 1991. Niacin revisited: Clinical observations on an important but underutilized drug. *The American Journal of Medicine.*

Hennekens, Charles, and Julie Buring, Richard Peto. 1994. Antioxidant vitamins: Benefits not yet proved. *The New England Journal of Medicine* 330 (no. 15): 1080–1081.

Henrich, J. B. 1992. The postmenopausal estrogen/breast cancer controversy. *JAMA* 268 (no. 14): 1900–1902.

Hofmann, J. 25–26 May, 1983. Ozone therapy in coronary heart disease. Paper presented at Sixth Ozone World Congress of the International Ozone Association, Washington, DC.

June 25, 1992. High cholesterol diet linked to sex problems. *Medical Tribune* 14.

Hoffmann, D. 1993. *The new holistic herbal.* MA: Element Books.

Holti, G. 1979. An experimentally controlled evaluation of the effect of inositol nicotinate upon the digital blood flow in patients with Raynaud's phenomenon. *J.Int.Med.Res.* 7: 473–83.

Howard, J. M. H. 1984. Clinical import of small increases in serum aluminum. *Clinical Chemistry* 30 (no. 10): 1722–3.

Huggins, Hal A. and Sharon A. Huggins. 1989. *It's all in your head.* Tacoma, WA: Life Sciences Press.

Hughes, E. G. 1992. Cigarette smoking: does it reduce fecundity? *Journal of the Society of Obstetricians and Gynecologists of Canada* 14 (no. 9): 27–37.

Hughes, J., and R. Norman. 1992. Diet and calcium stones. *Canadian Medical Association Journal* 146 (no. 2): 137–143.

Hunt, Douglas. 1987. *No more cravings.* New York: Warner Books .

Infante, M., et al. 1991. Laboratory evaluation during high dose vitamin A administration: a randomized study on lung cancer patients after surgical resection. *Journal of Cancer Research* 117: 156–62.

1991. *Is your family showing signs of stuttering?* New York, NY: The National Centre for Stuttering.
(200 East 33rd St., New York, NY 10016)

Iwasaki, Y., et al. 1992. Plasma amino acid levels in patients with amyotrophic lateral sclerosis. *Journal of Neurologic Sciences* 107: 219–222.

Jaffe, R., and O. Kruesi. 1992. *The biochemical-immunology window: A molecular view of psychiatric case management.* Journal of Applied Nutrition 44 (no. 2).

Jaffe, R. *Host defenses: An approach to risk identification and risk reduction in HIV+ individuals.* In press.

Janicijevic, Nenad. 1991. Numbness from aspartame. Cortlandt Forum 116: 36–49.

Johnson, Elizabeth, et al. 1992. Lack of an effect of multivitamins containing vitamin A on serum retinyl esters and liver function tests in healthy women. *Journal of the American College of Nutrition* 11 (no. 6): 682–686.

Johnston, Cameron. Nov. 1987. Malnutrition in hospitals is life-threatening. *The Medical Post* 17.

Juhlin, L. 1982. Blood glutathione-peroxidase levels in skin diseases: effect of selenium and vitamin E treatment. *Acta Derm. Venereol* (Stockh) 62 (no. 3): 211–14.

Kamen, Betty. 1993. *Hormone replacement therapy: Yes or no?* Novato, CA : Nutrition Encounter Inc.

Kaplan, H. K., et al. 1986. Behavioral effects of dietary sucrose in disturbed children. *American Journal of Psychiatry* 143 (no. 7): 944–45.

Karjalaimen J., and H. M. Dosch, et al. 1992. A bovine albumin peptide as a possible trigger of insulin-dependent diabetes mellitus. *The New England Journal of Medicine* 327 (no. 5): 302–307.

Kaufmann, Klaus. 1991. *Eliminating poison in your mouth.* Vancouver: Alive Books.

Kaufmann, Klaus. 1990. *The joy of juice fasting.* Vancouver: Alive Books.

Kaufmann, Klaus. 1990. *Silica: The forgotten nutrient.* Vancouver: Alive Books.

Kaufmann, Klaus. 1992. *Silica: The amazing gel.* Vancouver: Alive Books.

Kataoka, et al. 1990. Vitamin E status in pediatric patients receiving antiepileptic drugs. *Dev. Pharmacol.* Ther. 14: 96–101.

Keyser, A., and S. De Bruijn. 1991. Epileptic Manifestations and vitamin B1 deficiency. *European Neurology* 31: 121–125.

King, D. S. 1985. Statistical power of the controlled research on wheat gluten and schizophrenia. *Biol Psychiatry* 20 (no. 7): 785–7.

Kirk, Othmer. 1981. Ozone. *Encyclopedia of Chemical Technology* Vol. 16, 3rd ed. John Wiley & Sons, Inc.

Kirsch, M. 1990. Bacterial overgrowth. *American Journal of Gastroenterology.* Vol 85 (no. 3): 231-237.

Kirshon, B., and A. N. Poindexter. 1988. Contraception: a risk factor for endometriosis. *Obstetrics and Gynecology* 71: 829–31.

Kleijnen, Jos, and Paul Knipschild. 1992. Ginkgo biloba. *Lancet* 340: 1136—1139.

Kleiner, Susan M. 1992. Don't cook away those nutrients. *The Physician and Sports Medicine* 20 (no. 1): 15–16.

Klich, Barbara. March 19, 1991. Beware of the nasties in the kitchen. *The Medical Post*, p.19.

Knapp, Howard R. and Garrett Fitzgerald. 1989. The antihypertensive effects of fish oil. *New England Journal of Medicine* 320: 1037–1043.

Kohri, K., et al. 1989. Magnesium-to-calcium ratio in tap water and its relationship to geological features and the incidence of calcium-containing urinary stones. *Journal of Urology* 142: 1272–1275.

Kok, D.J., et al. 1990. The effects of dietary excesses in animal protein and in sodium on the composition and the crystallization of kinetics of calcium oxalate monohydrate in the urines of healthy men. *Journal of Clinical Endocrinology and Metabolism* 71 (no. 4): 861–867.

Kolate, Gina. April 17, 1994. Challenging the faith of the vitamin culture. *The New York Times.*

* Kolb, E. 1984. Recent knowledge concerning the biochemistry and significance of ascorbic acid. Z. *Gesamte Inn Med.* 39.

Konrad, Heinz. 25–26 May, 1983. Ozone vs. hepatitis and herpes: the choice. Paper presented at Sixth Ozone World Congress of the International Ozone Association, Washington, DC.

Koutsikos, D., et al. 1990. Biotin for diabetic peripheral neuropathy. *Biomed and Pharmacotherapy* 44: 511–514.

Kozlovsky, A. S., et al. 1986. Effects of diets high in simple sugars on urinary chromium losses. *Metabolism* 35 (no. 6): 515–18.

Kramer, Fritz. 25–26 May, 1983. Ozone in the dental practice. Paper presented at Sixth Ozone World Congress of the International Ozone Association, Washington, DC.

Krasinski, S. D., et al. 1989. Relationship of vitamin A and vitamin E intake to fasting plasma retinol, retinol-binding protein, retinyl esters, carotene, alpha-tocopherol and cholesterol among elderly people and young adults: increased plasma retinyl esters among vitamin A supplement users. *American Journal of Clinical Nutrition* 49:112–20.

Krueger, Guenther. February 11, 1992. Vancouver MD rocks the status quo about estrogen replacement therapy. *The Medical Post* p.30.

Kruis, W., et al. 1991. Effects of diets low and high in refined sugars on gut transit, bile acid metabolism and bacterial fermentation. *Gut* 32: 367–371.

Kuhne, T., et al. 1991. Maternal vegan diet causing a serious infantile neurologic disorder due to vitamin B12 deficiency. *European Journal of Pediatrics* 150: 205–208.

Kurpad, A. V., et al. 1989. Reduced thermoregulatory thermogenesis in undernutrition. *European Journal of Clinical Nutrition* 43: 27–33.

Lands, Lark. 1991. *Therapeutic basics for people living with HIV.* Washington, DC: Carl Vogel Foundation. (1413 K. St. NW, 14th floor, 20005; 202-289-4898; for phone consultations with the author, call 717-794-5471.)

Lands, Lark. 1991. *Dietary guidelines for people living with HIV.* Washington, DC: Carl Vogel Foundation. (1413 K. St. NW, 14th floor, 20005; 202-289-4898; for phone consultations with the author, 717-794-5471.)

Lands, Lark. 1992. *HIV treatment strategy, parts 1, 2 and 3: Drug information for people living with HIV.* Washington, DC: Carl Vogel Foundation. (1413 K. St. NW, 14th floor, 20005; 202-289-4898; for phone consultations with the author, 717-794-5471.)

Lands, Lark. *Positively well: AIDS as a chronic, manageable, survivable disease.* Washington, DC: Carl Vogel Foundation. (1413 K. St. NW, 14th floor, 20005; 202-289-4898; for phone consultations with the author, 717-794-5471.)

Lane, William I., and L. Comac. 1992. *Sharks don't get cancer: How shark cartiage could save your life.* Garden City, New York: Avery Publishing Group.

Langsjoen, P. H., and K. Folkers. 1990. Long-term efficacy and safety of coenzyme Q10 therapy for idiopathic dilated cardiomyopathy. *American Journal of Cardiology* 65: 521–523.

LaPerchia, P. 1987. Behavioral disorders, learning disabilities and megavitamin therapy. *Adolescence* (U.S.) 22: 729–38.

Lappe, Frances Moore. 1982. *Diet for a small planet,* 10th ed. New York: Ballantine.

Last, J. A., and D. L. Warren, E. Pecquet-Goad, H. Witschi. 1987. Modification by ozone of lung tumor development in mice. *J Natl. Cancer Inst.* 78 (no. 1): 149–54.

Laton, Thomas. (Sept.) 1990. Restless leg syndrome secondary to iron deficiency. *Journal of Osteopathic Medicine* 54.

Laurent, J., and G. Lagrue. 1989. Dietary manipulation for idiopathic nephrotic syndrome: A new approach to therapy. *Allergy* 44:599–603.

Leppert, J., et al. 1990. Lower serum magnesium level after exposure to cold in women with primary Raynaud's phenomenon. *J. Intern. Med.* 228: 235–9.

Lee, John R. 1990. Osteoporosis reversal: The role of progesterone. *International Clinical Nutrition Review* 10 (no. 3): 384–391.

Lee, John R. 1994. *Natural Progesterone.* Sebastopol, CA: BLL Publishing.

Lee, S. 1980. Ozone selectively inhibits growth of human cancer cells. *Science* 209: 931–932.

Lessoff, M. H., ed. 1983. *Clinical reactions to foods.* Chichester: Wiley & Sons.

Levinson, Paul D., et al. 1990. Effect of N-3 fatty acids in essential hypertension. *American Journal of Public Health* 13: 754–760.

Levy, Sheldon L., et al. 1990. An evaluation of the anticonvulsant effects of vitamin E. *Epilepsy Research* 6: 12–17.

Lin, David. Jan 1993. Esterified vitamin E acetate and succunate: therapeutically active, preferred - and well documented. *Townsend Letter for Doctors* 26–29

Li, J-Y, and P. R. Taylor, et al. 1993. Nutrition intervention trials in Linxian, China: Supplementation with specific vitamin/mineral combinations, cancer incidence and disease-specific mortality among adults with esophageal dysplasia. *J. Natl. Cancer Inst* 85 (no. 18): 1492–1498.

Lieb, J. 1979. Remission of recurrent herpes infection during therapy with lithium. *New England Journal of Medicine* 301: 942.

Lipski, P. S., et al. 1993. A study of nutritional deficits of long-stay geriatric patients. *Age and Aging* 22: 244–255.

Dec 21,1991. Lithium may relieve herpes. *Medical Tribune* 2.

Loomis, Donald. 1990. Fatal poisonings from vitamin supplements. *Preventive Medicine Update* 10 (no. 3).

Loomis, Donald C. 1993. Fatalities resulting from poisonings in the United States. *Health Action* (Summer) 6.

Lukaski, Henry C., et al. 1986. Validation of tetrapolar bioelectrical impedance method to assess human body composition. *Journal of Applied Physiology* 60:1327–32.

Lui, Edmund, et al. 1990. Metals and the liver in Alzheimer's disease: an investigation of hepatic zinc, copper, cadmium and metallothionein, *Journal of the American Geriatric Society* 38 (no. 6): 633–639.

MacKarness, R. 1976. *Not All in the Mind.* London, England: Pan Books.

Majumdar, S. K., and P. P. Kahad. 1981. Serum vitamin B-12 status in chronic schizophrenic patients. *Journal of Human Nutrition* 35.

Mandell, Marshall, and Fran Gare Mandell. 1983. *It's not your fault you're fat diet.* New York: Harper and Rowe.

Marson, A. R. 1984. Elevated retinol levels may play an important role in the development of some attacks of gouty arthritis. *Lancet* 1: 1181.

Martin, Jeanne Marie.1991. *All natural allergy cookbook, The.* Madeira Park, BC: Harbour Publishing.

Martin, Jeanne Marie. 1982. *For the love of food.* New York: Ballantine.

Martin, Jeanne Marie. 1989. *Hearty vegetarian soups and stews.* Madeira Park, BC: Harbour Publishing.

Martin, Jeanne Marie.1993. *Vegan delights.* Madeira Park, BC: Harbour Publishing.

Mattasi, R. M. D., et al. 25–26 May, 1983. Ozone as therapy in herpes simplex and herpes zoster diseases. Paper presented at Sixth Ozone World Congress of the International Ozone Association, Washington, DC.

Maurizi, C. 1985. Could supplementary dietary tryptophan and taurine prevent epileptic seizures? *Medical Hypothesis* 18: 411–15.

McCabe, Ed. 1988. *Oxygen therapies: A new way of approaching disease.* Morrisville, NY: Energy Publications.

McCain G. A., et al. 1988. A controlled study of the effects of a supervised cardiovascular fitness training program on the manifestations of primary fibromyalgia. *Arthritis Rheum* 31: 1135.

McConville, B. J., et al. 1991. Nicotine may help reduce the frequency in Tourette's. *American Journal of Psychiatry* 148: 793–794.

McDougall, John A., and Mary A. McDougal. 1983. *The McDougall plan.* New Jersey: New Century Publishers, Inc.

McDougall, John A. 1985. *McDougall's medicine: A challenging second opinion.* New Jersey: New Century Publishers, Inc.

McDougall, John A. 1992. *The McDougall report: Lifesaving facts your doctor never told you.* Seattle, WA: Trillium Health Products.

McGrady, Angele, et al. 1991. Sustained effects of biofeedback-assisted relaxation therapy in essential hypertension. *Biofeedback and Self-Regulation* 16 (no. 4): 399–410.

Menzies, I. C. 1984. Disturbed children: the role of food and chemical sensitivities. *Nutrition and Health* 3: 39–54 .

Milhorat, A. T., et al. 1945. Effect of wheat germ on creatinuria and progressive muscular dystrophy. *Proc. Soc. Exp. Biol. Med.* 58: 40–1.

Mills, Simon Y. 1988. *The dictionary of modern herbalism.* Rochester, VT: Healing Arts Press.

Mindell, E. 1992. *Earl Mindell's herb bible.* New York: Simon & Schuster.

Mitsuoka, T. 1990. Bifidobacteria and their role in human health. *Journal of Industrial Microbiology* 6: 263–268.

Mitchell, Braxton D. 1990. Cigarette smoking and neuropathy. *Diabetic Care* 13 (no. 4): 434–437.

Moldofsky, H. 1989. Sleep and fibrositis syndrome. *Rheum. Dis. Clin. North Am.* 15: 91.

Monti, D., et al. 1992. Apoptosis - programmed cell death: a role in the aging process? *American Journal of Clinical Nutrition* 55: 1208S–14S.

Moran, John P., et al. 1993. Plasma ascorbic acid concentrations relate inversely to blood pressure in human subjects. *American Journal of Clinical Nutrition* 57: 213–7.

Morris, David J., et al. 1990. Licorice, tobacco chewing and hypertension. *The New England Journal of Medicine* 322 (no. 12): 849.

Moss, Ralph W. 1991. *The Cancer Industry.* New York: Paragon House.

Moss, Ralph W. 1992. *Cancer therapy: The independent consumer's guide to non-toxic treatment and prevention.* New York: Equinox Press.

Moss, Ralph W. 1994. *The Cancer Chronicles Newsletter, serious consideration of alternative ideas.* New York: Equinox Press.
(For subscription, write to Equinoc Press, 144 St. John's Place, Brooklyn, NY 11217; or call 800-929-WELL.)

Murata, A. 1975. Virucidal activity of vitamin C: Vitamin C for prevention and treatment of viral diseases. Proceedings of the first Intersectional Congress of the international Association of the Microbiological Society 3: 432–42. Tokyo: Tokyo University Press.

Murty, G. E., et al. 1990. The etiology and management of glossodynia. *British Journal of Clinical Practice* 44 (no. 8): 389–392.

The National Council Against Health Fraud, Inc. Newsletter. Loma Linda, CA. The National Council Against Health Fraud, Inc.
(Write for subscriptions ($15.00US) PO Box 1276, Loma Linda, CA. 92534.)

Nault, Kate. Dec 1988. AIDS, cancer answer: Blowin' in the Wind. *Crosswinds*, p. 7–18.

Neu, H. C. 1992. The crisis in antibiotic resistance. *Science* 257:1064–1073.

Nityanand, S. et al. 1989. Clinical trials with gugulipid, a new hypolipidemic agent. *Journal of the Association of Physicians of India* 37: 321–8.

Norman, R.W., and W.A. 1990. Manette. Dietary restriction of sodium as a means of reducing dietary cystine. *Journal of Urology* 143: 1193–1194.

Ody, P. 1993. *The complete medicinal herbal.* New York: Dorling Kindersley.

Oishi, M. et al. 1990. Hair trace elements in amyotrophic lateral sclerosis. *Trace Elements in Medicine* 7 (no. 4): 182–185.

Okayama, H. et al. 1991. Treatment of status asthmaticus with intravenous magnesium sulfate. *Journal of Asthma* 28: 11–17.

Olson, Randall J. et al. 1991. Antioxidants and macular degeneration. *Journal of Cataract and Refractive Surgery* 17: 245–246.

Olson, Randall J. 1991. Supplemental vitamins and minerals in patients with macular degeneration. *Journal of the American College of Nutrition* 10 (no. 5; abstract 52): 550.

Ono, S., and Yamauchi, M. 1992. Glutamate and aspartate are decreased in the skin in amyotrophic lateral sclerosis. *ACTA Neurol. Scand.* 82: 481–484.

Orman, David J. May 1993. Letter to the editor. *Townsend Letter for Doctors.* 468–469.

Ornish, Dean et al. 1990. Can lifestyle changes reverse coronary heart disease? *Lancet* 336: 129–133.

Ornish, Dean. 1990. *Program for reversing heart disease.* New York: Ballantine Books.

Ovesen, L. 1984. Vitamin therapy in the absence of obvious deficiency. *DRUGS* 27.

Palacios, M., and R. A. Ingram. 1992. On the trail of burning feet. *Cortlandt Forum* 110: 49–11.

Patki, P. S. et al. 1990. Efficacy of potassium and magnesium in essential hypertension in a double-blind, placebo-controlled crossover study. *British Medical Journal* 301: 521–523.

Passwater, Richard A., and Elmer M. Cranton. 1983. *Trace elements, hair analysis and nutrition.* New Canaan, CT: Keats Publishing, Inc.

Pasquall R., and M. P. Cesari et al. 1987. Does ephedrine promote weight loss in low energy adapted obese women? *International Journal of Obesity* 11: 163–68

Pearson, D., and S. Shaw. 1982. *Life extension.* New York: Warner.

Peltz, James F. July 29, 1993. Alternative to surgery boosted: Mutual of Omaha to pay for heart therapy stressing diet, exercise. *The Sacramento Bee*, p. A8.

Perrone, L. et al. 1990. Impaired zinc metabolic status in children affected by idiopathic nephrotic syndrome. *European Journal of Pediatrics* 149: 438–440.

Petri, W .M., T. A. Ban, and J. V. Anath. 1981. The use of nicotinic acid and pyridoxine in the treatment of schizophrenia. *International Pharmacopsychiatry* 16.

Pfeiffer, C. C. 1984. Schizophrenia and wheat gluten enteropathy. *Biol Psychiatry* 19 (no. 3): 279–80.

Pfeiffer, C. C. 1975. *Mental and elemental nutrients.* New Canaan, CT: Keats Publishing, Inc.

Pfeiffer, C. C. 1978. *Zinc and other micronutrients.* New Canaan, CT: Keats Publishing, Inc.

Pfeiffer, Eric. 1988. What's new in Alzheimer's disease? *Postgraduate Medicine* 83 (no. 5): 107–115.

Philpott, W. H., and D. Kalita 1987. *Brain allergies: The psychonutrient connection.* New Canaan, CT: Keats Publishing.

Pizzorno, Joseph E. Jr., and Michael T. Murray. 1989. *Textbook of natural medicine.* Seattle, WA: John Bastyr College Publications.

Pizzorno, Joseph E. Jr., and Michael T. Murray. 1991. *An encyclopedia of natural medicine*. Rocklin, CA: Prima Publishing.

Plaitakis, A. 1990. Glutamate dysfunction and selective motoneuron degeneration in amyotrophic lateral sclerosis: a hypothesis. *Annals of Neurology* 28 (no. 1): 3–7.

Pritchard, Chris. Feb. 9. 1993. Vitamin A linked to birth defects. *Medical Post*.

Pogessi, L. et al. 1991. Effect of coenzyme Q10 on left ventricular function in patients with dilative cardiomyopathy. *Current Therapeutic Research* 49: 878–886.

Porikos, K.P., and T. B. Van Itallie. 1983. Diet-induced changes in serum transaminase and triglyceride levels in healthy adult men: Role of sucrose and excess calories. *American Journal of Medicine* 75: 624.

Portz, Douglas et al. 1991. Oxygen free radicals and pelvic adhesion formation: Blocking oxygen free radical toxicity to prevent adhesion formation in an endometriosis model. *International Journal of Fertility* 36 (no. 1): 39–42.

Prasad, A.S. 1982. Clinical, biochemical and nutritional aspects of trace elements. Current topics in nutrition and disease. Vol. 6. New York: Alan R. Liss.

April 30, 1993. Providers estimate one in four malnourished. *Nutrition Week*.

Pujalte, J. M. et al. 1990. Double-blind clinical evaluation of glucosamine sulfate in the basic treatment of osteoarthritis. *Curr. Med. Res. Opin.* 7: 110–114.

Puharich, H.A. May 25–26 1983. Successful treatment of neoplasms in mice with gaseous superoxide anion and ozone; with a rationale for the effect. Paper presented at Sixth Ozone World Congress of the International Ozone Association, at Washington, DC.

Q-L Choo, A.J., and L.R. Weiner, et al. Hepatitis C virus: the major causative agent of viral non-A, non-B hepatitis. *British Medical Bulletin* 46 (no. 2): 423–441.

Qadri, S. M. H. et al. (Nov.) 1989. Clinical significance of blastocystis hominis, *Journal of Clinical Microbiology* 2407–2409.

Rabinovitch, R. et al. 1951. Neuromuscular disorders amenable to wheat germ oil therapy. *J. Neurol. Neurosurg. Psychiat.* 14: 95–100.

Rai, G. S. et al. 1991. A double-blind, placebo-controlled study of ginkgo biloba extract in elderly outpatients with mild to moderate memory impairment. *Current Medical Research and Opinion* 12 (no. 6): 350–355.

Rachlis, Michael, and Carol Kushner. 1989. *Second opinion: What's wrong with canada's health-care system and how to fix it*. Toronto, ON: Collins.

Raloff, J. April 25, 1992. Microwaving can lower breast milk benefits. *Science News*, 141 261.

Randolph, T. G., and R. W. Moss. 1980. *Allergies: Your hidden enemy*. New York: Lippincott & Crowell.

Rapp, Doris J. 1979. *Allergies and the hyperactive child*. New York: Cornerstone Library (Simon & Schuster).

Rapp, Doris J. 1980. *Allergies and your family*. New York: Sterling Publishing.

Rappaport, E. M. 1955. Achlorhydria: associated symptoms and response to hydrochloric acid. *New England Journal of Medicine* 252 (no. 19): 802–5

Rasic, J.L., and J.A. Kurmann. 1983. *Bifidobacterium and their role*. Basel, Boston, Stuttgart: Birkhauser Verlag.

Rea, W. J. 1977. Environmentally triggered small vessel vasculitis. *Annals of Allergy* 38: 245–51.

Rea, W. J. et al. 1975. Environmentally triggered large vessel vasculitis. *Allergy: Immunology and medical treatment*. Chicago, IL: Symposia Specialists.

Rea, W. J. and C.W. Suits. 1980. Cardiovascular disease triggered by foods and chemicals. *Food allergy: New perspectives*, Springfield, IL: Charles C. Thomas.

Read, M.H., and G.C. Lauritzen. 1994. Supplementation recommendations by a sample of registered dietitians. *Top. Clin. Nutr.* 9: 67–72.

Reiser, S. Szepesi. 1978. SCOGS report on the health aspects of sucrose consumption. *American Journal of Clinical Nutrition* 31: 9–11.

Reynolds, E. H. 1992. Multiple sclerosis and vitamin B12 metabolism. *Journal of Neurology, Neurosurgery and Psychiatry* 55: 339–340.

Rilling, S., and R. Viebahn. 1987. *The use of ozone in medicine*. Heidelberg: Karl F. Haug Publishers.

Ring E. F. J. et al. 1981. Quantitative thermal imaging to assess inositol nicotinate treatment of Raynaud's syndrome. *J.Int. Med. Res.* 9: 393–99.

Riva-Sanseverino, E. May 25–26, 1983. The influence of ozone therapy on the remineralization of the bone tissue in osteoporosis. Paper presented at Sixth Ozone World Congress of the International Ozone Association, Washington, DC.

Robbins, John. 1987. *Diet for a new america.* Walpole, New Hampshire: Stillpoint.

Robbins, John. 1992. *May all be fed: Diet for a new world.* New York: William Morrow and Company.

Roberts, H. J. 1991. Does aspartame cause human brain cancer? *Journal Of Advancement of Medicine Winter* (no. 4): 231–241.

Rokitansky, O. 25–26 May, 1983. The clinical effects and biochemistry of ozone therapy in peripheral arterial circulatory disturbances. Paper presented at Sixth Ozone World Congress of the International Ozone Association, at Washington, DC.

Rodin, Donald O., and Clara Felix. 1987. *The omega-3 phenomenon.* New York: Rawson Associates.

Rona, Zoltan P. 1991. *Fertility control: The natural approach.* Toronto, ON: S.R. Vitamins.

Rona, Zoltan P. 1991. *The joy of health: A doctor's guide to nutrition and alternative medicine.* Toronto: Hounslow Press.

Rooney, James F. et al. 1991. Prevention of ultraviolet light-induced herpes labialis by sunscreen. *Lancet* 338: 1419–22.

Rose, G. A. Feb 1993. *Food sensitivity and epilepsy.* Journal of the Royal Society of Medicine 86: 119.

Rosenbaum, Michael, and Murray Susser. 1992. *Solving the puzzle of chronic fatigue syndrome.* Tacoma, WA: Life Sciences Press.

Rosenberg, I. H. et al. 1985. Nutritional aspects of inflammatory bowel disease. *Annual Review of Nutrition* 5: 463–84.

Rosenberg, I. H., and J. W. Miller. 1992. Nutritional factors in physical and cognitive functions of elderly people. *American Journal of Clinical Nutrition* 55: 123S–43S.

Rosmarin, Phillip C. et al. 1990. Coffee consumption and blood pressure: a randomized, crossover clinical trial. *The Journal of General Internal Medicine* 5: 211–213.

Rossner, S., G. Walldius, and H. Bjorvell. 1989. Fatty acid composition in serum lipids and adipose tissue in severe obesity before and after six weeks of weight loss. *International Journal of Obesity* 13: 603–612.

Rothstein, Jeffrey et al. 1992. Decreased glutamate transport by the brain and spinal cord in amyotrophic lateral sclerosis. *New England Journal of Medicine* 326 (no. 22): 1464–1468.

Rowland, David. *How to give nutritional advice legally.* Uxbridge, ON: Canadian Nutrition Institute.

(Canadian Nutrition Institute, PO Box 1650, Uxbridge, ON L9P 1T2; 416-852-6175)

Royal College of Physicians and the British Nutritional Foundation. April 1984. Food intolerance and food aversion. *Journal of the Royal College of Physicians* 18: 2.

Rudin, D. O. 1981. The major psychoses and neuroses as omega-3 essential fatty acid deficiency syndrome: substrate pellagra. *Biological Psychiatry* 16.

Rugg-Gunn, A. J. 1991. Empty calories? Nutrient intake in relation to sugar intake in English adolescents. *Journal of Human Nutrition and Dietetics* 4: 101–111.

Russell R. M., J. L. Boyer, S. A. Bagheri, et al. 1974. Hepatic injury from chronic hypervitaminosis A resulting in portal hypertension and ascites. *N. Engl. J.of Med.* 291: 435.

Russo, P. J. Dec. 15, 1992. NSAID-induced gastroenteropathy: A biochemical dissection. *Hospital Practice*: 123-132.

Sahakian, V. et al. 1991. Vitamin B6 is effective therapy for nausea and vomiting of pregnancy: a randomized, double-blind placebo-controlled study. *Obstetrics and Gynecology* 78: 33–36.

Salway, F. G. et al. Dec 16, 1978. Effect of myoinositol on peripheral nerve function in diabetes. *Lancet* 2: 1282–84.

Sanchez, A. Reeser et al. 1973. Role of sugars in human neutrophilic phagocytosis. *Am. J. Clin. Nutr.* 26: 1, 180–4.

Scanlon, Deralee. 1991. *Diets that work.* Los Angeles, CA: Contemporary Books.

Schauss, A. G. 1984. Nutrition and behavior: Complex interdisciplinary research. *Nutrition and Health* 3: 9–37.

Schmidt, M. A., L. H. Smith, and K. W. Sehnert. 1992. *Beyond antibiotics: Healthier options for families.* Berkeley, CA: North Atlantic Books.

Schorah, C. J., D. B. Morgan, and R. P. Hullin. 1983. Plasma vitamin C concentrations in patients in a psychiatric hospital. *Hum. Nutr. Clin. Nutr.* 37 (no. 6): 447–52.

Schwartz, A. G. Biological role of Dehydroepiandrosterone. *The Gerontologist* 32 (no. 3): 425. 1992.

Scott, F. W. Hypothesis. 1990. Cow milk and insulin-dependent diabetes mellitus: is there a relationship? *American Journal of Clinical Nutrition* 51: 489–91.

Scott, et al. 1988. Evidence for a critical role of diet in the development of insulin-dependent diabetes mellitus. *Diabetes Research* 7: 153–157.

Selye, Hans. 1974. *Stress without distress.* New York: Signet.

Selye, Hans. 1976. *Stress in health and disease.* Boston/London: Butterworths.

Sharon, Michael. 1989. Complete nutrition: How to live in total health. London: *PRION.*

Shklar, G., and J. Schwartz. 1993. Oral cancer inhibition by micronutrients: The experimental basis for clinical trials. *Oral Oncol. Eur. J. Cancer* 29B (no. 1): 9–16.

Siblerud, R. L. The relationship between mercury from dental amalgam and mental health. *American Journal of Psychotherapy* 58: 575–87.1989.

Siegel, Bernie S. 1986. *Love, medicine and miracles.* New York: Harper & Row.

Siegel, Bernie S. 1989. *Peace, love and healing.* New York: Harper & Row.

Siegel, Bernie S. 1993. *How to live between office visits: A guide to life, love and health.* New York: Harper-Collins.

Siegel, J. 1981. Inflammatory bowel disease: Another possible facet of the allergic diathesis. *Annals of Allergy* 47:92–94.

Siguel, Edward N. 1994. *Essential fatty acids in health and disease.* Brookline, MA: Nutrek Press.

Sinaiko, Alan R., et al. 1993. Effect of low sodium diet or potassium supplementation on adolescent blood pressure. *Hypertension* 21 (no. 6): 989–994.

Singh, R. B., et al. 1990. Dietary modulators of blood pressure and hypertension. *European Journal of Clinical Nutrition* 44: 319–327.

Singh, R. B., et al. 1990. Does dietary management of minerals prevent aggravation of hypertension in humans? *Trace Elements in Medicine* 7 (no. 3): 149–154.

Singh, R. B., et al. 1991. Dietary changes modulate blood pressure and blood lipids in hypertension. *Journal of Nutritional Medicine* 2: 17–24.

Skelton, William Paul, and Khouzman Skelton. 1990. Vitamin B deficiency and neuropathy: Case reports. *Journal of the American Podiatric Association* 80 (no. 5): 254–256.

Skinner, G., C. Hartley, A. Bucham, et al. 1980. The effect of lithium chloride on the replication of herpes simplex virus. *Medical Microbiology and Immunology* 168: 139–48.

Smith, L. H. 1991. Diet and hyperoxaluria and the syndrome of idiopathic calcium oxalate urolithiasis. *American Journal of Kidney Diseases* 17 (no. 4): 370–375.

Smith, L. 1983. *Feed yourself right.* New York: McGraw-Hill.

Smythe, H. A. 1989. Nonarticular rheumatism and psychogenic musculoskeletal syndrome. *Arthritis and allied conditions: A textbook of rheumatology.* 11th ed. Philadelphia: Lea & Febiger.

Snow, Sheila. *The essence of essiac.* (Sheila Snow, Box 396, Port Carling, ON P0B 1J0.)

Snowdon, D. A., and R. L. Phillips. 1985. Does a vegetarian diet reduce the occurrence of diabetes? *American Journal of Public Health* 75: 507–12.

Solomons, N. W., and I. H. Rosenberg. 1984. Absorption and malabsorption of mineral nutrients. *In Current topics in nutrition and disease.* New York: Alan R. Liss.

Stevens, C. E. et al. 1990. Epidemiology of hepatitis C virus: A preliminary study in volunteer blood donors. *Journal of the American Medical Association* 263 (no.1): 49–53.

Stryker, W. S., L. A. Kaplan, E. A. Stein, et al. 1988. The relation of diet, cigarette smoking and alcohol consumption to plasma beta-carotene and alpha-tocopherol levels. *Am. J. Epidemiol* 127: 283–296.

Sunderland, G. T. et al. 1988. A double blind randomised placebo controlled trial of hexopal in primary Raynaud's disease. *Clin. Rheumatol.* 7 (no. 1): 46–49.

Sunnen, Gerard U. Ozone in medicine: Overview and future directions. *Journal of Advancement in Medicine.* In press.

Suzuki, H. et al. 1986. Cianidanol therapy for HBe-antigen-positive chronic hepatitis: A multicentre, double-blind study. *Liver* 6: 35.

Swank, R. L. 1970. Multiple sclerosis: 20 years on a low fat diet. *Archives of Neurology* 23: 460–74.

Swank, R. L. 1987. *The multiple sclerosis diet book.* New York: Doubleday.

Swank, R. L., and B. B. Dugan. 1990. Effect of low saturated fat diet in early and late cases of multiple sclerosis. *Lancet* 336: 37–39.

Tanner, Caroline M., and William Langston. 1990. Do environmental toxins cause Parkinson's disease? *Neurology* 40 (suppl. 3): 17–28.

Taussig, S., M. Yokoyama, et al. 1975. Bromelain, a proteolytic enzyme and its clinical application: A review. *Hiroshima J. Med. Sci.* 24:185–193.

Taussig, S. 1980. The mechanism of the physiological action of bromelain. *Med. Hypothesis* 6: 99–104.

Taylor, A. Aug. 1985. Trace elements in human disease. *Clinics in Endocrinology and Metabolism* 14: 3.

Taylor, Joyal. 1988. *The complete guide to mercury toxicity from dental fillings*. San Diego, CA: Scripps Publishing.

Tenney, Louise. 1983. *Today's herbal health*. Provo, UT: Woodland Health Books.

Tenney, Louise. 1991. *Nutritional guide with food combining*. Provo, UT: Woodland Health Books.

Theiss, Barbara and Peter. 1989. *The family herbal*. Rochester, VT: Healing Arts Press.

Thornton, J. R. et al. Feb 2, 1980. Diet and ulcerative colitis. *British Medical Journal*: 293.

Tintera, John W. 1980. *Hypoadrenocorticism*. New York: Hypoglycemia Foundation Inc.

Treben, Maria. 1990. *Health through God's pharmacy*. 15th ed. Steyr, Austria: Ennsthaler.

Tryphonas, H., and R. Trites. 1979. Food allergy in children with hyperactivity, learning disabilities and/or minimal brain dysfunction. *Annals of Allergy* 42: 22–7.

Tyber, M. Lithium carbonate augmentation therapy in fibromyalgia. *Canadian Medical Association Journal* 143 (no. 9): 902–904. 1990.

Tyler, Allen N. Bromelain: Proven effective in trauma, injury and pain therapy. *Holistic Update*. (Thorne Research Distributing Ltd. Langley, BC; 800-663-6369.)

Tyler, V. E. 1993. *The honest herbal: A sensible guide to the use of herbs and related remedies*. Binghamton, NY: The Haworth Press.

Van Voorhees, Abby S., and Michelle Riba. 1992. Acquired zinc deficiency in association with anorexia nervosa: case report and review of the literature. *Pediatric Dermatology* 9 (no. 3): 268–271.

Various authors. 1992. *Scientific American Medicine Consult* (on compact disc), St. Paul: Scientific American Inc.

Varro, J. 25–26 May, 1983. Ozone application in cancer cases. Paper presented at Sixth Ozone World Congress of the International Ozone Association, Washington, DC.

Vaz, A. 1982. Double-blind clinical evaluation of the relative efficacy of glucosamine sulfate in the management of osteoarthritis of the knee in outpatients. *Curr. Med. Res. Opin.* 8: 145–149.

Vilaseca, J. et al. 1990. Dietary fish oil reduces progression of chronic inflammatory lesions in a rat model of granulomatous colitis. *Gut* 31: 539–544.

Voirin, J., et al. 1989. Vitamin and trace element status in children with progressive muscular dystrophy. *Trace Elements in Medicine* 6 (no. 4): 165–168.

Volicer, Ladislav, Peter B. Crino, et al. 1990. Involvement of free radicals in dementia of the Alzheimer type: A hypothesis. *Neurobiology of Ageing* 11: 567–571.

Wabner, Cindy L. 1992. Modification by food of calcium absorbability and physiochemical effects of calcium citrate. *Journal of the American College of Nutrition* 11 (no. 5): 548–552.

Walker, A. R. P. 1991. Sugar, a love/hate situation: What should the clinician's common nutritionist, dietitian tell patients and the public? *International Clinical Nutrition Review* 11 (no. 1): 10–23.

Walker, Martin J. 1993. *Dirty Medicine: Science, big business and the assault on natural health care*. London: Slingshot Publications. (Available from Citizens for Health, P.O. Box 368, Tacoma, WA 98401; 206-922-2457.)

Walker, Martin J. July 1994. Letter to the editor. *Townsend Letter for Doctors* 698–698.

Walker, W. R., and D. M. Keats. 1976. An investigation of the therapeutic value of the copper bracelet: dermal assimilation of copper in arthritic/rheumatoid conditions. *Agents Actions* 6: 454.

Walters, Richard. 1993. *Options: the alternative cancer therapy book*. New York: Avery Publishing Group.

Warburg, Otto. 1956. On the origin of cancer cells. *Science* 123: 309–315.

Ward, Neil I. et al. 1990. The influence of the chemical additive tartrazine on the zinc status of hyperactive children: A double-blind placebo-controlled study. *Journal of Nutritional Medicine* 1:51–57.

Warren, Tom. 1991. *Beating Alzheimer's*. Garden City Park, NY: Avery publishing Group.

Weide, M. et al. 1991. Study of immune function of cancer patients influenced by supplemental zinc or selenium-zinc combination. *Biological Trace Element Research* 28 (no. 1): 11–20.

Weiss, Gabrielle. 1990. Hyperactivity in childhood. *New England Journal of Medicine* 323 (no. 20): 1413–1414.

Wells, K. H., J. Latino, J. Gavalchin, and B. J. Poiesz. 1991. Inactivation of human immunodeficiency virus type 1 by ozone in vitro. *Blood* 78 (no. 7): 1882–90

Werbach, Melvyn R. 1989. *Nutritional influences on illness*. Northamptonshire, England: Thorsons.

Werbach, Melvyn R. 1993. *Nutritional influences on illness, 2nd ed*. Tarzana, CA:Third LinePress.

Werbach, Melvyn R. 1991. *Nutritional influences on mental illness.* Northamptonshire, England: Thorsons.

Werbach, Melvyn R. and Michael T. Murray. 1994. *Botanical influences on illness.* Tarzana, CA: Third Line Press.

Whiting, Susan, and Michelle Pluhator. 1992. Comparison of in vitro and in vivo tests for determination of availability of calcium from calcium carbonate tablets. *Journal of the American College of Nutrition* 11 (no. 5): 553–560.

Whitaker, Julian. 1985. *Reversing heart disease.* New York: Warner.

Whitaker, Julian. 1993. Reversing arthritis. *Health and Healing today.* Vol.3 (no.6).

White, James R. 1981. *Jump for joy.* San Diego: University of California.

Willard, Terry. 1992. *Edible and medicinal plants of the rocky mountains and neighbouring territories.* Calgary, Alberta: Wild Rose College of Natural Healing.

Willard, Terry. 1988. *Textbook of modern herbology.* Calgary, Alberta: Progressive Publishing.

Willard, Terry. 1991. *The wild rose scientific herbal.* Calgary, Alberta: Wild Rose College of Natural Healing.

Willard, Terry. 1992. *Textbook of advanced herbology.* Calgary, Alberta: Wild Rose College of Natural Healing.

Willard, Terry. 1985. *Feeling good with natural remedies.* Calgary, Alberta: Wild Rose College of Natural Healing.

Williams, Lynn, and Brian Haskins. 1993. *Breaking through the weight loss barrier with EverTrim.* Denver: Health Sciences.

Wilson, Denis E. 1991. *Wilson's syndrome: The miracle of feeling well.* Longwood, FL: Cornerstone Publishing.
(This book is available by calling 800-621-7006.)

Wilson, Nevin W. et al. 1990. Severe cow's milk induced colitis in an exclusively breast-fed neonate. *Clinical Pediatrics* 29 (no. 2): 77–80.

Winterberg, B., R. Korte, and A. E. Lison. Clinical impact of aluminum load in kidney transplant recipients. *Trace Elements in Medicine* 8 (suppl. 1): 46–48.

Wolfe, F. H. A. Smythe, M. B. Yunus, et al. 1990. The american college of rheumatology criteria for the classification of fibromyalgia: Report of the multicenter criteria committee. *Arthritis Rheum.* 33: 160.

Wright, J. 1983. *Dr. Wright's book of nutritional therapy.* Emmaus, PA: Rodale Press.

Wright, Jonathan V., Russell M. Jaffe, and Alan R. Gaby. 1991. *Laboratory diagnosis in nutritional medicine.* (Two-day seminar, 13–15 April, Orlando, FL. Available on audio cassette: Meridian Valley Clin. Lab., 24040 132nd Ave. S.E., Kent, WA 98042; 206-631-8922.)

Yamaguchi, T. et al. 1992. Selenium concentration and glutathione peroxidase activity in plasma and erythrocytes from human blood. *Journal of Clinical Biochemical Nutrition* 12: 41–50.

Yasui, M. et al. 1991. High aluminum deposition in central nervous system of patients with amyotrophic lateral sclerosis from the Kii Peninsula, Japan: two case reports. *Neurotoxicology* 12: 277–284.

Yasui, M. et al. 1992. Magnesium and calcium contents in CNS tissues of amyotrophic lateral sclerosis patients from the Kii Peninsula, Japan. *European Neurology* 32: 95–98.

Yntema, Sharon K. 1984. *Vegetarian baby.* Ithaca, NY: McBooks Press.

Youdim, M. B. H. et al. 1989. Is Parkinson's a progressive siderosis of substantia nigra resulting in iron and melanin induced neurodegeneration? *ACTA Neurologica Scandinavia* 126: 47–54.

Ylikorkala, O., and U. M. Makila. 1985. Prostacyclin and Thromboxane in gynecology and obstetrics. *Am. J. of Obs. and Gyn.* 152 (no. 93): 318–29.

Yudkin, J. 1987. Metabolic changes induced by sugar in relation to coronary heart disease and diabetes. *Nutrition and Health* 5: 5–8.

Yudkin, John. 1990. Report on the COMA panel on dietary sugars in human disease: discussion paper. *J. of the Royal Soc. of Med.* 83: 627–628.

Yunus, Muhammad B. et al. 1992. Plasma tryptophan and other amino acids in primary fibromyalgia: A controlled study. *Journal of Rheumatology* 19:90–94.

Zaman, C. et al. 1992. Plasma concentrations of vitamins A and E and carotenoids in Alzheimer's disease. *Age and Ageing* 21: 91–94

Ziegler, E. E. et al. 1990. Cow's milk feeding in infancy: Further observations on blood loss from the gastrointestinal tract. *J. of Ped.* 116: 11–18.

Zierdt, C. H. 1988. Blastocystis hominis: A long misunderstood intestinal parasite. *Parasitology Today* 4: 1.

Zondek, B. 1959. Arborization of cervical, nasal mucous and saliva. *J. of Obs. and Gyn.* 13 (no. 4): 477–81.

Zucker, D. K. et al. 1981. B12 deficiency and psychiatric disorders: Case report and literature review. *Biological Psychiatry* 16: 197–205.

Index

103, 107, 109, 112, 115, 117, 119-120, 125-128, 131, 133, 135-136, 139, 141, 153-154, 160, 165, 168, 178-179, 190-193, 198-202, 207, 209, 211-212, 223, 226-227, 231-232, 239-241, 243, 245-246, 248, 250, 253, 258-260, 265-266, 269-271, 273-278, 280-284, 286-287, 292, 296, 299-303, 305
Vitamin K, 126, 163, 165-166, 170, 230, 246, 298
Vitiligo, 147, 261

W

Warts, 92
Water retention, 59, 127, 219, 243, 268
Weight gain, 22, 48, 61, 63, 95, 197, 218, 225, 243
Weight loss, 59-62, 70, 111, 129, 134, 149, 152, 183, 190, 200-201, 305
Wheat germ oil, 126, 207-208
Wheat grass, 79, 86
Wheat, 62, 68, 79, 86, 88-89, 93-94, 98, 100, 112, 116, 118, 123, 126, 134, 137-138, 146, 166, 169, 171-172, 178, 185, 190, 193, 197, 207-209, 220, 232, 239, 249, 251, 257, 268, 270, 276-277, 281-282, 315, 317, 326-327, 332, 356-357, 364, 376
White willow, 23, 45, 55-56, 61, 94, 98, 102, 108, 122, 131, 136, 155, 174, 178, 213, 296, 299, 307
Whole grain pancakes, 322, 332, 354
Wild yam extract, 299
Wilson's syndrome, 32, 70, 75, 110, 122, 235, 244
Wintergreen, 92, 165, 213
Wood betony, 45, 191, 199-201, 203, 211
Wormwood, 36, 76, 87, 147-148, 158, 171, 178, 187, 278

Y

Yarrow, 72, 79, 86, 102, 131, 155, 159, 165, 174, 204, 213, 254, 287
Yeast syndrome, 34, 36, 95, 147, 218, 234
Yeast, 17-18, 33-37, 62-63, 87, 93, 95-97, 99-100, 116, 125, 134, 137-138, 146-150, 157-160, 165, 169, 171, 174, 178, 183, 185, 188, 191, 193, 198-203, 205, 209, 211, 218, 225-227, 232, 234, 239, 249-250, 258, 271, 277, 281-282, 291, 298, 301, 316-319, 323
Yerba maté, 56, 61, 72, 254, 288
Yohimbe, 61
Yucca, 74, 102, 132, 294, 296

Z

Zinc sulphate solution, 96
Zinc, 14-15, 18-20, 29-30, 32, 42, 44, 50, 52, 57, 62, 64, 71, 74, 76, 79-80, 82-84, 86, 89, 91-96, 98, 100, 102-110, 112, 116, 121, 124, 126-127, 129-131, 133, 135, 139, 141, 147, 150-151, 154, 157, 164, 167-168, 174, 179, 181-182, 185-188, 190-191, 194, 199-202, 205, 208-209, 211-213, 218, 220, 230, 232-233, 239-240, 243, 246, 248, 253, 257-258, 260, 262-267, 269-280, 282-284, 286-287, 292, 294, 296-297, 299-300, 303, 305

Other titles by Alive Books

Fats That Heal Fats That Kill
The complete guide to fats, oils, cholesterol and human health.
Udo Erasmus, 480 pp softcover

Healing with Herbal Juices
A practical guide to herbal juice therapy: nature's preventative medicine.
Siegfried Gursche, 240 pp softcover

Silica – The Forgotten Nutrient
Healthy skin, shiny hair, strong bones, beautiful nails. A guide to the vital role of organic vegetal silica in nutrition, health, longevity and medicine.
Klaus Kaufmann, 128 pp softcover

Silica – The Amazing Gel
An essential mineral for radiant health, recovery and rejuvenation.
Klaus Kaufmann, 176 pp softcover

The Joy of Juice Fasting
For health, cleansing and weight loss.
Klaus Kaufmann, 114 pp softcover

Making Sauerkraut and Pickled Vegetables at Home
The original lactic acid fermentation method.
Annelies Schoeneck, 80 pp softcover

Cancer – There Is Hope
Alternative treatments, testimonials of cures, the Essiac story and more.
Byrun F. Tylor, 128 pp softcover

The Breuss Cancer Cure
Advice for prevention and natural treatment of cancer, leukemia and other seemingly incurable diseases.
Rudolf Breuss (Translated from German), 112 pp softcover

Devil's Claw Root and Other Natural Remedies for Arthritis
A herbal remedy has helped free thousands of arthritis sufferers from crippling pain.
Rachel Carston (Revised by Klaus Kaufmann), 128 pp softcover

Allergies: Disease in Disguise
How to heal your allergic condition permanently and naturally.
Carolee Bateson-Koch DC ND, 224 pp softcover

International Health News Yearbook (Annual)
The latest, most important discoveries in nutrition, health and medicine.
Hans Larsen, 96 pp softcover

All books are available at your local health food store or from
Alive Books, PO Box 80055, Burnaby BC V5H 3X1